CARCINOGENESIS—
A COMPREHENSIVE SURVEY
VOLUME 8

Cancer of the Respiratory Tract

Predisposing Factors

Carcinogenesis—A Comprehensive Survey

Vol. 8: Cancer of the Respiratory Tract: Predisposing Factors, *edited by M. J. Mass, D. G. Kaufman, J. M. Siegfried, V. E. Steele, and S. Nesnow, 496 pp., 1985*

Vol. 7: Cocarcinogenesis and Biological Effects of Tumor Promotors, *edited by E. Hecker, N. E. Fusenig, W. Kunz, F. Marks, and H. W. Thielmann, 664 pp., 1982*

Vol. 6: The Nitroquinolines, *edited by T. Sugimura, 167 pp., 1981*

Vol. 5: Modifiers of Chemical Carcinogenesis, *edited by T. J. Slaga, 285 pp., 1980*

Vol. 4: Nitrofurans: Chemistry, Metabolism, Mutagenesis, and Carcinogenesis, *edited by G. T. Bryan, 243 pp., 1978*

Vol. 3: Polynuclear Aromatic Hydrocarbons, *edited by P. W. Jones and R. I. Freudenthal, 507 pp., 1978*

Vol. 2: Mechanisms of Tumor Promotion and Cocarcinogenesis, *edited by T. J. Slaga, R. K. Boutwell, and A. Sivak, 605 pp., 1978*

Vol. 1: Polynuclear Aromatic Hydrocarbons: Chemistry, Metabolism, and Carcinogenesis, *edited by R. Freudenthal and P. W. Jones, 465 pp., 1976*

Carcinogenesis ᵥ₅Z 4E6
A Comprehensive Survey
Volume 8

Cancer of the Respiratory Tract
Predisposing Factors

Editors

Marc J. Mass, Ph.D.
Carcinogenesis and Metabolism Branch
U.S. Environmental Protection Agency
Research Triangle Park, North Carolina

David G. Kaufman, M.D., Ph.D.
Department of Pathology
University of North Carolina
Chapel Hill, North Carolina

Jill M. Siegfried, Ph.D.
Environmental Health Research and
Testing, Inc.
Research Triangle Park, North Carolina

Vernon E. Steele, Ph.D.
Northrop Services, Inc.
Research Triangle Park, North Carolina

Stephen Nesnow, Ph.D.
Carcinogenesis and Metabolism Branch
U.S. Environmental Protection Agency
Research Triangle Park, North Carolina

Raven Press ■ New York

Raven Press, 1140 Avenue of the Americas, New York, New York 10036

Made in the United States of America

Library of Congress Cataloging in Publication Data
Main entry under title:

Cancer of the respiratory tract.

(Carcinogenesis—a comprehensive survey ; vol. 8)
Based on the symposium "Tumor Promotion and
Enhancement in the Etiology of Human and Experimental
Respiratory Tract Carcinogenesis," held June 18–20, 1984,
Williamsburg, Va., sponsored by the Carcinogenesis and
Metabolism Branch, Genetic Toxicology Division, Health
Research Laboratory, U.S. Environmental Protection Agency.
  Includes bibliographies and index.
  1. Respiratory organs—Cancer—Etiology—Congresses.
2. Cocarcinogenesis—Congresses.   3. Carcinogenesis—
Congresses.   I. Mass, Marc J.   II. Health Effects Research
Laboratory (Research Triangle Park, N.C.). Genetic
Toxicology Division. Carcinogenesis and Metabolism
Branch.   III. Series: Carcinogenesis—a comprehensive
survey ; v. 8.   [DNLM: 1. Carcinogens—congresses.
2. Respiratory Tract Neoplasms—chemically induced—
congresses.   W1 CA7624 v.8 / WF 450 C215 1984]
RC268.5.C36 vol. 8   616.99′4071 s   85-1920
[RC280.R38]   [616.99′42071]
ISBN 0-88167-109-6

Foreword

The contribution of airborne carcinogens to the human lung cancer burden is a matter of scientific investigation and controversy. The large contribution of smoking to the incidence of lung cancer tends to make smaller contributions from environmental sources difficult to measure. A recent estimate produced at a Karolinska Institute Symposium in 1982 was that combustion products of fossil fuels in ambient air possibly acting together with cigarette smoke contributed to approximately 10% of the observed lung cancer burden (2). The recent controversy in *Science* arising from an article by Bruce Ames in which he stated that most cancers are attributable to diet and smoking and less strikingly related to environment and occupation points to additional research needs in this area (1).

One of the goals of the Environmental Protection Agency is to assess the carcinogenic risk to humans from chemical exposure. A recent Office of Science and Technology Policy Report describes a set of principles to guide Federal Agencies in assessing these risks (3). These principles include the understanding that carcinogenesis is a multistage phenonemon and that these stages may be influenced to varying degrees by routes of exposure, hormonal status, diet, and intra- and interspecies variability. The document also recognizes the need for a firm understanding of the mechanisms by which chemicals induce cancer, and how they interact in combination to alter biological effects.

The goals of this book are to explore these mechanisms in order to understand the known interactive effects observed in the human population such as smoking and asbestos exposure or smoking and uranium exposure and also to explore other potential combinations of exposures which may be synergistic with regard to respiratory cancer. An additional goal is to investigate the extent of the contribution of tumor promoters and enhancers toward the incidence of lung cancer in humans. In this book, epidemiological studies are discussed as well as general pathologic states of the lung which might predispose an individual to respiratory cancer. Corroborating and exploratory studies using experimental *in vivo* and *in vitro* methodologies are also presented.

This book represents the thoughts of a diverse group of investigators who critically address the issues concerning the relevance of tumor promotion and enhancement in the etiology of human and experimental respiratory tract carcinogenesis.

Stephen Nesnow, Ph.D.

REFERENCES

1. Ames, B. N. (1984): *Science*, 221:1256–1264.
2. Holmberg, B., and Ahlborg, A. (1983): *Environ. Health Perspect.*, 47:1–30.
3. Office of Science and Technology Policy (1984): *Fed. Reg.*, 49:21594–21661.

Preface

The existence of substances that enhance or promote the yield of carcinogen-induced tumors in laboratory animals has been recognized for over 40 years. However, the existence of such agents in the etiology of human malignancies has not been positively affirmed, nor has this issue been seriously enough investigated to render the decision that tumor promoting/enhancing substances in the environment contribute to the incidence of cancer. The frequency of occurrence of bronchogenic carcinoma is relatively high, and epidemiologic research has unambiguously identified a major causative agent—cigarette smoke. Therefore, lung cancer is the malignancy of choice on which to begin the testing of hypotheses regarding the relevance of enhancers in human cancer. In order to arrive at a decision to monitor tumor enhancers or promoters or even to decide that their role is significant, the available evidence needs to be reviewed and assimilated within and correlated to the current data. This volume serves such a function.

In the first section of this volume, Askin and Kaufman provide the histopathologic basis for the recognition of human lung cancers and elucidate the distinguishing characteristics of these cancers. Kuschner provides the expertise of a clinical and experimental pathologist and has written a comprehensive perspective on predisposing conditions to the development of this disease. The observation of enhancement of lung cancer by exposure to radon daughters in cigarette-smoking uranium miners is given a new interpretation by Archer that integrates human and animal data. Wynder et al. review aspects of the etiology of bronchogenic carcinoma and comment upon the apparent shift toward adenocarcinomas seen in smokers, promoters in cigarette smoke, the issue of passive smoking, the low-yield cigarette, and issues in lung cancer prevention.

In the second section, Saffiotti and colleagues discuss the intratracheal instillation model that Saffiotti developed in hamsters and the factors that influence tumor incidence in the respiratory tract *in vivo*. The pioneering work of Saffiotti and that of Nettesheim and the group at the Oak Ridge National Laboratories, continues to be the foundation of the observation and insight that fuel current experimental respiratory carcinogenesis research. Feron and colleagues discuss intratracheal instillation of glass fibers and the inhalation of constituents of cigarette smoke as cofactors for lung cancer in hamsters. Klein-Szanto et al. review their work at the Oak Ridge National Laboratories including *in vivo* studies on the effect of chronic respiratory infection and immunosuppression on the development of lung cancer; they also discuss the demonstration of 12-O-tetradecanoylphorbol-13-acetate (TPA) and asbestos as tumor promoters in tracheal epithelium as well as the dynamics of neoplastic development and promotion in the *"in vivo–in vitro"* model for carcinogenesis in rat tracheal epithelium. Heinrich et al. discuss inhalation experiments in rodents and the detection of carcinogenic or cocarcinogenic emissions from vehicular combustion engines. Witschi presents the mouse lung adenoma model and discusses the use of butylated hydroxytoluene as a promoter in this tissue.

In the third section, Harris and colleagues discuss selective clonal expansion theory as it relates to promotion, and the induction of terminal differentiation by tumor promoters in cultured human bronchial epithelial cells. Mass et al. describe differences in early responses of cultured respiratory epithelial cells from three species and report interindividual variability in responses to TPA in specimens from humans. Work by Steele demonstrates that initiation-promotion experiments *in vitro* with rat tracheal epithelial cells designed like those initially performed *in vivo* with mouse skin yield analogous results; he also demonstrates the utility of measuring DNA content and keratin synthesis in identifying preneoplastic populations of cells exposed to tumor promoters *in vitro*. Dissimilarities in responses of normal and carcinogen-altered rat tracheal cells elicited by TPA are described by Nettesheim et al. The ability of asbestos and other minerals to induce biochemical events linked with promotion such as the induction of ornithine decarboxylase activity, and the inhibition of cell–cell communication is elaborated by Mossman, Cameron, and Yotti; effects of asbestos on the morphology of hamster tracheal epithelium are presented.

The fourth section compiles observations of promotion-like enhancement and enhancers as viewed in nonpulmonary experimental systems. Research on cocarcinogens such as catechol, nitrosamines of nicotine, and passive uptake of tobacco smoke components is presented by Hoffmann and associates. Nesnow et al. investigate the ability of several environmental effluents to act as initiators, promoters, and coinitiators on mouse skin. Using cultured human endometrial stromal cells, Siegfried et al. show that two-stage initiation-promotion protocols result in selection for carcinogen-altered cells. Trush et al. suggest that promoters such as TPA can enhance carcinogen activation in human polymorphonuclear leukocytes; these cells can accumulate in the lung during inflammatory processes. A review of the effects on metabolic cooperation in V79 hamster lung cells of selected compounds and their metabolites relevant to lung cancer is given by Malcolm et al. Initiation-promotion experiments in Syrian hamster cells are reviewed by DiPaolo and colleagues, and Boreiko examines similar experiments in C3H10T½ cells. Gindhart et al. thoroughly describe molecular aspects of effects of promoters in the JB-6 mouse epidermal cell culture system.

The last section contains presentations by Pelling and Slaga, and by Weinstein et al. that provide an encompassing view of possible mechanisms in tumor enhancement and promotion that may operate on the cellular and molecular level. In addition, Chu proposes a mathematical model for carcinogenesis that accounts for tumor promotion. Also included are short personal perspectives on issues in tumor promotion, progression, and enhancement as they relate to respiratory tract carcinogenesis by Barrett, Kennedy, Higginson, Albert, and Williams.

The investigations presented in this volume chronicle state-of-the-art endeavors in respiratory tract carcinogenesis. This volume will be useful to cancer researchers and experimental pathologists whose interests are in the fields of lung cancer and pulmonary diseases.

Marc J. Mass, Ph.D.

Introduction

Substantial progress has been made in the last decade in the experimental study of respiratory tract carcinogenesis, particularly in the development of *in vivo* and *in vitro* models for the study of pathogenetic mechanisms of lung cancer.

Lung cancer still remains the major cause of cancer deaths in the United States. When the first Gatlinburg Conference on respiratory carcinogenesis was held in October, 1969, the estimated lung cancer deaths for that year in the United States were 60,000, or 165 per day, or one every 8½ minutes (1). At the Seattle Conference, in June 1974, I remarked that the current estimates had risen to 75,000 lung cancer deaths, or 205 per day, or one every 7 minutes (2). Ten years later, at the time of this Williamsburg Conference in 1984, we are aware that the present National Cancer Institute estimates are 117,000 lung cancer deaths, or 320 per day, or one every 4½ minutes. While these increases are in part due to population increases in the United States, they also correspond to continuing increases in lung cancer morbidity and mortality rates, which have become particularly high in women.

No stronger motivation exists for us to continue the investigation of the causative and pathogenetic mechanisms of lung cancer and the development of suitable experimental models, using animal and human target tissues, than one that could lead to the control and prevention of this prevalent form of neoplastic disease.

It is, therefore, a most appropriate and timely initiative that has brought together an extensive review of the predisposing factors related to respiratory tract carcinogenesis, particularly of those factors that involve promoting or other enhancing mechanisms.

Carcinogenesis can be considered as a multifactorial, multiphasic, and multitargeted process. Many agents are known to be causative determinants of cancer in the respiratory tract, as shown by evidence derived both from human pathology and epidemiology and from experimental animal studies. Among the major categories of recognized respiratory carcinogens are polycyclic aromatic hydrocarbons carried by particulate matter, asbestos, ionizing radiation, alkylating agents, halo ethers, and certain metals (chromates, arsenic). Extensive experimental evidence has also been obtained with nitrosamines. In the human, exposures to respiratory tract carcinogens are usually complex, involving several individual carcinogens, cocarcinogens, promoters, and other modifying factors. Several carcinogens are also known to have interactive effects in the causation of respiratory carcinogenesis, sometimes with clearly synergistic mechanisms.

Many of these factors are active by exposure through the respiratory tract, but others are active by systemic routes. In addition to physical carcinogens and direct-acting chemicals, there are many chemicals that require metabolic activation, which in turn is regulated by both genetic and environmental factors. Host factors are responsible for a wide range of individual susceptibility levels, and even the most severe exposures to well established carcinogens only exceptionally have resulted in cancer incidences close to 100% in human populations (3).

Let us consider the multiplicity of factors that concur in the causation of respiratory cancers. *Genetic factors*, particularly somatic cell genetic mechanisms, are currently being investigated in great depth and reveal the complexities of genetically controlled mechanisms that are involved in the carcinogenic response of every individual. *Nutritional factors* are intrinsic to cell growth and appear involved in the modulation of cancer susceptibility and expression. Although their role is not as apparent for respiratory cancers as it is for some other types, they are a necessary component among the multiple factors that control the host response. The role of vitamin A deficiency and the mechanisms of action of retinoids in the modulation of respiratory carcinogenesis have been extensively studied. *Physical factors* are known to play a significant role in both human or experimental carcinogenesis. Ionizing radiation from such sources as radon and radon daughters, ^{210}polonium, and radioactive particulates have been extensively documented. Physical properties of asbestos and, as recently observed, of crystalline silica are critical in determining their carcinogenic activity. The role of particulate matter and of mechanical cellular injury as cofactors in respiratory carcinogenesis will be discussed in this volume. *Inhaled factors* represent a major source of causative agents for respiratory tract cancers, including most prominently cigarette smoke, as well as asbestos and a variety of chemical carcinogens, including occupational and environmental exposures. *Other sources* of respiratory carcinogens or modifying factors may derive from dietary contaminants (e.g., enzyme inducers such as chlorinated compounds), hormones, and possibly infectious agents, which may play an enhancing role. *Unknown factors* still have to be accounted for in the genesis of all cancers.

We are, therefore, faced with a wide range of multiple concurrent causative factors that interplay in the pathogenesis of respiratory cancers in all individuals. Thus, instead of attempting to attribute each cancer to a single factor, we are considering a wide overlap of causative factors, each of which may contribute to the origin of each cancer by a varying degree of intensity.

When new factors are recognized to be involved in the causation of certain cancers, should the estimated role of the previously known factors be correspondingly decreased? Not necessarily, if the wide overlap of different causative factors is considered. Each set of factors may affect a large proportion of the individual cases, even all of them, but to such a different level in different individuals as to range from a virtually absent to a highly prominent role. Each of the concurring factors can be viewed as contributing to a set of permissive conditions; some factors will be additive, some synergistic, some will be inhibitory, and some may act as nonspecific enhancing factors. Their balance will be the determining factor for each individual case.

A temporal multiphasic aspect also needs to be considered, because certain carcinogenesis mechanisms require a definite sequence of events to be effective. For example, classic promoting agents need to be preceded by an initiating stage; certain synergistic effects of carcinogens appear to require a specific sequence of exposures; agents inducing marked cell proliferation may contribute to the fixation and expression of a previously latent transformed genotype; the fully malignant, invasive, and metastasizing phenotype may be acquired through several stages of pretransformed and transformed phenotypes.

Especially when considering the complex interactions that regulate the response to carcinogens and to cofactors, it becomes apparent that the mechanisms of respiratory carcinogenesis (and of carcinogenesis in general) are also multi-targeted, involving not only mutational changes in DNA, but also other genomic alterations, such as gene amplification or repression, and chromosomal translocations and rearrangements, as well as nongenomic alteration, for example in membrane receptors, specific gene products, signal transduction mediators, and bioenergetic mechanisms.

The present volume illustrates not only the complexity of the pathogenetic mechanisms of lung cancer, but also the rapid progress that is being made in their investigation and elucidation by the imaginative use of *in vivo* and *in vitro* models studied by a wide array of research approaches.

Umberto Saffiotti, M.D.

REFERENCES

1. Saffiotti, U., and Baker, C. G. (1970): In: *Inhalation Carcinogenesis*, edited by M. G. Hanna, Jr., P. Nettesheim, and J. R. Gilbert, pp. 467–480. Atomic Energy Commission Symposium Series No. 18, Oak Ridge, Tennessee.
2. Saffiotti, U. (1974): In: *Experimental Lung Cancer: Carcinogenesis and Bioassays*, edited by E. Karbe and J. F. Park, pp. 1–5. Springer-Verlag, New York.
3. Saffiotti, U. (1973): In: *Host Environmental Interactions in the Etiology of Cancer in Man*, edited by R. Doll and I. Vodopija, pp. 243–252. International Agency for Research on Cancer, Lyon.

Acknowledgments

The symposium "Tumor Promotion and Enhancement in the Etiology of Human and Experimental Respiratory Tract Carcinogenesis" was held on June 18–20, 1984 in Williamsburg, Virginia, and it is from the proceedings of this conference that this volume is derived. The organizing committee for the symposium consisted of David G. Kaufman (University of North Carolina at Chapel Hill), Marc J. Mass (symposium chairman; U.S. Environmental Protection Agency), Stephen Nesnow (U.S. Environmental Protection Agency), Jill M. Siegfried (Environmental Health Research and Testing, Inc.), and Vernon E. Steele (Northrop Services, Inc.). The symposium was sponsored by the Carcinogenesis and Metabolism Branch, Genetic Toxicology Division, Health Effects Research Laboratory, U.S. Environmental Protection Agency.

On behalf of the organizing committee, I would like to thank Dan Tisch and Cathy Bollinger of Northrop Services, Inc. for their expertise in successfully coordinating all aspects of the symposium, including help in preparing the proceedings. Special sincere thanks to Linda Hesterberg of Northrop Services, Inc., for most skillful text processing and formatting of this volume.

On behalf of the editors, I express deep appreciation to the contributors for their superb efforts.

Marc J. Mass, Ph.D.

Contents

EXPERIMENTAL EVIDENCE FOR TUMOR ENHANCEMENT IN THE RESPIRATORY TRACT *IN VITRO*

TUMOR ENHANCEMENT AND ENHANCERS IN NON-RESPIRATORY TISSUES

MECHANISMS IN PROMOTION, COCARCINOGENESIS, AND TUMOR ENHANCEMENT

Perspectives on Tumor Promotion

Contributors

John D. Adams
*Naylor Dana Institute for Disease
    Prevention*
American Health Foundation
Valhalla, New York 10595

Roy E. Albert
Institute of Environmental Medicine
New York University Medical Center
550 First Avenue
New York, New York 10016

Victor E. Archer
*Rocky Mountain Center for Occupational
    and Environmental Health*
*Department of Family and Community
    Medicine*
Building 512
University of Utah
Salt Lake City, Utah 84112

John Arcoleo
*Division of Environmental Sciences and
    Cancer Center*
Institute of Cancer Research
Columbia University
New York, New York 10032

Frederic B. Askin
Department of Pathology
*University of North Carolina School of
    Medicine*
Chapel Hill, North Carolina 27514

J. Carl Barrett
*Laboratory of Pulmonary Function and
    Toxicology*
*National Institute of Environmental
    Health Sciences*
P.O. Box 12233
*Research Triangle Park, North Carolina
    27709*

Diane K. Beeman
Carcinogenesis and Metabolism Section
*Environmental Health Research and
    Testing, Inc.*
*Research Triangle Park, North Carolina
    27709*

Craig J. Boreiko
Department of Genetic Toxicology
Chemical Industry Institute of Toxicology
*Research Triangle Park, North Carolina
    27709*

Klaus D. Brunnemann
*Naylor Dana Institute for Disease
    Prevention*
American Health Foundation
Valhalla, New York 10595

G. S. Cameron
Department of Pathology
*University of Vermont College of
    Medicine*
Burlington, Vermont 05405

Kenneth C. Chu
Occupational Cancer Branch
National Cancer Institute
9000 Rockville Pike
Bethesda, Maryland 20205

Nancy H. Colburn
Laboratory of Viral Carcinogenesis
National Cancer Institute
Frederick, Maryland 21701

Joseph A. DiPaolo
Laboratory of Biology
National Cancer Institute
National Institutes of Health
Bethesda, Maryland 20205

Jay Doniger
Laboratory of Biology
National Cancer Institute
National Institutes of Health
Bethesda, Maryland 20205

Charles H. Evans
Laboratory of Biology
National Cancer Institute
National Institutes of Health
Bethesda, Maryland 20205

V. J. Feron
Institute CIVO—Toxicology and Nutrition
    TNO
P.O. Box 360
3700 AJ Zeist, The Netherlands

Sebastiano Gattoni-Celli
Division of Environmental Sciences and
    Cancer Center
Institute of Cancer Research
Columbia University
New York, New York 10032

Thomas D. Gindhart
Laboratory of Experimental Pathology
National Cancer Institute
Frederick, Maryland 21701

Marc T. Goodman
American Health Foundation
320 East 43rd Street
New York, New York 10017

Roland C. Grafstrom
Department of Toxicology
Karolinska Institutet
S-104 01 Stockholm, Sweden

Thomas E. Gray
Laboratory of Pulmonary Function and
    Toxicology
National Institute of Environmental
    Health Sciences
Research Triangle Park, North Carolina
    27709

Nancy J. Haley
Naylor Dana Institute for
    Disease Protection
American Health Foundation
Valhalla, New York 10595

Curtis C. Harris
Laboratory of Human Carcinogenesis
Division of Cancer Etiology
National Cancer Institute
Bethesda, Maryland 20205

Glenn A. Hegameyer
Laboratory of Viral Carcinogenesis
National Cancer Institute
Frederick, Maryland 21701

Uwe Heinrich
Fraunhofer-Institut für Toxikologie und
    Aerosolforschung
3000 Hannover 61, Federal Republic of
    Germany

John Higginson
Universities Associated for Research and
    Education in Pathology, Inc.
9650 Rockville Pike
Bethesda, Maryland 20814

Dietrich Hoffmann
Naylor Dana Institute for Disease
    Prevention
American Health Foundation
Valhalla, New York 10595

Wendy Hsiao
Division of Environmental Sciences and
    Cancer Center
Institute of Cancer Research
Columbia University
New York, New York 10032

Alan M. Jeffrey
Division of Environmental Sciences and
    Cancer Center
Institute of Cancer Research
Columbia University
New York, New York 10032

David G. Kaufman
Department of Pathology
University of North Carolina School of
Medicine
Chapel Hill, North Carolina 27514

Kevin P. Keenan
Department of Pathology
University of Maryland School of
Medicine
Baltimore, Maryland 21201

Ann R. Kennedy
Department of Cancer Biology
Harvard School of Public Health
Boston, Massachusetts 02115

T. W. Kensler
Johns Hopkins School of Hygiene and
Public Health
Baltimore, Maryland 21205

Paul Kirschmeier
Division of Environmental Sciences and
Cancer Center
Institute of Cancer Research
Columbia University
New York, New York 10032

A. J. P. Klein-Szanto
Science Park—Research Division
The University of Texas System Cancer
Center
P.O. Box 389
Smithville, Texas 78957

C. F. Kuper
Institute CIVO—Toxicology and Nutrition
TNO
P.O. Box 360
3700 AJ Zeist, The Netherlands

Marvin Kuschner
School of Medicine
Health Sciences Center
State University of New York at Stony
Brook
Stony Brook, New York 11794

Michael Lambert
Division of Environmental Sciences and
Cancer Center
Institute of Cancer Research
Columbia University
New York, New York 10032

Sharon A. Leavitt
Carcinogenesis and Metabolism Branch
Genetic Toxicology Division
Health Effects Research Laboratory
U.S. Environmental Protection Agency
Research Triangle Park, North Carolina
27711

A. Russell Malcolm
Biological Effects Division
Environmental Research Laboratory
U.S. Environmental Protection Agency
Narragansett, Rhode Island 02882

A. C. Marchok
Biology Division
Oak Ridge National Laboratory
Oak Ridge, Tennessee 37831

Marc J. Mass
Carcinogenesis and Metabolism Branch
Genetic Toxicology Division
Health Effects Research Laboratory
U.S. Environmental Protection Agency
Research Triangle Park, North Carolina
27711

Elizabeth M. McDowell
Department of Pathology
University of Maryland School of
Medicine
Baltimore, Maryland 21201

Assieh Melikian
Naylor Dana Institute for Disease
Prevention
American Health Foundation
Valhalla, New York 10595

Lesley J. Mills
Department of Microbiology
University of Rhode Island
Kingston, Rhode Island 02881

Ulrich Mohr
Institut für Experimentelle Pathologie
Medizinische Hochschule Hannover
3000 Hannover 61, Federal Republic of
Germany

B. T. Mossman
Department of Pathology
University of Vermont College of
Medicine
Burlington, Vermont 05405

Yoshiyuki Nakamura
Laboratory of Viral Carcinogenesis
National Cancer Institute
Frederick, Maryland 21701

Karen G. Nelson
Department of Pathology
University of North Carolina
Chapel Hill, North Carolina 27514

Stephen Nesnow
Carcinogenesis and Metabolism Branch
Genetic Toxicology Division
Health Effects Research Laboratory
U.S. Environmental Protection Agency
Research Triangle Park, North Carolina
27711

Paul Nettesheim
Laboratory of Pulmonary Function and
Toxicology
National Institute of Environmental
Health Sciences
P.O. Box 12233
Research Triangle Park, North Carolina
27709

Jill C. Pelling
Science Park—Research Division
The University of Texas System Cancer
Center
P.O. Box 389
Smithville, Texas 78957

Nicolae C. Popescu
Laboratory of Biology
National Cancer Institute
National Institutes of Health
Bethesda, Maryland 20205

Friedrich Pott
Medizinisches Institut für Umwelthygiene
4000 Düsseldorf, Federal Republic of
Germany

P. G. J. Reuzel
Institute CIVO—Toxicology and Nutrition
TNO
P.O. Box 360
3700 AJ Zeist, The Netherlands

Umberto Saffiotti
Laboratory of Experimental Pathology
National Cancer Institute
Frederick, Maryland 21701

Andrew J. Saladino
Baltimore Veterans Administration
Medical Center
Baltimore, Maryland 21218

J. L. Seed
Johns Hopkins School of Hygiene and
Public Health
Baltimore, Maryland 21205

Jill M. Siegfried
Carcinogenesis and Metabolism Section
Environmental Health Research and
Testing, Inc.
Research Triangle Park, North Carolina
27709

Thomas J. Slaga
Science Park—Research Division
The University of Texas System Cancer
Center
P.O. Box 389
Smithville, Texas 78957

Bonita M. Smith
Laboratory of Viral Carcinogenesis
National Cancer Institute
Frederick, Maryland 21701

B. J. Spit
Institute CIVO—Toxicology and Nutrition
TNO
P.O. Box 360
3700 AJ Zeist, The Netherlands

Vernon E. Steele
Pulmonary Carcinogenesis Laboratory
In Vitro Toxicology Program
Northrop Services, Inc.
Research Triangle Park, North Carolina
27709

Linda A. Stevens
Laboratory of Experimental Pathology
National Cancer Institute
Frederick, Maryland 21701

Sherman F. Stinson
Laboratory of Experimental Pathology
National Cancer Institute
Frederick, Maryland 21701

Werner Stöber
Fraunhofer—Institut für Toxikologie und
  Aerosolforschung
3000 Hannover 61, Federal Republic of
  Germany

M. Terzaghi
Biology Division
Oak Ridge National Laboratory
Oak Ridge, Tennessee 37831

Larry L. Triplett
Biology Division
Oak Ridge National Laboratory
Oak Ridge, Tennessee 37831

James E. Trosko
Department of Pediatrics and Human
  Development
College of Human Medicine
Michigan State University
East Lansing, Michigan 48824

M. A. Trush
Johns Hopkins School of Hygiene and
  Public Health
Baltimore, Maryland 21205

I. Bernard Weinstein
Division of Environmental Sciences and
  Cancer Center
Institute of Cancer Research
Columbia University
New York, New York 10032

Michael W. West
Program Resources, Inc.
Frederick, Maryland 21701

James C. Willey
Laboratory of Human Carcinogenesis
Division of Cancer Etiology
National Cancer Institute
Bethesda, Maryland 20205

Gary M. Williams
Naylor Dana Institute for Disease
  Prevention
American Health Foundation
Valhalla, New York 10595

H. P. Witschi
Biology Division
Oak Ridge National Laboratory
Oak Ridge, Tennessee 37831

R. A. Woutersen
Institute CIVO—Toxicology and Nutrition
  TNO
P.O. Box 360
3700 AJ Zeist, The Netherlands

Ernst L. Wynder
American Health Foundation
320 East 43rd Street
New York, New York 10017

L. P. Yotti
Department of Pathology
University of Vermont College of
  Medicine
Burlington, Vermont 05405

CARCINOGENESIS—
A COMPREHENSIVE SURVEY
VOLUME 8

Cancer of the Respiratory Tract

Predisposing Factors

Carcinogenesis, Vol. 8, edited by M. J. Mass et al.
Raven Press, New York © 1985.

Histomorphology of Human Lung Cancer

Frederic B. Askin and David G. Kaufman

*Department of Pathology, University of North Carolina School of Medicine,
Chapel Hill, North Carolina 27514*

Malignant neoplasms can arise in any of the structural, cellular components of the lung. The vast majority of cancers, however, are of epithelial origin and arise from the lining of the airways (bronchi and bronchioles). In attempting to define etiologic factors in the pathogenesis of lung cancer, the large number of these epithelial neoplasms leads one to consider them preferentially in terms of epidemiologic study (3). Diffuse mesotheliomas, malignant neoplasms of the pleural surfaces, represent another type of malignancy in the lung which occurs in sufficient numbers to allow epidemiologic study.

The common malignant epithelial neoplasms of the lung are listed in Table 1 along with their approximate distribution by type as derived from several large studies (1,2,7).

TABLE 1. Morphologic classification of principal lung cancers

Tumor type	% of all lung cancers
Squamous cell carcinoma	40
Small cell carcinoma	20
Adenocarcinoma	25
Large cell undifferentiated	15

SQUAMOUS CARCINOMA

Squamous, or "epidermoid", carcinoma is the most common form of lung cancer. These tumors tend to be located centrally or in the mid-zone of the lung. They generally arise from dysplastic squamous epithelium in a bronchus.

Histologically, tumors of this type consist of cells with squamous differentiation. Cytologic and nuclear features of atypia are present and stromal invasion is a histologic feature of malignancy. These cells express characteristics of squamous epithelium in that they contain keratin and they grow as if to form a mucosal or cutaneous surface in that they mature, forming keratin pearls (Fig. 1).

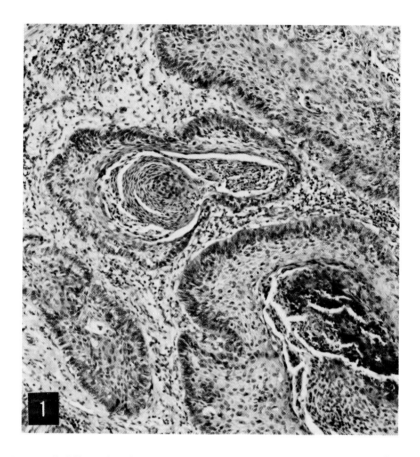

FIG. 1. Well-differentiated squamous carcinoma. The neoplasm grows in nests which invade fibrous stroma. Theses nests show central areas of partial maturation seen here as whorled masses of keratin ("keratin pearls"). Original magnification, 100×.

In other instances the tumors may be more poorly differentiated: the cells retain their polygonal mosaic pattern and they mature, somewhat; however, instead of keratinizing in the center or pseudosurface, the tumor cells simply undergo necrosis (Fig. 2).

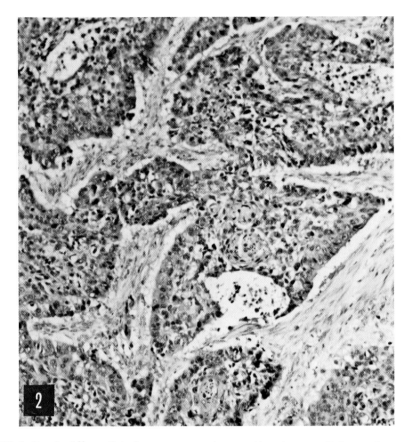

FIG. 2. Poorly differentiated squamous carcinoma. Here tumor cells have a less prominent nesting pattern and do not produce keratin pearls. Original magnification, 100 ×.

Since the lining of the respiratory tract is not normally composed of squamous cells, squamous carcinoma of the lung is presumed to arise in areas of squamous metaplasia and dysplasia in the bronchial epithelium. The abnormal squamous epithelium arises via irritation and consequent metaplasia. Cigarette smoke and environmentally and occupationally related inhalants are a probably source of irritation (3). The fact that this process occurs over a prolonged period of time leads to the possibility that we might be able to find very early or occult carcinomas of the lung. A great deal of attention is being aimed in this direction.

Figure 3 represents a specimen taken from a patient who presented to the hospital with a single episode of hemoptysis. There

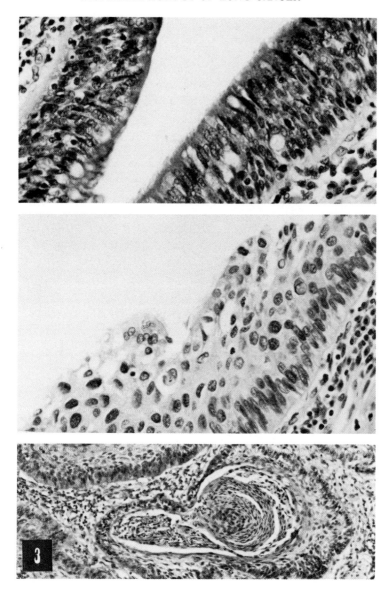

FIG. 3. Clinically occult squamous carcinoma. This section shows normal bronchial epithelium (top), dysplastic squamous epithelium (center) and invasive squamous carcinoma (bottom). The entire lesion was less than 2 cm in diameter. Original magnification, 100 ×.

were malignant cells in the sputum on cytologic examination, and a subsequent bronchoscopy gave the information that there was a ragged mucosal surface in one of the subsegmental bronchi. Dysplastic squamous epithelium and invasive carcinoma were seen contiguously. This patient had occult carcinoma. If we could identify more tumors at this stage, presumably we would be able to salvage a larger number of patients.

Squamous carcinoma of the lung may also be found in the mid-zone of the lung and may also be associated with a peculiar property of central necrosis and cavitation. Ninety percent of those carcinomas of the lung showing central cavitation are squamous carcinomas. The reason for this phenomenon is not clear but it may have something to do with the propensity of these tumors to undergo central maturation or necrosis. One problem associated with clinical and radiologic assessment of the actual size of any squamous cancer is the frequent association of an area of pneumonia distal to an obstructed bronchus.

SMALL CELL CARCINOMA

Kulchitsky cells (K-cells) are specialized neuroendocrine cells that appear in many organs. The K-cells in the lung are located in the bronchial and small airway mucosa and they are demonstrable by light microscopy only by use of special stain. Figure 4 shows a Grimelius stain for neurosecretory granules; the K-cells are seen as the darkly stained cells near the basement membrane. These cells are better seen by electron microscopy because K-cells show characteristic membrane bound cytoplasmic granules that have the appearance of neurosecretory granules.

K-cells in the lung can give rise to a wide spectrum of neoplasms (6). At the most benign end of the spectrum is the carcinoid tumor which may present as either a central, or peripheral mass in the lung. These carcinoid neoplasms may also present as endobronchial lesions, and can also grow into the lung parenchyma, giving rise to so called dumbell lesions that are partially endobronchial and partially parenchymal in location.

Carcinoid tumors in the lung are usually not malignant. There are, however, rare instances in which bronchial carcinoid tumors have metastasized to bone or other organs. Microscopically, the cells of these tumors have a fusiform or spindle-cell configuration especially if they are located in the periphery of the lung. Those lesions that are located

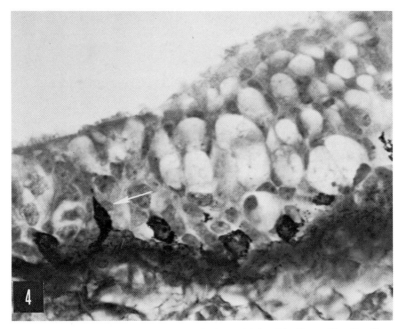

FIG. 4. Grimelius stain of Kulchitsky cells in bronchial epithelium. The K-cells are triangular dark cells (arrow) just above the basement membrane. Original magnification, 450 ×.

in the submucosa of the main bronchi tend to have an insular or trabecular pattern.

At the malignant end of the K-cell tumor spectrum lies the small cell anaplastic carcinoma or the so-called "oat cell" carcinoma. This type of tumor may be peripheral but it is most commonly a central, perihilar mass. The amount of tumor in the soft tissue around the hilar structures often greatly exceeds the amount discernable within the lung parenchyma itself. Figure 5 illustrates an autopsy specimen from a patient with oat cell carcinoma of the lung. The mucosa of the trachea and bronchus is generally smooth and free of disease. All of the firm tan-white tissue lying along the trachea and main-stem bronchus is metastatic carcinoma.

Microscopically, small cell carcinoma presents a variety of patterns. The classical "oat cell" carcinoma is illustrated in Fig. 6 which shows fusiform cells not unlike the carcinoid tumor at first glance. Further inspection reveals extensive mitotic activity and large foci of necrosis in these tumors. Another variety of oat cell carcinoma

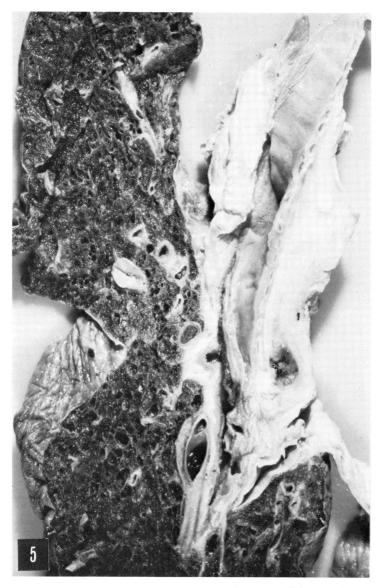

FIG. 5. Gross photo of small cell carcinoma. Note that most of the neoplasm seen here is growing in the tissue outside of the lung.

that is being increasingly more recognized is composed of larger "intermediate" cells. This neoplasm shows a pattern that could be confused with squamous carcinoma at first glance. However, the

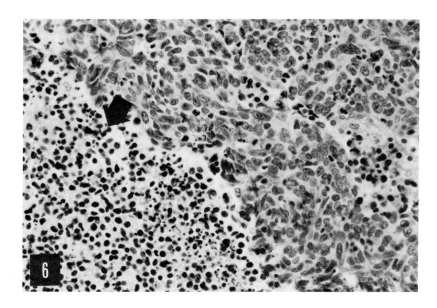

FIG. 6. Photomicrograph showing small cell carcinoma. The characteristic tumor cells are small and uniform. Necrosis (arrow) is a characteristic feature. Original magnification, 250×.

chromatin pattern of these cells with the very faint dusting of chromatin, lack of nucleoli, and the very high mitotic rate gives good evidence that this is a different sort of neoplasm. If one carefully examines most cases of oat cell carcinoma, and if one has a large enough specimen, it will be possible to see transitions between the small and intermediate sized cell components of the neoplasm.

It is also possible to have other cell types admixed with small cell carcinoma. Where there is a mixture of cell types in the neoplasm, the poor prognosis of the small cell neoplasm generally takes precedence in the biologic behavior of the neoplasm. There is no clearly convincing clinical evidence that the various forms of oat cell carcinoma (e.g., small cell versus intermediate cell) differ in prognosis or response to therapy.

ADENOCARCINOMA

Adenocarcinomas of the lung may present as either peripheral or central lesions. In the periphery of the lung the tumors presumably arise from the epithelium of small airways, although in some cases it is probably true that alveolar lining cells may play a role in the histogenesis of these lesions. There are some adenocarcinomas that arise centrally in the lung. These true adenocarcinomas must be distinguished from lesions of bronchial gland origin. Lesions of bronchial gland origin that are analogous to salivary gland neoplasms are rare, but do occur. They will not be discussed here.

Adenocarcinomas histologically show some evidence of gland formation (Fig. 7) or the ability to produce mucin (2). In some cases, there is no clear evidence of intracellular mucin, but gland formation may be demonstrated by light or electron microscopic study.

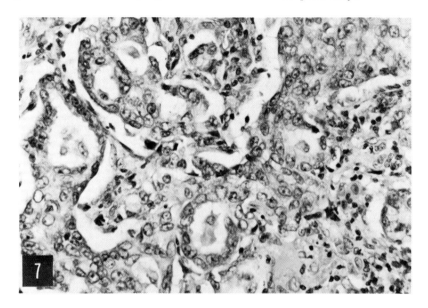

FIG. 7. Adenocarcinoma. This lesion shows malignant cells arranged in a glandular configuration. Original magnification, 100 ×.

In addition to the central and peripheral forms of adenocarcinoma, there is also a variant of adenocarcinoma called bronchioloalveolar carcinoma. This designation refers to a histologic growth pattern of these tumors. These tumors can occur in several forms, either a solitary, or multiple distinct lesions, or as massive consolidative lesions of the lung. The characteristic feature is growth along the alveolar septa without destruction of the underlying lung architecture (Fig. 8).

When considering adenocarcinomas in the lung, it is essential to consider and exclude the possibility that the tumor represents a metastatic adenocarcinoma to the lung from another organ.

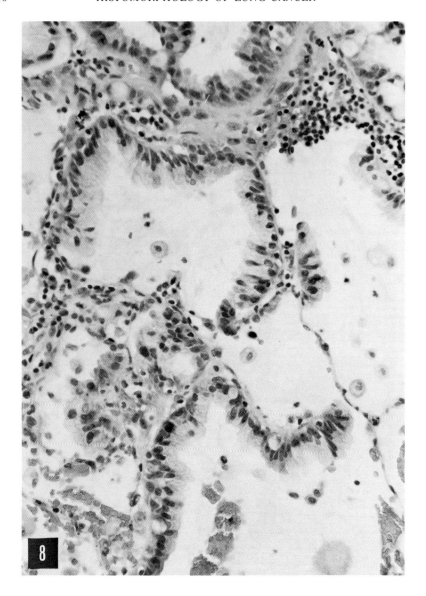

FIG. 8. Bronchoalveolar cell carcinoma. This adenocarcinoma is characterized by growth along the alveolar septa without obliteration of lung architecture. Original magnification, 250 ×.

Adenocarcinomas also arise in the scarred lung. These so-called "scar carcinomas" are controversial. Approximately 2/3 are adenocarcinomas, and the rest are squamous carcinomas. One of the major controversies concerns whether the scar produces the tumor or whether the tumor produces the scar. In specific cases, either one or the other of the two hypotheses may be correct (5).

LARGE CELL CARCINOMA

The last major classification of epithelial human lung cancers is the large cell undifferentiated carcinoma. This tumor has almost no differentiated histological features. The tumor is composed of large pleomorphic cells with prominent nucleoli (Fig. 9). There is no evidence of nesting as in squamous carcinomas, and by light microscopy there is no evidence of keratin or mucin formation. If one analyzes these tumors by electron microscopy with set criteria, up to 90% of these tumors can be distinguished as squamous or adenocarcinomas. Therefore, the number of large cell undifferentiated carcinomas in a particular clinical series depends on the care with which these cases were investigated and the criteria chosen (e.g., electron microscopy and histochemical staining versus light microscopy alone). Giant cell carcinoma of the lung is thought to be a related lesion. Again, a substantial fraction of these tumors can be distinguished as squamous or adenocarcinoma, if they are thoroughly studied.

PROGNOSIS OF LUNG CARCINOMA

Next, let us consider the prognosis of lung cancer, at least in those cases in which some form of primary surgical therapy is possible. Oat cell carcinoma is not considered here because it is generally thought to be an inoperable lesion. It is generally treated with a combination of radiation and chemotherapy and there are almost no two or three year survivors of this disease. There is a little more success with squamous and adenocarcinoma. Five year surival is described for patients with these tumors as a function of tumor type and stage at diagnosis. This staging is a matter of tumor bulk and whether the tumor has spread out of the lung (metastasis) before therapy was begun. An increasingly high stage represents more widespread disease. In early lung cancer, stage I, approximately half survive two years for both adeno- and squamous carcinoma. In stage II, the prognosis is a little better for squamous carcinoma than adenocarcinoma. In widespread disease the prognosis for either type tumor is quite dismal. Note that the overall prognosis is even less favorable since some inoperable cases have been excluded in the data noted above (1,2,7).

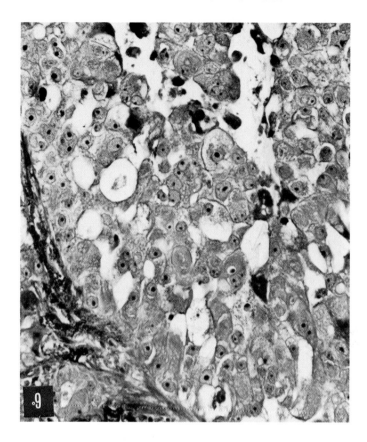

FIG. 9. Large Cell Carcinoma. These large malignant cells do not produce keratin or mucin as seen by light microscopy, and they form neither glands nor squamous nests. Original magnification, 250 ×.

Most of the patients dying of lung cancer have disseminated disease. Lung tumors have a particular pattern of spread. They often involve the hilar and mediastinal lymph nodes and even the contralateral lungs. Outside the thorax about 30-40% of metastatic lung tumors spread to the liver, 20-30% go to the adrenals, and 10-20% go to bone and brain.

OTHER TUMORS

We have discussed epithelial tumors of the lung. But tumors also arise in the soft tissues of the lung, and mixed tumors are also seen. For the most part these are rare biological oddities and cannot be considered in a brief review.

Another category of lesions that needs to be separated from lung carcinoma is that class of neoplasms that arise from the mesothelium or lining of the lung surface and pleural cavities: malignant mesotheliomas (4). Figure 10 shows thick white tumor growing on the surface of the lung and spreading in the lobar septa. Malignant mesothelioma is often a biphasic lesion composed of malignant spindle cell stroma and also some area of glandular differentiation. In any one area, one or the other of these forms of differentiation may predominate. Asbestos exposure has been implicated in the pathogenesis of these lesions.

SUMMARY

We have seen that neoplasms can arise at a number of sites through the lung. They arise from a variety of cells populating these sites. And, specific lesions of different cell types have a variety of biological behaviors. Some are very aggressive and spread rapidly throughout the body. Some are slower growing and are more amenable to therapy.

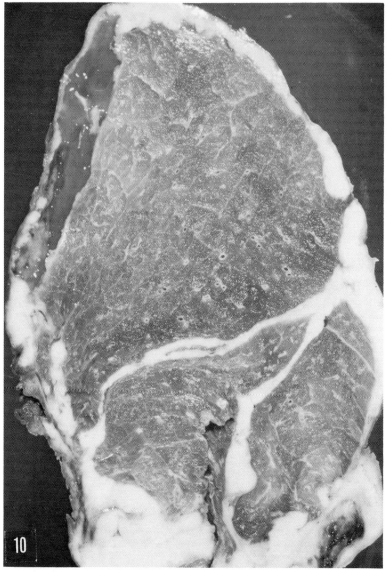

FIG. 10. Mesothelioma. In this photograph of a resected lung, tumor can be seen growing along pleural surfaces including those of the major fissures.

REFERENCES

1. Carr, D. T. (1981): *Hosp. Pract.*, 16:97-115.
2. Carter, D., and Eggleston, J. C. (1979): In: *Atlas of Tumor Pathology*, Second Series, Fascicle 17, Armed Forces Institute of Pathology, Washington.
3. Frank, A. L. (1982): *Clin. Chest Med.*, 3:219-228.
4. Griffith, M. H., Riddell, R. J., and Xipell, J. M. (1980): *Pathology*, 12:591-603.
5. Madri, J. A., and Carter, D. (1982): *Human Pathol.*, 15:625-631.
6. Tischler, A. S. (1978): *Semin. Oncol.*, 5:244-252.
7. World Health Organization (1981): In: *International Histological Classification of Tumours, No. 1: Histological Typing of Lung Tumors*, second edition. World Health Organization, Geneva.

Carcinogenesis, Vol. 8, edited by M. J. Mass et al.
Raven Press, New York © 1985.

Perspective on Pathologic Predisposition to Lung Cancer in Humans

Marvin Kuschner

School of Medicine, Health Sciences Center, State University of New York at Stony Brook, Stony Brook, New York 11794

In the late 1940's when lung cancer began to appear on the wards in alarming numbers, considerable interest developed in the morphogenesis and natural history of the lesions. These concerns were tied inextricably to the question of etiology. There was much speculation as to the possible role of remote (1918) influenza infection. In the course of observations made at the time of the flu epidemic, unusual proliferative responses had been noted in the bronchial lining and Winternitz (11) had suggested the possibility of a major increase in lung cancer that might follow an influenza at some time in the future. Of course, the brilliant retrospective and prospective epidemiologic studies that established the role of cigarette smoking soon submerged any possibility of a relationship between the developing epidemic of lung cancer and the remote pandemic of influenza (2-4). Nevertheless, a note had been struck and for those of us interested in the staged events that preceded frank cancer of the lung, proliferative changes of all sorts were to attract our attention and continue to do so.

At the outset, there were two major approaches to the illumination of the morphogenesis of lung cancer. One was the meticulous and detailed studies of multiple sections of the bronchial tree and correlations to smoking history performed by Auerbach (1). It seemed eminently reasonable to examine the entire bronchial tree, for the offending agent was an inhaled substance and although the tumors were primarily clinically unicentric, it was more than likely that the effects of an inhaled material would be widespread. Such was indeed the case and Auerbach presented us with an extraordinary series of lesions which he believed could be arrayed in sequential fashion. There was basal cell hyperplasia, stratification, squamous metaplasia, atypia, carcinoma-*in-situ*, and ultimately invasive cancer. I think it can be fairly stated that Auerbach's concept was that these were all stages in the progression to cancer, but more significantly that they were part of the process of malignant transformation.

The second approach to the study of morphogenesis involved the development of animal models in which the process might be interrupted by serial observations. Initial attempts at direct inhalation or intratracheal instillation of pure, potent, polycyclic hydrocarbons, were unsuccessful in the strains of rats then commonly used (5). It was found that implanting carcinogen impregnated pellets in the bronchus or transfixing the bronchus with carcinogen impregnated threads (9) would induce squamous carcinoma entirely comparable to human squamous cell carcinoma. These techniques demonstrated the carcinogenicity of other materials such as certain compounds of chromium and ionizing radiation (5,6). The key to the readiness with which tumors could be induced seemed to lie in the irritative, proliferative, and metaplastic changes induced by the trauma of pellet implantation or thread transfixion. The tumor yield with ionizing radiation was high enough that serial sacrifices could be performed with the assurance that animals observed were on their way to develop tumors. When this was done, the induction of squamous metaplasia was seen to precede carcinoma. The metaplastic epithelium, then, was the substrate on which tumor developed. It was possible to show that the two processes could be dissected. By combining exposure to a material which of itself produced proliferation and metaplasia, namely SO_2, with inhaled carcinogen, benzo(a)pyrene, one could now induce tumors which could not be produced by benzo(a)pyrene alone (6). This could be done in another species as well. Hamsters exposed by intratracheal intubation to benzo(a)pyrene or alternatively to methylcholanthrene, develop tumors only with the latter. If one combines the pure benzo(a)pyrene with inhalation of SO_2 one sees the development of squamous metaplasia and then squamous carcinoma. Our concept then became that squamous metaplasia preceded the development of cancer as Auerbach stated, but that it itself was not an intrinsic part of the process of cancerization. Rather, that the malignant change was superimposed on this peculiarly susceptible new lining.

The sequence of events was beautifully demonstrated in Saccomanno's cytologic studies (8) in which metaplastic cells were desquamated for a number of years before the malignant change occurred. But was the malignant alteration already present? This question had been asked as early as 1949 when Niskanen saw metaplasia preceding cancer (7) and asked whether the metaplasia was "cancerous or non-cancerous." Considerable support was given to the belief that hyperplasia and metaplasia was not in itself predetermined to go on to malignant change by the epidemiological evidence for diminished risk with cessation of smoking, and by Auerbach's demonstration of the reduction in abnormalities in ex-smokers, and in those who smoked filter cigarettes. Perhaps most convincing was Nettesheim's (10) splendid series of studies that involved extracting cell lines at different times in the development of tumor in tracheal explants showing that considerable time and numerous pasages were required until a truly malignant cell line merged as evidenced by loss of anchorage dependence and tumorgenicity on reimplantation.

I believe we may be seeing the same combination of separable but reinforcing phenomena that one sees in the regenerating nodules of liver after exposure to carcinogens in which a few cells are ultimately transformed.

Thus, I believe one set of alterations induced by any number of non-specific irritants producing bronchial injury and subsequent repair, regeneration, and metaplasia may furnish the ideal substrate for the more specific action of carcinogens. Is this true of infectious agents as well? The original concern regarding influenza does not appear justified but there are now well documented instances of cancer developing at broncho-cavitary junctions in tuberculosis, in the lining of chronic lung abscesses, and in bronchiectasis--all instances in which reparative and metaplastic alterations in respiratory epithelium occurs.

Now we have concerned ourselves so far with tumors arising in central bronchi. There is another group of interesting changes in the lung which bear on susceptibility to cancer. I call your attention first to the phenomenon known as scar cancer. The literature old and new is replete with reports of cancer developing at the site of scars in the lung. Most reports call attention to the possible confusion that may result from the tendency of some tumors to undergo central cell death with attendant scarring and persistent peripheral growth. These may simulate scar cancers to a remarkable degree, and indeed they may be difficult to distinguish from true scar cancers. Nevertheless, all pathologists will have seen instances in which the age of scar is testified to by the presence of dysplastic bone, or old caseous remnants of tuberculosis, or evidences of old infraction, at the periphery of which tumors develop. Here, too, the principal predisposing change would appear to be the proliferating, regenerating, sometimes metaplastic epithelium trapped in the interstices of the extending fingers of scar. It would appear that these cases make a small--less than 10%--but real contribution to the universe of lung cancer. Of more interest, is the light these cancers in areas of focal scar, shed on the origin of tumors arising in association with more generalized scarring, that is in association with a variety of forms of interstitial fibrosis. In surveys of cases of peripheral carcinoma, a significant proportion, perhaps as many as 25%, have been found to occur superimposed on interstitial fibrosis which predates the tumor and involved portions of the lung other than the tumoral area. This association is well described by a number of authors all of whom ascribe the etiology, in part, to the particular susceptibility of the proliferating and often metaplastic epithelium in the air spaces entrapped in the zones of scarring. The reactivity of this epithelium can be appreciated even in association with resolving or organizing acute bacterial pneumonias. In chronic fibrosing disease or fibrosing alveolitis that is seen in "so-called" acute interstitial fibrosis of the Hamman-Rich type, in berylliosis, in "rheumatoid lung disease," in progressive systemic sclerosis, and most importantly perhaps in terms of numbers, asbestosis. In these, the tumor originates in the florid and often atypical proliferation associated with scarring.

It is important to recognize that the predilection for the development of cancer in the asbestotic lung does not differ from that seen in other forms of interstitial fibrosis. Asbestos fiber is not a carcinogen in the sense that it itself is not "genotoxic". This is testified to by the absence of any *in vitro* evidence of DNA interaction but most tellingly, by the failure of asbestos entrapped in scar for many, many years, to produce sarcomas of the lung.

If asbestos increases the hazard of lung cancer development by virtue of its ability to induce fibrosis, then we can profitably interest ourselves in what properties of asbestos fibers render them fibrogenic. It seems to be increasingly clear that the durability of asbetos and fiber dimension are the principal determinants of fibrogenicity and hence of contribution to cancer. It is the long, (longer than 10 µm and perhaps longer than 20 µm fibers) which are fibrogenic. This seems to be by virtue of its particualr reaction with macrophages and the ability of the long fiber to cause release of fibroblast stimulating substances.

REFERENCES

1. Auerbach, O., Stout, A. P., Hammond, E. C., and Garfinkel, L. (1962): *New Engl. J. Med.*, 267:119-125.
2. Doll, R., and Hill, A. B. (1952): *Brit. Med. J.*, 2:1271-1286.
3. Hammond, E. C. (1966): In: *National Cancer Institute Monograph 19*, pp. 127-204. U.S. Government Printing Office, Washington.

4. Kahn, H. A. (1966): In: *National Cancer Institute Monograph 19*, pp. 1-125. U.S. Government Printing Office, Washington.
5. Kuschner, M. (1968): *Am. Rev. Resp. Dis.*, 98:573-590.
6. Laskin, S., Kuschner, M., and Drew, R. T. (1970): In: *Inhalation Carcinogenesis*, edited by M. G. Hanna, P. Nettesheim, and J. R. Gilbert, pp. 321-351. U.S. Atomic Energy Commission, Oak Ridge, TN.
7. Niskanen, K. O. (1949): *Acta Pathol. Microbiol. Scand., Suppl.*, 80:1-80.
8. Saccomanno, G., Saunders, R. P., Archer, V. J. E., Auerbach, O., and Kuschner, M. (1965): *Acta Cytol.*, 9:413-423.
9. Stevenson, J. L., and von Haam, E. (1963): *Acta Cytol.* 7:126-128.
10. Terzaghi, M., and Nettesheim, P. (1979): *Cancer Res.*, 39:4003-4010.
11. Winternitz, M. C., Wason, J. M., and McNamara, F. P. (1920): *The Pathology of Influenza.* Yale University Press, New Haven, CT.

Carcinogenesis, Vol. 8, edited by M. J. Mass et al.
Raven Press, New York © 1985.

Enhancement of Lung Cancer by Cigarette Smoking in Uranium and Other Miners

Victor E. Archer

Rocky Mountain Center for Occupational and Environmental Health, Department of Family and Community Medicine, University of Utah, Salt Lake City, Utah 84112

It has been repeatedly noted when persons are exposed to occupational carcinogens such as asbestos or radiation that an interaction of the agents with cigarette smoke occurs. The nature of this interaction is a matter of dispute for uranium miners (1,3,31). Since cigarette smoke contains both cancer-initiating and cancer-promoting agents (8,33), it is possible that, when cigarette smoke is added to industrial carcinogens, the result could be additive, synergistic, promotive, or a combination of effects. In epidemiological studies on man, it is difficult to sort out these different possibilities because of multiple exposures and limited time period for observation. Since these possibilities have been explored in animal experiments, the best approach appears to be to start with what we have learned from animal experiments. If human data are consistent with the animal data, then it is reasonable to assume that the same interactions apply to human occupational cancers.

ANIMAL EXPERIMENTS

A number of animal experiments have explored the interaction between cigarette smoke or its components with ionizing radiation. These experiments (summarized in Table 1) have used both alpha and beta radiation; some have used rat or mouse skin as the test object, while others have used the lungs of living animals. Some have used cigarette smoke directly; others used a cigarette smoke condensate (tar), and one experimental series used benzo(a)pyrene (BP), one of the carcinogens identified in cigarette smoke. These diverse experiments have given surprisingly consistent results. In general, when the two agents are administered together, resultant cancers appear at earlier ages. In some cases, resultant cancers are directly additive, and in others they are more than additive. When cigarette smoke or BP is administered prior to the radiation, it has little effect. The effect of BP, tar or smoke appears to be greatest when administered several months after the radiation (9,10,18,22). In some cases, the early appearance of cancers or the greater number of cancers have led investigators to apply the word "synergism" to the interaction between radiation and the cigarette smoke agents (9,22,32). However, further follow up, plus the fact that the cigarette smoke, tar, or BP controls had few or no cancers, usually led the investigators to conclude that the interaction was mainly one of cancer promotion (10,11,23). This conclusion was buttressed by the observation that the cancer-promoting activity of cigarette smoke is much greater than its cancer-initiating activity (33).

There was one experiment that indicated a protective effect by cigarette smoke (12). In this experiment, a cigarette-smoking period preceded each daily radon daughter exposure. It is likely that in this sequence there was extra mucus production stimulated by smoke. This could form a protective layer that persisted long enough to stop most of the alpha radiation of radon daughters before it could reach the critical basal cells.

EPIDEMIOLOGICAL REPORTS

When the first lung cancer in a nonsmoking U.S. uranium miner was observed in 1965, there had already been 80 lung cancer deaths among cigarette smoking U.S. uranium miners. Since about one-third of the miners did not smoke cigarettes, the discrepancy was so striking that it led some observers to blame cigarette smoking for the problem and to conclude that, if uranium miners did not smoke, they would rarely get lung cancer. The reasoning was that most of the cancers resulted from a strong synergism between radiation and smoking (31).

A second lung cancer among a nonsmoking uranium miner had been observed when a mortality analysis of the U.S. uranium miner cohort was published in 1969 (19). This analysis pointed out that these two cases represented a four fold excess of lung cancers (only 0.5 case was expected among nonsmokers)--the same relative risk noted for cigarettes smokers (15 vs. 60). Since the U.S. uranium miners were known to smoke at a somewhat higher rate than other U.S. males, an analysis was done to see how much extra cancer could be due to this extra smoking (20). It was concluded that this extra smoking could account for no more than a 50% increase, certainly not a five- to ten-fold increase as had been observed. This discrepancy indicated an

TABLE 1. Animal experiments with radiation and cigarette smoke components

Reference	Animals	Type of experiment	Results
Suntazeff et al. (32)	Mice	Tar and β-radiation applied to skin	At 18 months, there were so many extra skin cancers among the mice with combined tar and radiation that it was called synergism.
Cowdry et al. (11)	Mice	Tar and β-radiation applied to skin (same experiment)	When all had died, it was simple additive effect. Cancers appeared 6-7 months earlier in combined group, giving early illusion of synergism.
McGregor (23)	Rats	Tar and β-radiation applied to skin together and sequentially	At 21 weeks, there were five times as many skin cancers in the combined group as in either tar or beta groups. By 32 weeks, this ratio was 1:5. When tar followed beta, cancers were earlier and more abundant. Promotion.
McGandy et al. (22)	Hamsters	Benzo(a)pyrene (BP) and α-radiation injected into trachea--together and sequentially.	Interaction greatest when the two agents given simultaneously. Synergism.
Little et al. (18)	Hamsters	BP and α-radiation injected into trachea--together and sequentially (same experiment)	When simultaneous, effects were additive. When BP given first, little interaction. When BP given 4-5 months later, effects appeared synergistic. When alpha was followed by NaCl lung injections, cancer increased. Therefore, chronic irritation by agents yields cancer promotion.

(continued)

TABLE 1. Continued

Reference	Animals	Type of experiment	Results
Nenot (25)	Rats	Inhaled smoke + α from Americium-241	Smoke increased yield of lung cancers and made them appear earlier. Promotion.
Cross et al. (12)	Dogs	Daily cigarette smoke inhalation followed by radon daughter inhalation	Seven lung cancers among 20 nonsmoking dogs vs. one among 20 smoking dogs. Protection.
Chameaud et al. (9, 10)	Rats	Inhaled cigarette smoke given prior to or after a series of radon daughter inhalations	Smoke prior to alpha had little effect. Smoke subsequent to alpha made cancers appear earlier and doubled yield. Interaction was promotion or synergism.

interaction between the two agents. A later analysis (Fig. 1) confirmed this analysis.

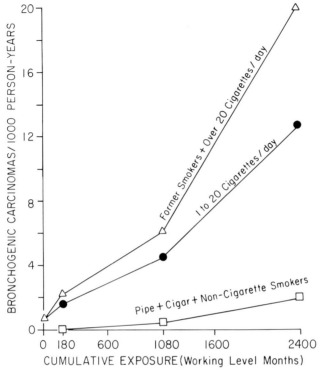

FIG. 1. Incidence of bronchogenic carcinoma among U.S. uranium miners by radiation exposure and cigarette smoking. Adapted from Archer et al. (3).

The distribution of histological types of cancer appearing among uranium miners has been repeatedly studied (4,29,30). This distribution is clearly different from that found among the general population. This distribution is approximately the same for smoking and nonsmoking uranium miners (2,26,29). This finding indicates that the major cause of the cancers among both smoking and nonsmoking uranium miners must be the same. It must be radiation, since the histological types differ from those found among the general population, which is largely attributed to cigarette smoking. Interaction of radiation and smoking is apparently not involved in determining the histological types.

There is one additional report that is pertinent here (27). It illustrated a drop in the absolute incidence of lung cancer at advanced ages among U.S. uranium miners (Fig. 2). Since the lung cancer rate in this group is dominated by lung cancers among smokers, it means that the lung cancer rate among smoking uranium miners declines markedly after about age 65 or 70. This point would be more clear, however, if this analysis had also included data on smoking and radiation exposure. Figure 2 does, however, confirm the age dependence of the induction-latent period. The decline in lung cancer rate among older smokers is consistent with the report of Axelson (6), who found that most of the lung cancers in his mining group occurred among nonsmokers at advanced ages.

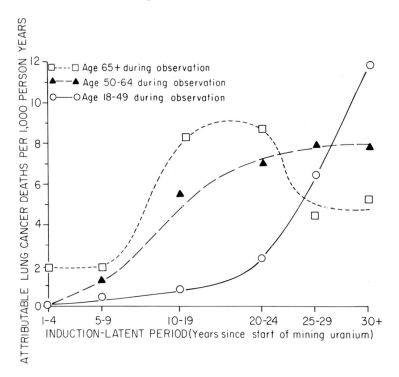

FIG. 2. Incidence of lung cancer attributable to uranium mining by induction-latent period and by age at observation for white U.S. miners.

Many of the other analyses of lung cancer among mining populations exposed to elevated levels of radon daughters do not bear out the initial impression of synergism obtained from the U.S. data (Table 2). A protective effect from cigarette smoking, a simple additive effect, and multiplicative effects (synergism) have all been reported from other groups.

DISCUSSION

There are a number of different ways in which cigarette smoke could interact with radiation in cancer production. One is that chronic smoking results in metaplasia of bronchial epithelium. The metaplastic cells might be more susceptible to cancer induction than normal epithelial cells. In addition, since metaplastic cells do not have cilia, there might be a pile up of mucus and radon daughters in such areas, leading to higher local radiation doses. Temporary paralysis plus loss of cilia could reduce dust clearance rates. Another effect of cigarette smoke is to stimulate mucus production. This effect appears to have several components. The irritation of smoke induces a prompt outpouring of mucus. In chronic exposure situations, there is an increase in number of goblet cells and size of mucus glands. It is likely that the viscosity of the mucus is also altered. This extra mucus, if thicker than normal, might slow particle clearance rates. If it coats the epithelium prior to and during radon daughter exposure, it might give some protection, as the α-particles can penetrate only about 70 μm in mucus or tissue. The diffuse pulmonary injury from tobacco smoke might cause smoking miners to breathe more deeply or faster when doing physical work in a mine. This could result in a larger bronchial radiation dose than would be received by nonsmoking fellow workers. The carcinogens in tobacco smoke might act in a synergistic manner with the radiation. The cancer-promoting agents in tobacco smoke might act to speed up the appearance of cancer induced by all chemical and physical agents.

In view of the contradictory results noted in Table 2, must we reject some of the epidemiological studies and embrace others? Perhaps all of the observations are correct, but some are sufficiently misleading as to result in erroneous conclusions. Study of the results suggest that they may not really be contradictory, but that they may be looking at the situation at different points in time along the path of carcinogenesis among the miners. Those studies that suggested synergism, such as the early observations among U.S. uranium miners, were clearly looking at the earliest cancers appearing among an exposed group. By contrast, the study of Axelson (6), which suggested that smoking was protective, was looking mainly at lung cancers among retired miners--the last cancers to appear among an exposed group. Those that suggested an

TABLE 2. Epidemiological reports on lung cancer and smoking among underground miners

Reference	Group studied	Results
Saccomanno et al., 1967 (31)	U.S. uranium miners (case collection)	One cancer among nonsmokers vs. 80 cancers among smokers. Synergism.
Lundin et al., 1969 (19)	U.S. uranium miners (cohort analysis)	Smokers had 10 × more lung cancer than nonsmokers. Definite interaction.
Lundin et al., 1971 (20)	U.S. uranium miners (cohort analysis)	Interaction is more likely cancer promotion than synergism.
Archer et al., 1973 (5)	U.S. uranium miners (case-control)	Induction-latency shorter among smokers. Histologic-type distribution same in smokers and nonsmokers. Interaction must be tumor promotion or co-carcinogenesis.
Hornung et al., 1981 (17)	U.S. uranium miners (Cox regression)	Smoking and radiation effects are additive.
Gottlieb et al., 1981 (16)	U.S. Navajo uranium miners (case collection)	Smoking played little role in the Navajo lung cancers.
Damber et al., 1982 (14)	Swedish miners (case-control);	Induction-latency is shorter in smokers. Effects are multiplicative.

Edling, 1982 (15)	Swedish iron miners (case-control)	Induction-latency is shorter in smokers. Effects are additive.
Whittemore et al., 1983 (34)	U.S. uranium miners (Cox regression)	Effects are multiplicative.
Radford et al., 1982 (26)	Swedish iron miners	Little difference in induction-latency. Effects are additive.
Axelson et al., 1978 (6,7)	Swedish lead-zinc miners	Smokers had shorter induction-latency. Smoking protected against radiation.

additive effect were either looking at an intermediate point or were looking at the full spectrum of early, intermediate, and late cancers.

If the above interpretation is correct, then it follows that the mean induction-latent periods for lung cancer among smokers and nonsmokers must be different; that is, the lung cancers must appear earlier among smokers, just as they did in experimental animals. Most of the studies that have investigated this point have concluded that the lung cancers do, indeed, appear earlier among smokers (at younger ages and with shorter induction-latent periods). This is strongly supported by a recent analysis by Archer (1), which showed that the average induction-latent period is strongly dependent on both age at start of exposure and on smoking history. It may also be dependent on rate and magnitude of exposure, as well as length of follow up. However, one recent report failed to find a significant difference betwen smokers and nonsmokers in the age at cancer development (28). Most of the above reports on smoking-nonsmoking differences failed to take into account differences between smokers and nonsmokers in follow-up time, in age at start of mining, and magnitude or rate of exposure. If such differences between smokers and nonsmokers were present, results could be misleading. Since smoking habits were known to be changing while these studies were underway, such differences were likely to have been present.

PRESENT ANALYSIS

To settle the disputed points about differences in induction-latent periods and age at lung cancer for smokers and nonsmokers, a case-control analysis was done on U.S. uranium miners.

The cases were nonsmoking underground uranium miners who developed lung cancer. Nonsmokers were defined as men who had smoked a total of less than four pack-years of cigarettes and had not smoked within 10 yr of cancer diagnosis. A few of them had smoked a pipe or cigars. Two controls were chosen for each case from 334 smoking U.S. uranium miners who were known to have developed lung cancer before January 1984. The controls were matched on birthdate ($\pm$ 3 yr), on year when their mining started ($\pm$ 5 yr), on magnitude ($\pm$ 50%) and rate of exposure to radiation ($\pm$ 80%). All potential controls were compared, and those that matched best on all four matching parameters were chosen. The results of the matching and the differences in age at lung cancer and length of induction-latent period are given in Table 3. The high degree of significance obtained from a

TABLE 3. Case-control study of induction-latent period of smokers vs. nonsmokers

	Nonsmoking uranium miners with lung cancer (35 cases)	Matched smoking uranium miners with lung cancer (70 controls)	P-value of paired differences
Mean induction-latent period	23.8 yr	18.5 yr	<0.001
Mean age at death	54.7 yr	50.2 yr	<0.001
Mean year of birth	1920	1920	--
Mean age at start of uranium mining	31.2 yr	32.0 yr	--
Mean radiation exposure (WLM)	1723	1794	--
Mean exposure rate (WL)	10.6	12.6	--

paired t-test (21) leaves no doubt that, when other factors are equal, smoking miners have shorter induction-latent periods and develop lung cancer at an earlier age than do nonsmoking miners. Judging from Axelson's data (6), it appears likely that the magnitude of the observed difference would become greater with longer follow up.

HYPOTHESIS

We are now in a position to propose an hypothesis that integrates both the animal and human data. We postulate that any given alpha radiation dose from radon daughters induces a finite number of lung cancers in any radiated group. In the absence of cigarette smoking, these cancers will have a long latent period and may or may not be fully expressed among the population, depending on the force of competing causes of death among the older members of the population and the presence or absence of promoting agents. In the presence of cigarette tar, these radiation-induced cancers will appear at an earlier date (and at younger ages) than among groups not exposed to cigarette tar.

According to our hypothesis, the lung cancers that would normally be induced by cigarette smoke would still be present and added to those induced by radiation in the mining population. The hypothesis is best understood by reference to Fig. 3. In this hypothetical graph, we assume that an equal number of smoking and nonsmoking miners of the same age are exposed at age 20 to the same amount of radon daughters. The resultant curves of lung cancer incidence then reflect the distribution in time of the appearance of induced cancers. It is evident, after examining these curves, that investigators who examine lung cancer mortality data at different points in time after start of mining could obtain data indicating synergism, additivity, or a smoking protective effect. The only piece of human or animal data that is not consistent with this hypothesis is the smoking dog data, which showed a protective effect. It is probably the consequence of a different type of interaction.

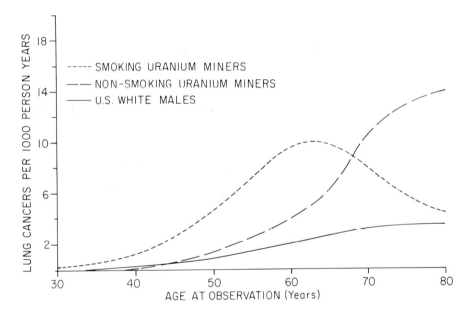

FIG. 3. Hypothetical incidence of lung cancer by time after initial exposure to radon daughters at age 20, for smoking and nonsmoking men. The general population lung cancer mortality for white males was adapted from NCI Monograph Number 59 (24).

If the radiation dose is sufficiently high, or the life span of the species sufficiently short, or with short observation periods in human studies, many of the radiation-induced cancers might not be observed without the addition of the cigarette tar or other promoting agent. In such situations, the effect of a promoting agent might appear to be multiplicative. If, however, the competing causes of death are not too great and follow up continues until most of a human group has died, most of the cancers would be expressed, even without the presence of a promoting agent.

A mortality analysis of radon daughter-exposed miners within 25 yr after they started mining would then give an impression of synergism, just as the early observations of Sunzteff and McGandy (22,32) did in the animal experiments. However, in the human studies, the radiation-induced cancers may be sufficiently exhausted in smoking miners by the time most reach the age of 70 that the incidence of lung cancer among smokers would fall below that of nonsmoking miners. If viewed late in the course of carcnogenesis, a finding like that of Axelson et al. (6), "apparent protection by smoking," would not be surprising.

SUMMARY

There are substantial animal and epidemiological data related to cigarette smoking and lung cancer among miners exposed to elevated levels of radon daughters that appears to be in disagreement. An hypothesis is advanced that explains most of this disagreement as being derived from temporal differences of cancer expression. The hypothesis is that a given radiation exposure induced a finite number of lung cancers, which have shorter latent periods due to the cancer promotion activity of smoke among cigarette smokers. According to this hypothesis, the life-shortening effect is greater among smoking miners than nonsmoking miners, and the ultimate number of lung cancers among smoking miners will be only a little larger than among nonsmokers. The greater number will derive from the additive effect of radiation and smoking, plus the greater force of competing causes of death among elderly nonsmokers.

REFERENCES

1. Archer, V. E. (1981): *J. Occup. Med.*, 23:502-505.
2. Archer, V. E., Gillam, J. D., and Wagoner, J. K. (1976): *Ann. N.Y. Acad. Sci.*, 271:280-293.
3. Archer, V. E., Gillam, J. D., and James, L. A. (1979): In: *Proceedings of the Third International Symposium on Detection and Prevention of Cancer*, edited by H. E. Nieburgs, pp. 1689-1710. Marcel Dekker, New York.
4. Archer, V. E., Saccomanno, G., and Jones, J. H. (1974): *Cancer*, 34:2056-2060.
5. Archer, V. E., Wagoner, J. K., and Lundin, F. E. (1973): *J. Occup. Med.*, 15:204-211.
6. Axelson, O., and Sundell, L. (1978): *Scand. J. Work Environ. Health*, 4:46-52.
7. Axelson, O., and Sundell, L. (1980): *Scand. J Work Environ. Health*, 6.227-231.

8.   Bock, F. G. (1968): *Cancer Res.*, 28:2363-2368.

9.   Chameaud, J., Perraud, R., Chretien, J., Masse, R., and Lafuma, J. (1982): In: *Early Detection and Localization of Lung Tumors in High Risk Groups*, edited by P. R. Baud, pp. 11-20. Springer-Verlag, Heidelberg.

10. Chameaud, J., Perraud, R., Masse, R., and Lafuma, J. (1981): In: *Radiation Hazards in Mining*, edited by M. Gomez, pp. 228-235. Society of Mining Engineers of the American Institute of Mining, Metallurgical and Petroleum Engineers, New York.

11. Cowdry, E. V., Croninger, A., Solerie, S., and Suntzeff, V. (1961): *Cancer*, 14:344-352.

12. Cross, F. T., Palmer, R. F., Filipy, R. E., Dagle, G. E., and Stuart, B. O. (1982): *Health Phys.*, 42:33-52.

13. Dahlgren, E. (1979): *Lakartidningen*, 76:4811-4814.

14. Damber, L., and Larsson, L. G. (1982): *Acta Radiol. Oncol.*, 21:305-313.

15. Edling, C. (1982): *Am. J. Ind. Med.*, 3:191-199.

16. Gottlieb, L. S., and Husen, L. A. (1982): *Chest*, 81:449-452.

17. Hornung, R. W., and Samuels, S. (1981): In: *Radiation Hazards in Mining*, edited by M. Gomez, pp. 363-368. Society of Mining Engineers of the American Insitute of Mining, Metallurgical and Petroleum Engineers, New York.

18. Little, J. B., McGandy, R. B., and Kennedy, A. R. (1978): *Cancer Res.*, 38:1929-1935.

19. Lundin, F. E., Lloyd, J. W., Smith, E. M., Archer, V. E., and Holaday, D. A. (1969): *Health Phys.*, 16:571-578.

20. Lundin, F. E., Wagoner, J. K., and Archer, V. E. (1971): *Radon Daughter Exposure and Respiratory Cancer: Quantitative and Temporal Aspects.* NIOSH-NIEHS Joint Monograph No. 1, National Technical Information Service, Springfield, VA.

21. Mather, K. (1965): *Statistical Analysis in Biology*, pp. 55-60. Methuen and Company, London.

22. McGandy, R. B., Kennedy, A. R., Terzaghi, M., and Little, J. B. (1974): In: *Experimental Lung Cancer: Carcinogenesis and Bioassays*, edited by E. Karbe and J. F. Park, pp. 485-491. Springer-Verlag, Heidelberg.

23. McGregor, J. F. (1982): *J. Natl. Cancer Inst.*, 68:605-611.

24. National Cancer Institute Monograph No. 59. *Cancer Mortality in the United States 1950-1977.* NIH Publication No. 82-2435, Government Printing Office, Washington.

25. Nenot, J. C. (1977): In: *Proceedings of the International Atomic Energy Agency Symposium*, pp. 228-234. International Atomic Energy Agency, Chicago.

26. Radford, E. P., and Renard, K. G. St. C. (1984): *New Engl. J. Med.*, 310:1485-1494.

27. Roscoe, R. J., Waxweiler, R. J., and Archer, V. E. (1983): Presented at Conference on Epidemiology Applied to Health Physics. Health Physics Society, January 9-13, 1983, Albuquerque, NM.

28. Saccomanno, G. (1982): In: *Early Detection and Localization of Lung Tumors in High Risk Groups*, edited by P. R. Band, pp. 43-52. Springer-Verlag, Heidelberg.

29. Saccomanno, G., Archer, V. E., Auerbach, O., Kuschner, M., Egger, M., Wood, S., Mick, R. (1981): In: *Radiation Hazards in Mining*, edited by M. Gomez, pp. 675-679. Society of Mining Engineers of the American Institute of Mining, Metallurgy and Petroleum Engineers, New York.

30. Saccomanno, G., Archer, V. E., Auerbach, O., Kuschner, M., Saunders, R. P., and Klein, M. (1971): *Cancer*, 27:515-523.
31. Saccomanno, G., Saunders, R. P., and Scott, J. (1967): Bull. Pathol., 8:226-227.
32. Suntzeff, V., Cowdry, E., and Croninger, A. (1959): *Proc. Am. Assoc. Cancer Res.*, 3:68.
33. Van Duuren, B. L., Sivak, A., Katz, C., and Melchione, S. (1971): *J. Natl. Cancer Inst.*, 47:235-240.
34. Whittemore, A., and McMillan, A. (1983): *J. Natl. Cancer Inst.*, 71:489-500.

Carcinogenesis, Vol. 8, edited by M. J. Mass et al.
Raven Press, New York © 1985.

Lung Cancer Etiology: Challenges of the Future

Ernst L. Wynder, Marc T. Goodman, and Dietrich Hoffmann

American Health Foundation, New York, New York 10017

In a recent review of the etiology of lung cancer we discussed several questions (61). These were: [1] the reported shift toward an increasing proportion of adenocarcinoma compared to squamous cell carcinoma of the lung in men, [2] the probable protective effect of green vegetables and fruits, especially ß-carotene and vitamin A, against the induction of lung cancer, and [3] the possibility of a tumor enhancing effect of dietary fats. Other aspects considered were [4] the relative contribution of tumor initiators and tumor promoters in tobacco carcinogenesis, [5] the effect of the low-yield cigarette on the reduction of the risk of cancer of the larynx and lung, and [6] the risk of the "passive smoker" to develop lung cancer. Finally, we discussed current and future efforts toward reducing the number of smokers among the adolescent and adult population and educational methods for preventing young people from starting the smoking habit. In this communication we will focus on the question of the low-yield cigarette and on the epidemiology of lung cancer in nonsmokers.

RECOMMENDATIONS FOR FUTURE STUDIES

Histologic Pattern

An examination of pathology reports after lung cancer surgery demonstrates a noticeable lack of uniformity among pathologists as to their classification of the lesions (65,70). Changes in diagnostic techniques and classification systems, improvements in treatment, as well as the aggressiveness of the physician may all contribute to secular differences in histologic patterns (41,53,54,61). For instance, some pathologists who are interested in a specific type of lung cancer will employ various histological techniques for the identification of that lesion, whereas other pathologists will be satisfied with reporting the cancer as a "bronchiogenic carcinoma." When a pathological diagnosis has both etiologic and prognostic implications, minimum standards should be followed regarding an acceptable histologic definition. An organized body of pathologists should set up a list of criteria, such as a refinement of the *Atlas of Tumor Pathology* already in use (2), to be used as a guide in interpreting slides.

Our findings, based in large part on data obtained from Memorial Sloan-Kettering Cancer Center, which has uniform standards of diagnosis, suggest a significant trend towards glandular lung cancer, especially in males (Table 1), the natural history of which requires investigation. One possible source of this shift might be the general decline in the sales-weighted tar yield of cigarettes sold on the market since about 1964 (46). Smokers who switch to lower yield cigarettes tend to compensate for the low nicotine delivery by smoking more intensely and inhaling more deeply (51). This may have an effect on the incidence of peripherally located lesions.

Metabolism Studies

Currently, there is an increased interest regarding the role of dietary fat, vitamin A, retinoids and other micronutrients in the etiology of lung cancer (7,21). A recent report indicating that dietary fat enhances benzo(a)pyrene-induced lung cancer in rats provides an experimental basis for its role in the etiology of this cancer (3). Differences in the tumor promoting effects of various types of dietary fat should be studied experimentally as we have done for breast and colon cancer (11,32). In the case of mammary cancer, the risk associated with the consumption of unsaturated fats in rats is higher than that associated with the consumption of saturated fats (9). No increase in the risk of breast or colon cancer is linked to the use of monounsaturated fats (11,42). There are many conceivable mechanisms for the enhancement of carcinogenesis by fat, and these may vary by cancer site. Although it appears that cholesterol does not play a role in the etiology of lung cancer (58), it is possible that changes in the ratio of saturated to unsaturated fatty acids may increase cell membrane permeability, rendering the cells more susceptible to carcinogenic stimuli (16). Lipoproteins of all classes suppress the immunologic capacity of lymphocytes (16), and may saturate macrophages in the lung (19), thus impairing immunologic host-defenses against carcinogens. These hypotheses need to be explored by both the epidemiologist and the laboratory scientist.

TABLE 1.A. Ratio of Kreyberg type I to type II lung cancer: Men[a][1,5] (37)

Series	Type I: type II[b]	Lung cancer incidence	Sources of material
Italy (Ferrari and Kreyberg; 17)	3.21:1 [71]		86% necropsy, remainder surgical
Finland (Kreyberg and Saxen; 35)	12.10:1 [528]	70.0	14% necropsy, remainder surgical
Norway (Kreyberg and Saxen; 35)	3.39:1 [522]	16.5	6.5% necropsy, remainder surgical
Birmingham, United Kingdom (Shinton; 44)	17.10:1 [626]	73.3	27.8% necropsy, remainder surgical[c]
St. Louis, MO, USA (Vincent et al.; 54)	3.05:1 [1140]	20.8-47.8	unknown
Israel (Cahansky et al.; 8)	1.32:1 [77]	26.4	Surgical material
South Africa (Uys; 52)			
White patients	9.30:1 [246]	44.7	42% netropsy, remainder surgical[c]
Coloured patients	5.10:1 [171]	42.8	34% necropsy, remainder surgical[c]
Bantu patients	4.58:1 [33]	26.9	40% necropsy, remainder surgical[c]
Singapore, China (Law et al.; 37)	4.58:1 [476]	56.1	10.8% necropsy, remainder surgical
Buffalo, NY, USA (Vincent et al.; 53)	2.82:1 [1404]		42% necropsy, remainder surgical
United States (TNCS[d]) (Ernster et al.; 15)	1.40:1 [5074]	43.7	Composition unknown
American Health Foundation			
(1)	3.21:1 [1441]		100% surgical
(1)	1.80:1 [2004]		100% surgical

(continued)

TABLE 1.B. Ratio of Kreyberg type I:type II lung tumors: Women[a] (37)

Series	Type I: type II[b]	Lung cancer incidence	Sources of material
Finland (Kreyberg and Saxen; 35)	0.47:1 [27]	4.4	14% necropsy, remainder surgical
Birmingham, United Kingdom (Shinton; 44)	4.25:1 [63]	8.4	27.8% necropsy, remainder surgical[c]
St. Louis, MO, USA (Vincent et al.; 54)	0.34:1 [141]	6.1-9.0	10.4% necropsy, remainder surgical
Israel (Cahansky et al.; 8)	0.75:1 [23]	8.7	Surgical material only
South Africa (Uys; 52)			
White patients	1.93:1 [41]	5.3	42% necropsy, remainder surgical[c]
Coloured patients	1.10:1 [21]	4.2	34% necropsy, remainder surgical[c]
Singapore, China (Law et al.; 37)	1.12:1 [154]	17.0	10.6% necropsy, remainder surgical
Buffalo, NY, USA (Vincent et al.; 54)	2.01:1 [278]		42% necropsy, remainder surgical
United States (TNCS[d]) (Ernster et al.; 15)	0.57:1 [1556]	9.5	Composition unknown
American Health Foundation			
(1)	1.40:1 [438]		100% surgical
(1)	1.31:1 [2004]		100% surgical

[a] Histologic lung cancer types according to Kreyberg (34). Type I squamous and large and small cell carcinomas. Type II bronchiolar cell carcinomas and benign and malignant adenomas and salivary gland type tumors.

[b] Numbers in brackets indicate number of cases of lung tumors.

[c] Percentage of cases in both sexes.

[d] Third National Cancer Survey, 1969-1971.

A major epidemiologic lead in the area of nutrition and lung cancer is the relatively low rate of lung cancer in Japan compared to that in the United States. It appears that the comparatively low intake of green vegetables and fruits in Japan in the past would not be consistent with a causal association of lung cancer among Japanese males. Any international comparisons of nutrition and lung cancer rates would have to adjust for the effects of tobacco smoking and smoke uptake by the smoker.

In the United States, investigations of macro- and micronutrients especially of carotenoids on lung cancer risk are indicated. However, it has to be recognized that the disease itself may have a profound effect on the current biochemical status of individuals with lung cancer. Therefore, case-control studies of tobacco-related cancer and nutrition must be conducted carefully, especially since it is presently not possible to obtain reliable lifetime dietary histories of cancer patients. Prospective studies with large scale blood collection and storage for later analysis appears more promising (58).

Tobacco-Tumor Initiators and Promoters

Experimental studies have shown that tobacco smoke contains tumor initiators, tumor promoters, and cocarcinogens (31,59). Tobacco smoke represents a sufficient agent in the causation of cancer in that tumors have been produced with tobacco smoke particulates irrespective of the experimental protocol. Of great concern is the relative importance of these three types of tumorigenic agents to tobacco carcinogenesis and the extent to which either of these groups of components have changed over the last three decades through cigarette modification. When the first experimental studies on mouse skin in the 1950's were reported (20,60,63,64,66), the rate of conversion from papilloma to cancer was faster than that observed in more recent skin painting tests. Such findings suggest that the concentration of initiating carcinogens has been reduced. In fact, some reduction in polynuclear aromatic hydrocarbons has been observed. It might also suggest some changes in the concentration of tumor promoting agents and cocarcinogens in cigarette smoke. This is an area where further analysis is needed.

Epidemiology has yet to contribute to an evaluation of the relative importance of initiating carcinogens, cocarcinogens, and tumor promoting agents in tobacco carcinogenesis. It appears that for lung cancer, both initiation and promotion influence tumor development. If the decline of lung cancer among exsmokers is rapid, it might be postulated that tumor promoters play a predominant role. However, this is not the case. Among long-term heavy smokers, prospective as well as retrospective studies have not shown a major decline in the first four years after giving up smoking. This persistent increased risk of lung cancer may be an expression of the latent effects of long-term heavy smoking in association with preclinical stages of the disease and symptoms of an incipient lung cancer at the time of smoking cessation. Another possibility is that tobacco smoke also contains tumor inhibitors which might keep some initiated cancer cells temporarily in check. The gradual decline in lung cancer risk among exsmokers over time indicates, of course, that although initiation has probably occurred, the initiated "precancerous" cell lies dormant without the added effect of promotion. Aging and nutritional factors are also associated with the initiating process, although mechanisms have yet to be clearly defined.

Passive Smoke Exposure

A review of the literature regarding passive smoke exposure and lung cancer is summarized in Table 2. A hallmark of a causal association is the internal and external consistency of data. The divergent findings from prospective studies by Hirayama in Japan (25,26) and Garfinkel in the United States (18), and the inconsistencies of retrospective studies in this area (10,12,32,33,47) may be due to: [1] cultural differences between nations which bias exposure information; [2] major differences in methodology which affect the analyses; [3] differences in the histologic type of lung cancer studied; and [4] the degree of histologic confirmation.

Information bias may confound exposure levels obtained from cases and controls in retrospective studies. Nonsmoking lung cancer patients, aware of the fact that this disease may be tobacco-associated, may perceive questions regarding exposure to the smoke of others with a different concern than do persons in the control group. In terms of consistency, it is incumbent, as Cochran suggested in the first Surgeon General's Report on Smoking and Health (50), that we examine the causal significance of the current epidemiologic evidence regarding passive smoke exposure using a "criterion for judgement." Several questions regarding lung cancer remain unanswered: [1] Has there been a real increase in the rate of nonsmokers with lung cancer? [2] Is the risk of lung cancer among non-inhaling cigar and pipe smokers significantly greater than that of nonsmokers since this is the group

TABLE 2. Summary of studies of the role of passive smoke exposure in lung cancer in nonsmokers (32)

Author/type of study/ population	Number of cases	Histology	Findings	Comments
Hirayama T., 1981, 1983 (25,26)/ prospec- tive/ Japanese nonsmok- ing wives aged 40 + .	200 deaths in married non- smoking females with lung cancer among 91540 nonsmoking married women.	Out of a sample of 23 cases, 17 were adenocarcinoma.	A dose-response relation- ship was seen between the nonsmoking wives' risk and the husband's smoking habit: wives of exsmokers or of 1-13 cigs/day smokers had RR = 1.42; wives of smokers of 15-19 cigs/day RR = 1.53; of ≥ 20 cigs/day had RR = 1.91; and of exsmokers RR = 1.36.	Exposure index was based on husbands' smoking habits.
Garfinkel L., 1981 (18)/ Analysis of data from 2 prospec- tive stud- ies/ACS popula- tion. Dorn study of veterans.	195 deaths from lung cancer among male nonsmokers; 564 deaths from lung cancer among female non- smokers (ACS). 168 lung cancer deaths among nonsmokers (Dorn).	Histologic confirmation of diagnosis in 69% of cases in first 6 yr of ACS study. Among lung cancer cases with con- firmed detailed his- tology, 46% of male and 59% of female non- smokers had adeno- carcinoma compared to 23% of male and 46% of female smokers (personal communi- cation).	No significant increase in lung cancer risk seen in nonsmoking wives of smoking husbands compared to non- smoking wives of nonsmoking husbands.	Exposure index was based on husbands' smoking habits.

(continued)

TABLE 2. (continued)

Author/type of study/ population	Number of cases	Histology	Findings	Comments
Trichopoulos D., et al., 1981, 1983. Case-control/ female caucasian residents of Athens.	77 female non-smokers with lung cancer other than adeno or terminal bronchiolar.	14 cases were histological-ly confirmed; 19 were cytologically confirmed; 18 were clinically confirmed. Excluded adeno and terminal bronchiolar.	RR of lung cancer associated with having a husband who smokes <1 pack/day was 2.4; RR associated with having a husband who smokes >1 pack/day was 3.4. (χ^2 for linear trend = 6.45; p < 0.02).	Exposure index was based on smoking habits of husbands and former husbands.
Chan W. C., (10), Fung, S. C. (10). Case-control/ Hong Kong Chinese.	There were only 2 nonsmokers out of 208 male lung cancer cases; 84 nonsmokers out of 189 female lung cancer patients.	15 of the 84 female cases were squamous or epidermoid cancer; 38 were adenocarcinoma; 15 had no histologic verificat on.	Among nonsmoking females the proportion of cases whose spouse smoked was slightly lower than that of controls (34 out of 84 or 40.5% vs. 66 of 139 or 47.5%). Among nonsmoking females, there was no significant difference in the proportion of cases who used kerosene fuel in cooking compared to controls.	It is unclear what question was used to get information since in an earlier paper (Chan et al., 1979), the question is given as "Are you exposed to the tobacco smoke of others at home or at work?" whereas here reference is made only to "smoking habits of spouses". No information is given on how many subjects were married.

Correa P., et al., (12), case-control/ Louisiana.	1338 cases and 1393 controls. Bronchioalveolar carcinomas were excluded. Only 10 out of 1036 male cases were nonsmokers. There were 25 nonsmoking, ever-married female cases out of 302 female cases.	97% of the cases had histologic confirmation.	Nonsmokers of both sexes married to heavy smokers had an increased risk of lung cancer (RR = 1.0, 1.48, 3.11 for nonsmokers married to spouses smoking 0, 1-40, ≥41 pack-years, respectively). In the total study population, subjects whose mothers smoked were also at increased risk, but no effect of paternal smoking was found.	The numbers of non-smokers are extremely small (8 male and 22 female cases used in analysis). Although the authors give a p-value of <0.05 for OR of 3.11, the 95% confidence interval is 0.56-22.27.
Koo, L., et al., (33), case-control/ Hong Kong Chinese women.	120 female cases and equal numbers of controlls. 56 cases were never-smokers.	63% of cases had histologic confirmation.	There were no significant differences between cases and controls on proportions with environmental smoke exposure, on total hr of exposure, or years of exposure.	

with heaviest exposure to sidestream smoke from tobacco products? [3] Is the incidence of lung cancer among individuals in occupations likely to be heavily exposed to environmental tobacco smoke, such as waiters, bartenders and train conductors, significantly elevated compared to nonsmokers? [4] Why is it that adenocarcinoma of the lung predominates among nonsmokers? [5] How are we to interpret pathological studies showing that among nonsmokers there is virtually no hyperplastic or metaplastic change in the bronchial epithelium?

These questions require careful consideration before we can conclude that passive smoke exposure is causally related to lung cancer (and/or other types of cancer).

The American Health Foundations' investigation of the effect of exposure to environmental smoke uses a detailed questionnaire to obtain information on such current and past exposure in the home, at work, on transportation, and in social settings. This questionnaire is reproduced in the Appendix. A preliminary analysis of our data demonstrated no significant differences between lung cancer cases and controls, with the exception of a greater frequency of exposure to environmental smoke at work among male cases, although it is premature to draw any definite conclusions from this sample (32). Our case-control study is closely integrated with biochemical assessments of the smoke uptake by nonsmokers (29). Biochemical assessment is made by determining levels of nicotine and its major metabolite cotinine in saliva and urine and, if feasible, in blood with radioimmunoassay techniques. So far, these studies have shown that nicotine and cotinine concentrations in these physiological fluids amount merely to a few percent of the levels recorded for active cigarette smokers (22,29).

If an association of passive smoke exposure and lung cancer were to be established, nitrosamines should be considered as etiological agents. It is of importance to note that the sidestream smoke of tobacco products contains higher amounts of volatile nitrosamines (N-nitrosodimethylamine 0.35-1.0 μg/cigarette) and of the carcinogenic nicotine-derived N-nitrosamines (0.34-2.1 μg/cigarette) than does mainstream smoke (0.001-0.02 μg and 0.2-1.2 μg/cigarette respectively; 28). Although sidestream smoke is quickly diluted by air, nitrosamines can reach measurable concentrations in certain enclosed environments (6). Furthermore, indoor environments polluted with tobacco smoke can be relatively rich in nitrogen oxides, agents which, in cigarette smokers, are known to induce the endogenous formation of nitrosamines (30). In summary, however, an association between long-term passive smoke exposure and lung cancer can, at present, only be considered as a working hypothesis and requires in-depth epidemiological and biochemical studies.

The Low-Yield Cigarette

There have been conflicting reports in the literature regarding the effect of the introduction of the filter cigarette, with the concomitant lowering of smoke yields, on the risk of lung cancer (5,13,23,24,36,38,39,43,55-57,67,68). The divergent findings may be partially explained by differences in analytic techniques, the gradual reduction in sales-weighted tar contained in the smoke of filter and nonfilter cigarettes, and the relative duration that these cigarettes have been smoked. It is postulated that smoking of filter cigarettes represents a lower risk of lung cancer if their tar yield differs significantly from that of nonfilter cigarettes. An analysis of the effects of tar and nicotine exposure on disease risk must include a consideration of the duration of smoking by brand to insure a sufficient interval of exposure. In future epidemiological surveys, notations of brand at any given time can be supplemented by available Federal Trade Commission data for smoke yields to afford an approximation of exposure. Exact exposure assessment, however, can be deduced only from reliable biochemical indicators of smoke uptake (22,27,51).

That individuals in currently recorded cohorts with lung cancer have generally started the smoking habit with nonfilter cigarettes is an important analytic consideration. In addition, although there has been an overall decline in the tar yield of both filter and nonfilter cigarettes over the years, as smokers shift from a higher to a lower yield cigarette, they tend to compensate for the reduction in nicotine through the practice of more frequent puffing, deeper inhalation, and longer smoke retention compared to the puff-drawing and inhalation practices associated with the higher yield cigarette (22,27,51). Thus, *a priori*, one would expect to find similar risk estimates for individuals smoking nonfilter cigarettes averaging 22 mg of tar and for individuals smoking high-yield filter cigarettes averaging 18 mg tar, a type of cigarette smoked by 35% of the United States' male cigarette smokers (49).

An analysis of data from a long-term case-control study of lung cancer conducted at the American Health Foundation demonstrates some decline in risk by tar yield for long-term smokers of filter cigarettes (62). While the decline in risk was expected to be greatest in individuals smoking cigarettes yielding ≤ 10 mg tar, we were surprised to find this not to be the case. In investigating why this occurred, we found that some smokers who do switch from a high- to a low-yield cigarette dramatically increase the number of cigarettes they smoke. Our findings indicate that patients with lung cancer increase the number of cigarettes smoked per day to a greater extent than do their controls. Subjects developing lung cancer may thus represent the more habituated smokers, adjusting their daily nicotine dosage through increased cigarette consumption. Thus, among lung cancer patients, there tends to be a strong inverse association between quantity of cigarettes smoked per day and the smoke yield and, especially the nicotine delivery of the preferred brand. This was not observed for the controls (Table 3).

TABLE 3. Means and standard errors (SE) of the average quantity of cigarettes smoked per day by lung cancer patients (Kreyberg type I) and their controls by average tar yield (62)

Tar Yield	Nicotine Yield	Cases		Controls		Difference in mean number of cigarettes
		N	Mean (± SE)	N	Mean (± SE)	
A. Men						
< 10 mg	0.8 mg	27	45.8 (3.3)	18	30.6 (3.5)	+ 15
10-14 mg	0.8-1.1 mg	55	40.3 (1.8)	63	29.7 (1.9)	+ 10
≥ 15 mg	≥ 1.2 mg	151	37.1 (1.2)	146	30.1 (1.3)	+ 7
Nonfilter		180	37.0 (1.2)	134	28.7 (1.0)	+ 8
B. Women						
< 10 mg	0.8 mg	24	36.4 (3.0)	17	21.5 (3.4)	+ 15
10-14 mg	0.8-1.1 mg	60	31.1 (2.0)	46	25.9 (2.1)	+ 5
≥ 15 mg	≥ 1.2 mg	81	31.9 (1.6)	40	21.1 (1.7)	+ 10
Nonfilter		59	30.6 (1.6)	35	25.4 (2.2)	+ 5

Evidence based upon American data suggests marginal differences in the risk of lung cancer among older smokers who have predominantly smoked nonfilter or high-yield filter cigarettes compared to long-term smokers of the lower-yield filter cigarettes. In the case of the younger male cohorts in the United Kingdom and the United States, their reduced mortality rate may be at least partially explained by the fact that their smoking habit was predominantly started with the low-yield cigarette. The younger smokers appear also to compensate less for the low nicotine delivery than the older smokers. This concept finds support when we study the comparative lung cancer mortality rates in different cohorts, as has been done by Doll and Peto in Great Britain, and from United States SEER data (Table 4). The British data show that the younger cohorts smoke 20% fewer cigarettes than the older cohorts - differences that cannot account alone for a 50% difference in lung cancer rates. The data suggest, therefore, that a reduced tar yield of cigarettes, particularly <10 mg, may have some impact on lung cancer risk. Additional support for this hypothesis lies in the finding that younger women have a lower rate of lung cancer than younger men. This may be partially due to the fact that women smoke cigarettes with lower tar yields than men in the same cohorts (51).

Smoking Cessation and Smoking Prevention

One final issue with grave social implications remains the continued smoking by a large segment of our society, particularly among women, minorities and adolescents. On the positive side, there is a growing population of exsmokers, particularly among educated, white males. The majority of them have been able to give up smoking by themselves rather than depending on specific smoking cessation therapies. Nonetheless, we should have smoking cessation clinics as part of every health care facility since smokers who would like to give up but cannot do so independently, should be offered readily accessible support services.

It is of particular public health importance to make certain that young people do not begin to smoke. We have developed a "Know Your Body (KYB)" school health promotion program to provide school-aged children with a program that enhances health knowledge, positively affects their health attitudes and behaviors, and helps them make appropriate decisions in terms of avoiding clinical risk factors (4,69). This type of curriculum should be started as early as the first grade.

By and large, our society has neglected the field of school health education. This represents a significant oversight and omission with

TABLE 4. Decreases in lung cancer, comparing 1978 data with data for the worst-affected[a] generations of men in England and Wales and in the United States (14)

Age (year)	Worst-affected[a] generation (born ca. 1910-1911)		Rates for 1978 compared with those for worst-affected generation		Worst-affected[a] generation (born ca. 1910-1911)		Rates for 1978 compared with those for worst-affected generation	
	Mortality/ million men	Period of observation	Mortality/ million men in 1978	Decrease[b]	Mortality/ million men	Period of observation	Mortality/ million men in 1978	Decrease[b]
30-34	40	1941-45	17	58%/35 yr	24	1958-62	17	30%/18 yr
35-39	98	1946-50	63	36%/30 yr	63	1963-67	62	15%/13 yr
40-44	253	1951-55	138	45%/25 yr	219	1968-72	192	12%/8 yr
45-49	597	1956-60	385	36%/20 yr	502	1973-77	480	4%/3 yr
50-54	1,234[c]	1961-65	1,047	15%/15yr	?	1980	1,021	--[e]
55-59	2,219[d]	1966-70	1,912	14%/10 yr	?	1985	1,647	--[f]

60-64	3,577[d]	1971-75	3,315	7%/5 yr	?	1990	2,625	--[g]
65-69	5,018	1978	5,018	--	?	1995	3,557	--[g]

[a] These are the generations with the highest death rates at ages 35-44, when substantial effects of smoking first became evident. However, if in the future the number of cigarettes smoked/individual will decrease, or the effective dose of noxious chemicals/cigarette will decrease, the benefits at some particular attained age to these two worst-affected generations may be greater than to the immediately previous generations. The maximum American lung cancer rates in old age may therefore be seen, at around the turn of the century, in the generation born in a few years before this "worst-affected" generation.

[b] Percentage decrease, comparing age-specific mortality in 1978 with that for the worst-affected generation (born 1910-11 in England and Wales, born 1927-28 in the United States).

[c] Might have been materially larger but for changes in cigarette composition.

[d] Would have been materially larger but for changes in cigarette composition.

[e] U.S. mortality at ages 50-54 should reach a maximum by ca. 1980.

[f] U.S. mortality at ages 55-59 is still rising.

[g] U.S. mortality at ages 60-64 and 65-69 is still rising rapidly.

respect to the long-term health of our young people. Our studies have shown that more than one-third of 12-year-old students have one or more known risk factors for chronic disease including cigarette smoking. It has been shown that the risk of smoking can be reduced substantially through an organized school health promotion program (4,40,45). We hope that school health education programs, like KYB, will become an integral component of the school curriculum in the United States and elsewhere.

Children are receptive to behavioral modification provided they are presented the opportunity to change. They are also ready to affect the health behavior of their parents if they are given the chance. Involving both children and parents will have an impact on the entire community. Thus, we regard appropriate school health education, properly evaluated and monitored, as a key component of a national strategy toward the prevention of avoidable illness. If we succeed in preventing young people from starting to smoke, most of the unresolved issues in this document will not require any further elucidation.

SUMMARY

The 1982 Report of the Surgeon General of the U.S. Public Health Service concluded that "cigarette smoking is the major single cause of cancer mortality in the United States" and that "85 percent of lung cancer cases are due to smoking" (51). Thus, major emphasis should be placed on school health education programs designed to prevent young people from smoking. Those students who are already cigarette smokers should be provided with an opportunity to attend smoking cessation courses with the hope that they stop. However, as long as society condones tobacco usage, millions of people will smoke, and millions of others with be involuntarily exposed to tobacco smoke. In this communication we have discussed the need for future research on the etiology of lung cancer. This includes the observation of a shift toward an increasing proportion of adenocarcinoma compared to squamous cell carcinoma of the lung in men, more detailed knowledge of the effects of macro- and micronutrients in the etiology of lung cancer, a clear delineation of the impact of tumor initiators, tumor promoters, and cocarcinogens in the development of lung cancer in cigarette smokers, and a study of the effects of the low-yield cigarette on the lung cancer risk of smokers.

Finally, we reviewed the present knowledge as to the possible association of passive smoke exposure and lung cancer. Here we have placed major emphasis on the need for a close cooperation between epidemiologists and clinical biochemists in risk assessment.

REFERENCES

1. American Health Foundation (1983): unpublished data.
2. Armed Forces Institute of Pathology (1952): *Atlas of Tumor Pathology, Fasc. 17*, edited by A. A. Lieban, 182 pp. Washington.
3. Beems, R. B., and van Beek, L. (1984): *Carcinogenesis*, 5:413-417.
4. Botvin, G. J., and Eng, A. (1982): *Prev. Med.*, 11:199-211.
5. Bross, I. J., and Gibson, R. (1968): *Am. J. Public Health*, 58:1396-1403.
6. Brunnemann, K. D., and Hoffmann, D. (1978): *IARC Sci. Publ.*, 19:343-356.
7. Byers, T., and Graham, S. (1984): *Adv. Cancer Res.*, 41:1-69.
8. Cahansky, G., Powzer, Y., and Kalter, Y. (1969): *J. Isr. Med. Assoc.*, 77:547-550.
9. Carroll, K. K., Hopkins, J. G., and Kennedy, T. J. (1981): *Prog. Lipid Res.*, 20:685-690.
10. Chan, W. C., and Fung, S. C. (1982): In: *Cancer Campaign, Vol. 6: Cancer Epidemiology*, edited by E. Grundmann, pp. 199-202. Gustav Fischer Verlag, Stuttgart.
11. Cohen, L. A., and Thompson, D. O. (1984): *Fed. Proc.*, 43:614.
12. Correa, P., Pickle, L. W., Fontham, E., Lin, T., and Haenszel, W. (1983): *Lancet*, 2:595-597.
13. Dean, G., Lee, P. N., and Todd, G. F. (1977): *Tobacco Research Council, Research Paper No. 14*. Tobacco Research Council, London.
14. Doll, R., and Peto, R. (1981): *J. Natl. Cancer Inst.*, 66:1191-1308.
15. Ernster, V. L., Selvin, S., and Sacks, S. T. (1982): *J. Natl. Cancer Inst.*, 69:773-776.
16. Feinleib, M. (1982): *Prev. Med.*, 11:360-367.
17. Ferrari, E., and Kreyberg, L. (1960): *Brit. J. Cancer*, 14:604-611.
18. Garfinkel, L. (1981): *J. Natl. Cancer Inst.*, 66:1061-1066.
19. Ghaffer, A. (1981): In: *Manual of Macrophage Methodology: Collection, Characterization, and Function. Immunology Series No. 13*, edited by H. B. Herscowitz, H. I. Holden, and J. A. Bellantini, pp. 441-446. Marcel Dekker, Inc., New York.
20. Graham, E. A., Croninger, A. B., and Wynder, E. L. (1957): *Cancer Res.*, 17:1058-1066.
21. Graham, S. (1983): *Rev. Cancer Epidemiol.*, 2:1-45.
22. Haley, N. J., Axelrad, C. M., and Tilton, K. A. (1983): *Am. J. Public Health*, 73:1204-1207.
23. Hammond, E. C., Garfinkel, L., Seidman, H., and Lew, E. A. (1976): *Environ. Res.*, 12:263-274.
24. Hawthorne, V. M., and Fry, J. S. (1978): *J. Epidemiol. Community Health*, 32:260-266.
25. Hirayama, T. (1981): *Brit. Med. J.*, 282:183-185.
26. Hirayama, T. (1983): *Lancet*, 2:1425-1426.
27. Hoffmann, D., Adams, J. D., and Haley, N. J. (1983): *Am. J. Public Health*, 73:1050-1053.
28. Hoffmann, D., Brunnemann, K. D., Adams, J. D., and Hecht, S. S. (1984): *IARC Sci. Publ.*, in press.

29.   Hoffmann, D., Haley, N. J., Adams, J. D., and Brunnemann, K. D. (1984): *Prev. Med.*, in press.
30.   Hoffmann, D., Hecht, S. S., Haley, N. J., Brunnemann, K. D., Adams, J. D., and Wynder, E. L. (1983): In: *Human Carcinogenesis*, edited by C. C. Harris, and H. N. Autrup, pp. 809-832. Academic Press, New York.
31.   Hoffmann, D., Hecht, S. S., and Wynder, E. L. (1983): *Environ. Health Perspect.*, 50:247-257.
32.   Kabat, G. C., and Wynder, E. L. (1983): *Cancer*, 53:1214-1221.
33.   Koo, L. C., Ho, J. H. -C., and Saw, D. (1983): *J. Exp. Clin. Cancer Res.*, 4:367-375.
34.   Kreyberg, L. (1962): *Histological Lung Cancer Types: A Morphological and Biological Correlation*. Norwegian Universities Press, Oslo.
35.   Kreyberg, L., and Saxen, E. (1961): *Brit. J. Cancer*, 15:211-214.
36.   Kunze, M., and Vutuc, C. (1980): In: *A Safe Cigarette? Banbury Report 3*, edited by G. B. Gori and F. G. Bock, pp. 29-60. Cold Spring Harbor Laboratory, New York.
37.   Law, C. H., Day, N. E., and Shanmugaratnam, K. (1976): *Int. J. Cancer*, 17:304-309.
38.   Lee, P. N., and Garfinkel, L. (1981): *J. Epidemiol. Community Health*, 35:16-22.
39   Lubin, J., Blot, W. J., and Berrino, F. (1984): *Int. J. Cancer*, 33:569-576.
40.   Luepker, R. V., Johnson, C. A., Murray, D. M., and Pechacek, A. (1982): *J. Behav. Med.*, 6:53-62.
41.   Matthay, R. (1982): *Clin. Chest. Med.*, 3:217-454.
42.   Reddy, B. S., and Maeura, Y. (1984): *J. Natl. Cancer Inst.*, 72:745-750.
43.   Rimington, J. (1981): *Environ. Res.*, 24:162-166.
44.   Shinton, N. K. (1963): *Brit. J. Cancer*, 17:222-230.
45.   Telch, M. J., Killen, J. D., McAlister, A. L., Perry, C. L., and Maccoby, N. (1982): *J. Behav. Med.*, 5:1-8.
46.   Tobacco Institute (1984): *Tobacco Industry Profile 1984*, pp. 4. Tobacco Institute, Washington.
47.   Trichopoulos, D., Kalandidi, A., and Sparros, L. (1981): *Int. J. Cancer*, 27:1-4.
48.   Trichopoulos, D., Kalandidi, A., and Sparros, L. (1983): *Lancet*, 2:677-678.
49.   U.S. Department of Health and Human Services (1981): *The Health Consequences of Smoking. The Changing Cigarette. A Report of the Surgeon General*, 252 pp. Department of Health and Human Services, Public Health Service, Publication No. 81-50156.
50.   U.S. Public Health Service (1964): *Smoking and Health: Report of the Advisory Committee of the Public Health Service*, 387 pp. U. S. Department of Health Education and Welfare, Center for Disease Control, Public Health Service Publication No. 1103.
51.   U.S. Public Health Service (1982): *The Health Consequences of Smoking - Cancer. A Report of the Surgeon General*, 322 pp. Department of Health and Human Services, Public Health Service Publication 82-50179.
52.   Uys, C. J. (1970): *S. Afr. Cancer Bull.*, 14:8-14.
53.   Vincent, R. G., Pickren, J. W., Lane, W. L., Bross, I., Takita, H., Houten, L., Gutierres, A. C., and Raepha, T. (1977): *Cancer*, 39:1647-1655.
54.   Vincent, T. N., Satterfield, J. V., and Ackerman, L. V. (1965): *Cancer*, 18:559-570.
55.   Vutuc, C., and Kunze, M. (1982): *Prev. Med.*, 11:713-716.
56.   Vutuc, C., and Kunze, M. (1983): *J. Natl. Cancer Inst.*, 71:435-437.

57. Wald, N. J. (1976): *Lancet*, 1:136-138.

58. Wald, N., Idle, M., Boreham, J., and Biley, A. (1980): *Lancet*, 2:813-815.

59. Wynder, E. L. (1983): *Environ. Health Perspect.*, 50:15-21.

60. Wynder, E. L., Fritz, L., and Furth, N. (1957): *J. Natl. Cancer Inst.*, 19:361-370.

61. Wynder, E. L., and Goodman, M. T. (1983): *Epidemiol. Rev.*, 5:177-207.

62. Wynder, E. L., and Goodman, M. T. (1984): in preparation.

63. Wynder, E. L., Graham, E. A., and Croninger, A. B. (1953): *Cancer Res.*, 13:855-864.

64. Wynder, E. L., Graham, E. A., and Croninger, A. B. (1955): *Cancer Res.*, 15:445-448.

65. Wynder, E. L., and Hecht, S. S., editors (1976): *Lung Cancer*, 170 pp. UICC Technical Report Serial 25.

66. Wynder, E. L., Lupberger, A., and Grener, C. (1956): *Brit. J. Cancer*, 10:507-509.

67. Wynder, E. L., Mabuchi, K., and Beattie, E. J. (1970): *J. Am. Med. Assoc.*, 213:2221-2228.

68. Wynder, E. L. and Stellman, S. D. (1979): *J. Natl. Cancer Inst.*, 62:471-477.

69. Williams, C. L., Arnold, C. B., and Wynder, E. L. (1977): *Prev. Med.*, 6:344-357.

70. Yesner, R., Gerstl, B., and Auerbach, O. (1965): *Ann. Thorac. Surg.*, 1:33-49.

APPENDIX. Passive smoke exposure questionnaire

ID#:　| 1 | 4 | | | | | | | | |
　　　　1　2　3　4　5　6　7　8　9　10

Case-control: _____
Sex: _____
Dx: _____
Date: _____

Childhood exposure to other people's smoke at home

1. When you were a child (up to 21 yrs old), did anyone in your household smoke in your presence? (Include parents, other relatives, roomers).
   1 = yes (go to Q.A); 2 = No (go to Q.6); V = Don't know (go to Q.6)

□ 11

A	2	3	4	5
Who was it?	What type of tobacco did ____ smoke in your presence?	How many yrs did _____ smoke in your presence during child-hood?	During those yrs, how many hrs/day were your exposed to _____'s smoke on average?	Would you describe your exposure to _____'s smoke as:
	1 = Cigs only	V = Don't know	V = Don't know	0 = None
	2 = Cigs & cigars			1 = Light
	3 = Cigs & pipes			2 = Moderate
Check but do not code.	1 = Cigars only			3 = Heavy
	4 = Cigars & pipes			V = Don't know
	6 = Pipes only			
	7 = All three			
	V = Don't know			
____ Mother	□ 12	□□ 13	□□ 15	□ 17
____ Father	□ 18	□□ 19	□□ 21	□ 23
____ Other	□ 24	□□ 25	□□ 27	□ 29
____ Other	□ 30	□□ 31	□□ 33	□ 35
____ Other	□ 36	□□ 37	□□ 39	□ 41
____ Other	□ 42	□□ 43	□□ 45	□ 47

6. Do you happen to know if your mother smoked when she was pregnant with you?
1 = yes; 2 = No; V = Don't know

□ 48

Adulthood exposure to other people's smoke at home

7. In your adult years (>21 yrs old) has there ever been anyone living in your home who smoked <u>in your presence</u>? Include spouse (codes 01-09), children (codes 10-29), other relatives and roomers (codes 30-49).
1 = yes (go to Q.8); 2 = No (if no, code yrs of no exposure in Q.10-11);
V = Don't know

□ 49

8	9	10	11	12	13	14
Who is it?	How many cigarettes, cigars or pipes did _____ smoke in your presence? V = Don't know BLANK = Not exposed	Yr start- ed	Yr stopp- ed	How many hrs/day did ____ smoke in your presence? V = Don't know	Would your describe your exposure as: 1 = None 1 = Light 2 = Moderate 3 = heavy V = DK	If spouse smokes does he/she smoke in your bedroom: 1 = Yes 2 = No V = DK

Cigar-
ettes Pipes Cigars

□□ □□ □□ □□ □□ □□   □□   □ 64   □ 65
50   52   54   56   58   60   62

□□ □□ □□ □□ □□ □□   □□   □ 80
66   68   70   72   74   /6   78

ID#: 2 4 ☐☐☐☐☐☐☐☐   □ 11
      1 2 3 4 5 6 7 8 9 10

□□ □□ □□ □□ □□ □□   □□   □ 26   □ 27
12   14   16   18   20   22   24

□□ □□ □□ □□ □□ □□   □□   □ 42   □ 43
28   30   32   34   36   38   40

[boxes row 1: 44 46 48 50 52 54 56 58 59]

[boxes row 2: 60 62 64 66 68 70 72 74 75]

ID #: | 3 | 4 | | | | | | | | |
1 2 3 4 5 6 7 8 9 10

[boxes row 3: 11 13 15 17 19 21 23 25 26]

Exposure to other people's smoke at work

15. In your current, or most recent job, are/were you exposed to other
   people's tobacco smoke in enclosed areas ? (Only code jobs of 1 yr or
   more). _____ (write in job)
   1 = yes; 2 = No (code yrs of no exposure Q.17-18, go to Q.21);
   V = Don't know

27

16	17	18	19	20
How many hrs/week are you exposed in this way?	Yr started	Yr stopped	What was the average # of smokers within 10 ft. of you during these periods (i.e. at desk, during break)?	Would you say your exposure was: 0 = None 1 = Light 2 = Moderate 3 = Heavy V = Don't know

[boxes: 28] [boxes: 30] [boxes: 32] [boxes: 34] [box: 36]

21. At the job you held before that, were you exposed to other people's tobacco smoke in enclosed areas? _____

    (write in job)

    ☐ 37

    1 = yes; 2 = No (code yrs of no exposure Q.23-24, go to Q.27);
    V = Don't know

22	23	24	25	26
Hrs/week	Yr started	Yr stopped	Number of smokers	Quality of exposure
☐☐ 38	☐☐ 40	☐☐ 42	☐☐ 44	☐☐ 46

27. At the job before that, were you exposed to other people's tobacco smoke in enclosed areas? _____

    (write in job)

    ☐ 47

    1 = yes; 2 = No (code yrs of no exposure Q.29-30, go to Q.33);
    V = Don't know

28	29	30	31	32
Hrs/week	Yr started	Yr stopped	Number of smokers	Quality of exposure
☐☐ 48	☐☐ 50	☐☐ 52	☐☐ 54	☐☐ 56

33. At the job before that, were you exposed to other people's tobacco smoke in enclosed areas? _____

    (write in job)

    ☐ 57

    1 = yes; 2 = No (code yrs of no exposure Q.35-36, go to Q.39);
    V = Don't know

34	35	36	37	38
Hrs/week	Yr started	Yr stopped	Number of smokers	Quality of exposure
☐☐ 58	☐☐ 60	☐☐ 62	☐☐ 64	☐☐ 66

Exposure to other people's smoke on any form of transportation

39. As an adult (>21 yrs. old), how often (on the average) are you or
    have you in the past been exposed to other people's smoke in cars?
    _____ hrs/week   00 = Never exposed

67

40. For how many yrs have you been exposed in this way?
    _____ yrs   00 = Never exposed

69

41. As an adult (>21 yrs old), how often (on the average) are you or
    have you in the past been exposed to other people's smoke on
    commuter trains, buses, or other forms of transportation?
    _____ hrs/week   00 = Never exposed

71

42. How many years have you been exposed in this way?
    _____ yrs (leave blank if Q.41 = 00)

73

Exposure to other people's smoke socially

43. How often (on the average) are you, or have you been, exposed to
    other people's smoke on social occasions, i.e. at parties, card games,
    dinners in the home or in public areas restaurants, theaters, bingo
    games, etc.?
    _____ hrs/week   00 = Never exposed

75

44. How many years are you, or have you been, exposed in this way?
    _____ yrs (leave blank if Q.43 = 00)

77

Carcinogenesis, Vol. 8, edited by M. J. Mass et al.
Raven Press, New York © 1985.

Tumor Enhancement Factors and Mechanisms in the Hamster Respiratory Tract Carcinogenesis Model

Umberto Saffiotti, Sherman F. Stinson, *Kevin P. Keenan, and
*Elizabeth M. McDowell

*Laboratory of Experimental Pathology, National Cancer Institute, Frederick, Maryland 21701;
*Department of Pathology, University of Maryland School of Medicine,
Baltimore, Maryland 21201*

Until the present time, little was known concerning enhancement or promotion during tumor induction in the respiratory epithelium, in spite of the fact that such mechanisms may be significant contributors to human respiratory carcinogenesis as indicated, for example, by the role of promoter-like factors in cigarette smoke.

Cell proliferation is an essential phenomenon for the fixation and expression of neoplastic changes and, therefore, it plays an important role in chemical carcinogenesis in general, and specifically in the mechanisms of tumor promotion as seen in skin and liver epithelia (23,28,30,131). The requirement for cell proliferation in chemical carcinogenesis has important implications in many organ systems, reflecting the nature of different target cells capable of cell proliferation and neoplastic transformation.

In tissues which normally replicate very slowly, including the respiratory epithelium, an important rate limiting step in the carcinogenic process may be cell proliferation. Cell death and cell renewal are predominant features of most toxicologic injuries to the respiratory epithelium (27). Thus, concomitant cell necrosis induced by various injuries, followed by regeneration, could be a major determinant in chemical carcinogenesis in the respiratory epithelium, as it is in the liver (28).

In the skin, wound healing represents a potent promoting factor (3,20,31,47), as are several specific chemicals. Relatively little, however, has been known until recently concerning the effects of cocarcinogens and promoters in the tracheobronchial epithelium (81). Nevertheless, a number of factors have been reported as suspected or identified cocarcinogens or promoters in human and experimental animal bronchial neoplasia (36), and these mechanisms are discussed in the present volume.

In order to clarify the nature and mechanisms of complete carcinogens, cocarcinogens, promoting agents, and other enhancing factors for the respiratory tract, their effects need to be characterized in appropriate experimental model systems.

A distinction should be made, at the outset of this review, between promoting agents and other enhancing factors. Promoting agents have biological effects and mechanisms closely similar to those of phorbol esters on mouse skin epithelium, while other factors may stimulate the expression of latent neoplastic changes by a wider range of temporal and functional mechanisms.

Generalizations from studies on mouse epidermis may not be applicable to other tissues having distinct pathways for cell renewal and differentiation, such as the respiratory epithelium. The normal tracheobronchial epithelium is pseudostratified columnar. This means that cells of all types rest on the basal lamina but not all cell types reach the lumen. The secretory (mucous) cells and the ciliated cells are tall columnar cells and reach to the lumen, but the basal cells and some of the endocrine cells are short and do not. This simple fact is often overlooked in humans because there are relatively few normal areas in the bronchi of adults, even in putatively healthy individuals. It has been demonstrated that the basal cells of adult human bronchi contain keratins of intermediate and high molecular weight (105). In the epidermis, these keratins are only found in the suprabasal differentiating cell layer, but not in the basal cells (8,126). This pattern suggests that bronchial basal cells are more highly differentiated than the basal cells of the epidermis.

We shall review our present understanding of experimental models and mechanisms involving the role of enhancing factors in the pathogenesis of respiratory tract neoplasia, as investigated in the hamster model.

It has been a long-standing tenet of our research that in order to correlate mechanisms of carcinogenesis at the molecular and biochemical levels with the corresponding events in human and animal tissues and organs, it is important to connect the different levels of observation in a series of biological model systems of decreasing complexity, which are closely related to each other in a step-by-step sequence. Thus, having started with the study of the human pathology of respiratory cancers, we first sought an animal model where such pathology could be induced experimentally by carcinogens in a way that would closely resemble the human counterpart. Subsequent developments included: (a) organ culture methods for the maintenance of the target tissue, namely the respiratory tract mucosa, and (b) cell culture methods for respiratory epithelial cells. The pathology induced by carcinogens and by enhancing or modifying factors can thus be studied by a variety of methods correlating different levels of biological organization in the target tissue. The phases of this sequential development of biological models for respiratory carcinogenesis will be discussed below and related to the role of enhancing factors.

DEVELOPMENT OF THE HAMSTER MODEL IN VIVO AND IN CULTURE

In Vivo Animal Model

The first goal, the establishment of an animal model closely related to human pathology, was well met by the development of the hamster model for respiratory carcinogenesis induced by carcinogens carried by inorganic particulates (99,100). This model was initially selected because the hamster has no spontaneous pulmonary tumors and because this species was found to be highly resistant to pulmonary infections and inflammatory reactions, even after intratracheal instillations. Effective delivery of carcinogens, such as polycyclic aromatic hydrocarbons, was obtained by attaching them to fine particles of inorganic carriers suspended in saline and administered by intratracheal instillation. The most commonly used treatment consists of benzo(a)pyrene (BP) attached to particles of ferric oxide (Fe_2O_3), and suspended in saline. This model has the advantage of avoiding the kind of deep and extensive tissue damage and scar reaction induced by pellets and threads, and can be closely related to the conditions of human exposure to inhaled carcinogens carried by dust or smoke particles. A degree of epithelial injury is induced, however, by intratracheal cannulation (58-60,62); the possible role of such focal injury is discussed below. Previous experience with the intratracheal instillation method acquired in studies on the cellular pathogenesis of silicosis in rats showed lack of toxic or fibrogenic response to certain particulates including Fe_2O_3 (93,94,98,104).

The hamster model was further validated when it was found to give rise to a carcinogenic response that closely resembles its human counterpart not only in terms of tumor pathology (97,100,101,103), but also in its histogenesis and ultrastructural morphology (11-13,46,68,72,100,129).

In Vitro Epithelial Culture Models

The next step in our experimental approach was to develop culture methods for the hamster tracheobronchial epithelium. With appropriate culture conditions, it was shown that this tissue could be maintained effectively in short-term organ cultures for coordinated biochemical and morphological studies on the effects of carcinogens and modifying factors applied directly to the epithelium (19,33,55,113).

The development of specialized methods for obtainment and culture of human tissues made it possible to extend the organ culture studies to the corresponding human target tissue, the bronchus (9,37-40,42,102,130). This major advance opened the way to the direct experimental investigation of the interactions and effects of carcinogens and cofactors on human tissues, and has generated substantial progress in the last decade (37). Studies on respiratory epithelia in organ culture further confirmed the analogy of the hamster model with its human counterpart.

Major accomplishments were obtained in other laboratories towards the establishment of epithelial cell cultures from the respiratory epithelium. Cell culture methods were developed for the hamster tracheal epithelium (66,78,135). More extensive work was devoted, however, to studies on the trachea of the rat, which was used by Nettesheim and coworkers to develop a series of imaginative model systems *in vivo*, *in vitro*, or with combined *in vivo/in vitro* methods (79-81). This approach has recently led to the induction of neoplastic transformation by carcinogens applied directly to isolated rat tracheal epithelial cells in culture (83), and to the characterization of epithelial cell populations with different potentials for preneoplastic or neoplastic growth (127). Methods for the growth of isolated human bronchial epithelial cells were also developed (63-65,124).

Current work in our laboratories includes the characterization of the culture requirements of hamster tracheobronchial epithelial cells in primary and secondary culture with serum-free media (54). These cells are investigated to identify their optimal requirements for factors capable of supporting growth and transformation. Similar methods were recently established for mouse epidermal keratinocyte cultures using a serum-free medium (14).

Comparative Studies In Vivo and In Vitro

The development of inbred strains of hamsters has made it possible to use this species for the study of model systems requiring *in vitro/in vivo* experiments. The battery of models can presently be used to investigate biochemical and molecular mechanisms of carcinogenesis and gene activation and to determine which mechanisms are shared by isolated epithelial cells, their tissues of origin in culture, the same tissues *in vivo* and the corresponding target organs in the whole organism, when exposed to various carcinogenic factors. At all these levels, except carcinogenesis *in vivo*, comparative experimental studies with the corresponding human tissues and cells are now feasible.

Studies on the metabolic activation of carcinogens and their binding (6) have further confirmed the close comparability of the hamster model and the human counterpart with the major distinction that quantitative interindividual variability appears to be much more marked in the human tissues. It is interesting that in comparative studies on the binding of BP to DNA from respiratory epithelia of various species, hamster tracheal tissue showed a particularly high level of binding (6).

CARCINOGENS FOR THE HAMSTER RESPIRATORY TRACT

Different types of carcinogens and various modes of administration have been shown to induce carcinogenic responses in the hamster respiratory tract. The induced epithelial tumors differ by degree of malignancy, types of cellular differentiation, and the site of prevalent localization.

Polycyclic Aromatic Hydrocarbons

The most extensive data have accrued with the repeated intratracheal administration of polycyclic hydrocarbons, usually BP, carried by inorganic particulates in saline suspension. The treatment results in a prevalence of carcinomas from the larynx, trachea, and extralobar and intralobar bronchi. The carcinomas can show various types of differentiation, often combining varying degrees of epidermoid and mucous differentiation in the same tumor. The highest incidence was found for prevalently epidermoid carcinomas (notably in the trachea), followed by poorly differentiated carcinomas (often with areas of partial or mixed differentiation), and by adenocarcinomas. Among the peripheral lung tumors which arise from the bronchiolar-alveolar epithelium, the majority of tumors are adenomas, followed by adenocarcinomas, and epidermoid carcinomas, and a few anaplastic carcinomas. Benign papillary tumors are relatively frequent in the larynx and trachea, and rare in the bronchi. No tumors are induced in the nasal mucosa (77,96,97).

The effects of polycyclic aromatic hydrocarbons in this hamster carcinogenesis system, alone or in combination with several other carcinogens and cofactors, were recently reviewed (123).

N-Nitroso Compounds

Many experimental studies have been conducted in the hamster with compounds of this category. The nitrosamide, N-methyl-nitrosourea (MNU), a water-soluble direct-acting alkylating agent, is a very effective carcinogen when instilled directly into the hamster respiratory tract; most of the induced tracheobronchial carcinomas show epidermoid differentiation (44,45,50,56). Combined treatment with MNU and with BP/Fe_2O_3 can be synergistic (56).

Topical intratracheal application of MNU to a limited segment of the tracheal mucosa was obtained by Schreiber et al. (108) by means of a double-walled cannula. The histogenesis of the tracheal lesions at the site of application of MNU could thus be effectively analyzed (108,121,122).

Systemic administration of diethylnitrosamine (DEN) and of other nitrosamines to hamsters gives rise to a wide range of tumor types. The tumor localization varies with different nitrosamines (Table 1).

Autoradiographic studies with radioactively labelled nitro-samines (90) showed that they bind mostly in metabolically active epithelial cells, namely the mucous cells of the trachea and large bronchi and the Clara cells of the small bronchi and bronchioles.

Combined treatments with intratracheal BP/Fe_2O_3 and systemic DEN were studied in the hamster (76,77). When BP/Fe_2O_3 was given at a low effective schedule (2 mg BP with 2 mg Fe_2O_3 every 2 weeks for 15 applications), no epidermoid carcinomas were induced in the tracheobronchial tract; subcutaneous administration of DEN (1 mg once weekly for 12 weeks) by itself also induced no carcinomas (only polyps or papillomas typical of DEN); however, when these treatments

TABLE 1. Incidence of respiratory tumors in Syrian golden hamsters induced by nitrosamines[a]

Nitrosamine	Dose	Nasal cavities	Larynx	Trachea	Bronchi	Lungs	Reference
Diethylnitrosamine	4 mg (×12)[b]	75	72	97	8	3	(75)
Di-n-propylnitrosamine	60 mg/kg[c]	92	27	100	50	67	(87)
2,2'-Dimethyldipropyl-nitrosamine	500 mg/kg[c]	5	15	30	5	0	(2)
2,2'-Dihydroxydi-n-propylnitrosamine	500 mg/kg[c]	45	8	41	0	45	(86)
2-Oxypropyl-n-propyl-nitrosamine	120 mg/kg[c]	84	0[e]	95[f]	11	16	(85)
Methyl-n-propylnitrosamine	50 mg/kg[c]	95	16	89	0	53	(88)
N-Nitrosohexamethy-leneimine	16 mg/kg[c]	15	8	58	0	3	(1)
2,6-Dimethylnitroso-morpholine	37 mg/kg[d]	34	13[g]	23	0	38	(91)

[a] Percent of effective number of animals.
[b] s.c. once weekly for 12 weeks.
[c] Approximately 0.1 LD_{50}, s.c. once weekly for life.
[d] Intragastric once weekly for life.
[e] A few laryngeal polyps at lower doses.
[f] Estimated.
[g] 25% in males and 0% in females.

were given sequentially (BP followed by DEN), a 31% incidence of carcinomas was induced (76). When subcutaneous DEN was given first (1 or 0.5 mg once weekly for 12 weeks), followed by intratracheal instillation, the prevailing combined response was shifted to the peripheral lung, with the development of adenomas and adenocarcinomas. This enhanced response was found to be induced not only by repeated instillations of BP/Fe_2O_3 (2 mg each, every 2 weeks, 10 to 15 times), but equally well by Fe_2O_3 without BP (77). This effect was observed, at a somewhat lower level, even when the DEN treatment was followed by saline treatment alone (115). No tumors were induced by Fe_2O_3/saline treatment alone in many control groups (77).

The enhanced induction of peripheral lung tumors in DEN treated hamsters, brought about by repeated intratracheal instillations of Fe_2O_3 in saline or even of saline alone, was the first indication we had that non-specific factors, that are not carcinogenic *per se*, could have an enhancing role. A similar enhancing effect was demonstrated when intratracheal administration of [210]Po, which induces peripheral lung tumors in hamsters, was followed by intratracheal instillations of saline (67,110).

Arsenic

Recent findings shed new light on the effects of arsenic in respiratory carcinogenesis, that suggests that arsenic may act through some enhancing mechanism.

Arsenic was known from epidemiologic studies to be a causative factor for human lung cancer, but evidence in animals was lacking. Therefore, arsenic was considered to be an exception in the list of agents known to be carcinogenic from both direct human evidence and animal evidence. Pershagen et al. (84) treated hamsters with 15 weekly intratracheal instillations of arsenic trioxide (As_2O_3) mixed by grinding with carbon particles, and suspended in a saline solution that also contained 2 mM sulfuric acid. Parallel groups were treated with As_2O_3 together with BP, with the same carrier. In groups of 48 hamsters, the "arsenic alone" group resulted in 3 carcinomas (1 squamous-cell carcinoma of the larynx, 1 bronchiolar adenocarcinoma and 1 bronchiolar small cell anaplastic carcinoma); in the "BP alone" group 42% of the animals had carcinomas, and in the group with combined treatment with arsenic and BP, 48% of the animals had carcinomas. These results suggest no overall enhancing effect of arsenic on carcinoma induction; however, if all the tumors with glandular differentiation (adenomas and adenocarcinomas) are considered together, the respective incidences are 6% for "arsenic alone", 35% for "BP alone" (for a sum of 41%), and 61% for the combined treatment, suggesting an increase due to synergism. These results (84) need further confirmation, but they suggest that arsenic may play a role in experimental respiratory carcinogenesis both as a carcinogen and as a synergistic cofactor.

The Role of Silica in Respiratory Carcinogenesis

At a meeting held at the University of North Carolina in April, 1984 (34), new evidence was presented on the role of silica in carcinogenesis, on the basis of both epidemiologic and experimental studies. Several occupational groups exposed to silica showed increased relative risks for lung cancer. Experimental administration of crystalline silica as quartz was found to induce not only pulmonary fibrosis, but also carcinomas of the lung, probably of bronchiolo-alveolar origin. This was demonstrated in rats of two strains and both sexes, treated either by inhalation or by intratracheal instillation (24,35,51). In hamsters, however, the intratracheal administration or inhalation of silica produced a macrophagic reaction, but no extensive necrosis of macrophages, no subsequent development of fibrosis, and moreover, no carcinogenic response (51,82). When silica was combined with BP for intratracheal instillation in the hamster, it produced the same type of response that was seen with Fe_2O_2 and BP, and in that respect it acted as a cofactor (82).

The species-specific response to silica, in which the fibrogenic and carcinogenic effects appear closely associated, was examined in view of possible pathogenetic mechanisms (98). The complex reticulo-endothelial reaction to silica in rat lungs was previously shown to involve phagocytosis by interstitial and alveolar macrophages and necrosis of macrophages with subsequent recruitment of other macrophages and proliferation of immature B-lymphocytes (differentiating into plasmacells), T-lymphocytes, mast cells (actively degranulating), polymorphonuclear leukocytes and, of course, fibroblasts, with production of a collagen network and deposition of immunoglobulins (93,94,104). In the hamster this complex reaction is absent and silica remains phagocytized in clusters of macrophages that do not appear to undergo extensive necrosis. This quiescent reaction is found also for non-fibrogenic dusts in both rats and hamsters.

The reticuloendothelial cells, so actively stimulated by silica in rats, as well as in the human lung, are known to produce and release a number of mediators acting on other target cells, as recently reviewed (98). Macrophages and polymorphonuclear leukocytes produce reactive oxygen species; macrophages release interleukin-1, plasminogen activator, components of complement, arachidonic acid, leukotrienes and prostaglandins, acid hydrolases, proteases, elastase, collagenase, factors stimulating the recruitment, attachment and proliferation of fibroblasts, fibronectin and alveolar macrophage derived growth factor. T-lymphocytes, activated by macrophages through antigen-presentation, release interleukin-2, monocyte chemotactic factor, macrophage migration inhibition factor, B-cell growth factor and B-cell differentiation factor.

Very little is known of the effects of such an array of mediators on adjacent epithelial cells, but some of these mediators, such as reactive oxygen species, are already known to induce genotoxic and mitogenic effects in epithelial cells systems. Review of these complex interactions resulted in the working hypothesis (98) that (a) mediators released by macrophages and other reticular cells during the process of fibrogenesis may act on the adjacent epithelial cells of the distal airways; (b) the effects on the epithelia are prolonged throughout the duration of the fibrogenic response; and (c) these effects, combined with direct genetic damage (possibly at the chromosomal level) induced by silica particles that penetrated into the epithelial cells in the early phases of the pulmonary response, are sufficient to account for the full carcinogenic activity of silica on the epithelia of susceptible species. The hamster provides a negative counterpart to the rat as model for the study of the carcinogenic mechanisms of silica.

ROLE OF PARTICULATES IN RESPIRATORY CARCINOGENESIS

In studies on carcinogens carried by particulates (e.g., BP/Fe_2O_3), an important note of caution needs to be emphasized. Since the carcinogens are administered in fine particulate form, adherent to the carrier particles, their distribution and retention in the target tissues largely depends on their physical characteristics, especially their particle size and their adhesion to the carrier particles. The importance of the particle size distribution for the retention rate of the carcinogen in the lung was demonstrated in the early studies with this system (96,99). When particles of BP considerably larger than 10 μm are present in the preparation, deposition and retention rates differ considerably from those obtained with particle sizes mostly below 5 μm, and the effects may be in part due to large BP crystals trapped in the mucociliary layer of the larger airways (29,82,117). Fine dispersion of BP on the surface of the carrier particles is effectively obtained by precipitation from an acetone solution slowly dropped into a large volume of water containing the carrier particles in suspension (95). The fine particle size and distribution of the BP/carrier preparation needs to be verified microscopically. Mere mixing of separately prepared suspensions of carcinogen and of inorganic particles does not ensure comparable tissue transport and distribution of the carcinogen.

In general, a marked carcinogenic response was reproducibly obtained in the hamster respiratory tract by intratracheal administration of carcinogens attached to inorganic particulates suspended in saline, while a much lower response was obtained when the same carcinogens were administered without the carrier particles. This generalization is subject to a number of experimental variables due to the physical characteristics of the particles and of the suspension. Effective dosage at the target tissue level should be considered when interpreting the biological responses.

Administration of BP by inhalation without carrier particles was demonstrated to be sufficient to induce respiratory tumors in hamsters (128), but the induced tumors were localized mostly in the pharynx and larynx, some in the nasal sinuses and in the trachea, and none in the bronchi and lungs. These results demonstrate a carcinogenic effect independent from the carrier particles, but the pattern of deposition and of target effects was quite different from that obtained by intratracheal administration.

Particle size characteristics are critical in determining the tissue retention rates of the carcinogens instilled intratracheally (48,49,96).

A variety of particulate carriers have been used in experiments of this type. Much of our work was done with Fe_2O_3, which effectively contributes to a high level of carcinogenic response. Similar levels of effect were reported for other particulates such as magnesium oxide, titanium dioxide, iodine and talc. On the other hand, other particulates were reported to yield lower levels of effect (aluminum oxide, carbon and ferric chloride). These comparisons are summarized in Table 2.

Niemeier et al. (82) recently reported the effects of silica and several silica substitutes used for metal casting in foundries; samples of these materials (mass median aerodynamic diameter from 5 to 10 μm) and of the control Fe_2O_3 (1.37 μm), were added to a suspension of BP in

TABLE 2. Respiratory tumors in Syrian golden hamsters induced by intratracheal instillations of benzo(a)pyrene attached to particulate carriers

Particulate carrier (dose)[a]	Benzo(a) pyrene dose[a]	No. of doses	No. of hamsters autopsied	Animals with respiratory tumors		Total number of tumors					Reference
				No.	(%)	Respiratory tract	Larynx	Trachea	Bronchi	Lungs	
Fe_2O_3 (3 mg)	3 mg	15	79	60	(76)	82	2	37	40	3	(96)
	3 mg	10	110	42	(38)	47	–	20	12	15	(96)
	3 mg	5	100	15	(15)	17	–	5	7	5	(96)
Fe_2O_3	different doses		887	253	(29)	359	14	115	181	49	(77)
Fe_2O_3 (3,6,9 mg)	3 mg	10	197	80	(41)	145	28	48	41	31	(109)
Fe_2O_3 (3 mg)	3 mg	15	44	31	(70)	64	14	22	24	4	(120)
Fe_2O_3 (3 mg)	3 mg	15	44	?		63	9	31	19	4	(119)
MgO (1 mg)	2 mg	20	45	32	(71)	63	14	27	19	3	(120)
TiO_2 (3 mg)	3 mg	15	48	?		52	16	18	17	1	(119)
Carbon particles (3 mg)	3 mg	15	45	?		13	2	7	4	0	(119)
Al_2O_3 (3 mg)	3 mg	15	45	?		6	1	3	0	2	(119)
I_2 (0.2 mg)	0.5 mg	20	48	17	(35)	29	2	21	4	2	(116)
$FeCl_3$ (0.16 mg)	0.5 mg	20	48	6	(12)	6	0	6	0	0	(116)
Talc (3 mg)	3 mg	18	45	33	(73)	120	9	12	7[b]	56[c]	(117)

[a] Each dose.
[b] Only extrapulmonary bronchi.
[c] Intralobar bronchi and lungs.

saline for instillation. The BP suspension in saline (20% of the particles > 10 µm) gave a fairly high yield of respiratory tumors, but addition of the particluates consistently increased the carcinogenic response in a range comparable to that obtained with Fe_2O_3. The results are summarized in Table 3.

The enhancing role of particulates in respiratory carcinogenesis, characteristic of the hamster model, can be interpreted considering several mechanisms discussed below.

Carrier Effect and Carcinogen Elution

An immediately apparent role of the particulates is their transport function, carrying carcinogens that have been attached to their surface into the interstitial tissues of the lungs. After instillation, the particles rapidly penetrate through the bronchiolar/alveolar epithelium and are phagocytized by macrophages that aggregate in clusters in the interstitial spaces or in the alveolar lumina. Soluble organic carcinogens are then eluted out and diffuse throughout the surrounding lung parenchyma. Physical characteristics of particle size and surface properties are important determinants of carcinogen retention rates. Exposure to carcinogens carried by particulates is highly relevant to human exposures to smoke and air pollutants.

Important species differences must be considered in the response. Comparable intratracheal treatments of hamsters and rats with BP/Fe_2O_3 were studied by Schreiber et al. (107); they observed a marked tracheobronchial epithelial hyperplasia (with later tumors) only in the hamster, while no such response occurs in the rat, which develops an initial granulomatous response and epidermoid metaplasia in the peripheral lung near the sites of particle deposition, followed by peripheral epidermoid lung tumors with massive keratinization. Studying the distribution of BP fluorescence under these conditions of treatment, Schreiber et al. (107) reported that the tracheal epithelium of the hamster showed marked and extensive fluorescence, accompanied by fluorescence in the underlying submucosa, peaking at two days after treatment. In contrast, the tracheobronchial epithelium and submucosa of the rat showed no fluorescence at all. Both species showed BP-containing macrophages in the tracheobronchial lumen. Schreiber et al. (107) interpreted their findings by suggesting that, in the hamster, BP diffuses from the luminal macrophages through the mucociliary layer into the tracheobronchial epithelium but that in the rat some mechanism prevents this diffusion completely. They

TABLE 3. Respiratory tumors in Syrian golden hamsters induced by intratracheal instillations of benzo(a)pyrene mixed with particulates[a]

Particulate carrier (dose)[a]	Benzo(a) pyrene dose[a]	No. of doses	No. of hamsters autopsied	Animals with respiratory tumors		Total number of tumors			
				No.	(%)	Respiratory tract	Larynx	Trachea	Bronchi & Lungs
None (saline) (0.2 ml)	3 mg	15	47	22	(47)	34	5	3	26
Fe$_2$O$_3$ (3 mg)	3 mg	15	48	35	(76)	80	5	6	69
Silica, Ottawa (1.1 mg)	3 mg	15	50	36	(77)	99	13	13	73
Quartz (Min-U-Sil) (0.7 mg)	3 mg	15	50	44	(90)	123	10	2	111
Quartz (Min-U-Sil) + Fe$_2$O$_3$ (0.7 mg) + 3 mg)	3 mg	15	50	38	(81)	95	11	4	84
Zirconium silicate (Australia) (0.9 mg)	3 mg	15	50	43	(88)	113	8	8	97
Zirconium silicate (Florida) (0.9 mg)	3 mg	15	50	36	(77)	94	9	9	76
Chromite sand (2.1 mg)	3 mg	15	48	37	(80)	87	12	13	62
Olivine (NC) (2.1 mg)	3 mg	15	50	40	(85)	104	14	7	83
Olivine (WA) (1.2 mg)	3 mg	15	50	39	(85)	82	8	11	63
Aluminum silicate (Remasil 48) (1.4 mg)	3 mg	15	50	38	(76)	103	12	12	79
Aluminum silicate (Remasil 60) (1.4 mg)	3 mg	15	50	31	(63)	68	13	7	48
Aluminum silicate (Remasil 70) (1.4 mg)	3 mg	15	50	37	(82)	78	11	8	59

[a] Benzo(a)pyrene (80% < 10 μm, 50% < 5 μm, 7% < 1 μm) suspended in saline and mixed with aliquot of particulate calculated to have a surface area equivalent to that of the Min-U-Sil sample.
All data from Niemeier et al. (82).

recognized, however, that their findings did not exclude a diffusion through the interstitial tissue from the lungs upwards to the bronchi and trachea in the hamster as previously suggested by Saffiotti et al. (100). The latter pathway would be consistent with the observed fluorescence in the tracheal submucosa in hamsters. It may be speculated that the granulomatous reaction in the lung periphery, present in the rat but not in the hamster, contributes to localizing carcinogen metabolism at the peripheral level, where epidermoid metaplasia and tumors are induced in rats but not in hamsters. The possible role of the induced granulomatous reaction on epithelial responses is discussed below. Further work is underway to clarify these issues.

Carrier Surface Effects on Metabolic Activities

The questions just mentioned also relate to the possible role of the carrier particles on the metabolic activation and degradation of the carcinogens, especially through mechanisms mediated by the macrophages and the surrounding cells. Human pulmonary alveolar macrophages have been demonstrated to metabolize BP (4,43) and to phagocytize BP/Fe_2O_3 particulates with the consequent release of BP and its metabolites (5). Cocultivation of human pulmonary alveolar macrophages with Chinese hamster V79 cells, which are susceptible to mutagenesis, showed that macrophages could provide the metabolic activation of BP needed to induce ouabain resistant mutations and sister chromatid exchanges in the adjacent susceptible V79 cells (52). The marked recruitment of macrophages with active phagocytosis, stimulated by particulates, should therefore contribute to carcinogen metabolism; their localization and accumulation are likely to contribute in the selection of the target tissue response. No studies have yet been carried out on the relative role of different types of particulates and different surface properties in the induction of carcinogen metabolism and binding in this system.

Role of Carriers on Carcinogen Interactions with Macrophages, with Other Reticuloendothelial Cells, and with Target Epithelial Cells

The cells that initially receive the highest amounts of carcinogens carried by particulates are the pulmonary macrophages. As the carcinogen diffuses in the lung, many reticuloendothelial cells of different types are also exposed. Yet practically no sarcomas derive from these cells. Injection of the same carcinogen/particulate suspensions directly into connective tissues (e.g., peritracheal or subcutaneous) however, readily produces sarcomas. In hamsters treated with polycyclic hydrocarbons and particulates, the vast majority of tumors derive from the epithelium of the bronchi (including intrapulmonary bronchi) and of the trachea, some from the epithelium of the larynx, and only a few from the bronchiolar/alveolar epithelium, in spite of the fact that the latter is directly in contact with carcinogens instilled into the lung and with carcinogen-laden macrophages.

Factors responsible for differential cellular susceptibilities to carcinogens need to be identified; they are likely to include specific factors for the metabolic activation and binding of carcinogens, but they may also include factors related to the proliferative capacity or mitogenic stimulation of the target cells. Many of the cells initially exposed to the carcinogen are cells that do not proliferate, such as the terminally differentiated ciliated cells of the larger airways, or many of the macrophages that are shed into the airways or die.

The differential response of the rat and hamster lung to the carcinogen/particulate instillation (107) acquires a new interest in view of the differential response to silica particles observed in rats and hamsters, and recently discussed in relation to reticuloendothelial cell mediators (98). The macrophagic and granulomatous reaction induced in the rat by BP/Fe_2O_3, with topical metaplasia and tumor formation, but not observed in the hamster, suggests that not only direct carcinogen-induced damage, but also a number of enhancing factors, some possibly mediated through the activation of reticuloendothelial cells, may play a topical role in carcinogenesis on the rat peripheral airway epithelium. Fe_2O_3 alone induces a simple macrophagic reaction with minimal cell toxicity or reticuloendothelial activation in rats (93,94,104). It was suggested (98) that in the case of BP carried on Fe_2O_3 particles, the carcinogen itself provides the toxic mechanism that starts the recruitment of reticuloendothelial cells for a granulomatous reaction. It may also induce cell-cell signals capable of contributing to the expression of a transformed state in the peripheral lung epithelium in the rat, but not in the hamster where macrophage toxicity and granulomatous reaction do not occur. This hypothesis (98) warrants further study. The respiratory epithelial cells that respond with neoplastic transformation and tumor growth may be those that not only interact with the carcinogen, but which also receive persistent stimuli capable of inducing cell proliferation and/or specific expression of neoplastic properties.

Role of Focal Mechanical Injury and Instilled Particulates or Saline on Epithelial Proliferation

We are currently investigating this problem in order to elucidate the role of non-carcinogenic enhancing stimuli on the process of carcinogenesis in the hamster respiratory epithelium that has been initiated with different chemical carcinogens such as BP, MNU, or DEN. We want to know if the proliferative stimuli to the respiratory epithelium induced by wounding or by the administration of Fe_2O_3 particles in saline, or by saline alone, act through mechanisms similar to those of skin promoting agents or by other mechanisms, so far less well defined. Epithelial wounding by intratracheal intubation has been shown to induce proliferative responses in the conducting airways (58-60,62). Since intratracheal instillation methods used in carcinogenesis studies produce similar microtrauma to the airways, we are attempting to determine whether wounding *per se* constitutes a stimulus for tumor enhancement or promotion in the respiratory epithelium. In addition, we are studying the role of instilled Fe_2O_3 particles in saline, or of saline alone, since the latter has been demonstrated to stimulate airway proliferation and to enhance the carcinogenic effect of DEN and of [210]Po on the pulmonary epithelium (67,110,115).

Preliminary studies have been performed on Syrian golden hamsters intubated with a 19-gauge cannula inserted intratracheally to the level of the carina, or only to the level of the larynx (61) (Fig. 1). Through the cannula, the animals received an instillation of 0.2 ml of either saline alone, or saline containing Fe_2O_3 or nothing. Dosing at the level of the larynx with saline or nothing resulted in no detectable effect on mitotic rates of the epithelium of any airway segment distal to the larynx. However, dosing with Fe_2O_3 in saline at the same level resulted in increased mitotic rates in the intrapulmonary bronchi and bronchioles, but not in the trachea. Dosing at the level of the carina resulted in an increased mitotic rate in the trachea associated with microtrauma from the cannulation; both saline and Fe_2O_3 in saline given at this level resulted in a significant increase in the mitotic rates of the intrapulmonary bronchi and bronchioles. These findings confirm the effects of intratracheal, but not laryngeal, cannulation trauma in elevating tracheal mitotic rates. They also show that mitogenic effects of Fe_2O_3 particulates in saline on the intralobar bronchi and bronchioles occur with both levels of cannulation, but the mitogenic effects of saline alone occur only when cannulation is extended to the carina (Fig. 1).

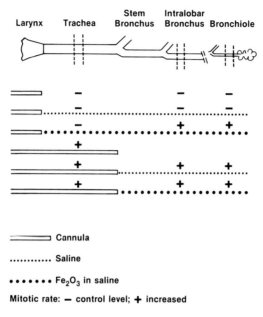

FIG. 1. Mitogenic stimulation of hamster respiratory tract epithelia by intralaryngeal or intratracheal cannulation with or without instillation of saline, or Fe_2O_3 in saline.

The vast majority of the mitotic figures observed in the tracheobronchial epithelium were seen in secretory cells, not basal cells. All the mitoses in the bronchioles were in secretory cells (Clara cells). This suggests that the enhanced regional response to certain carcinogens induced by cannulation trauma, or by Fe_2O_3 in saline, or by saline alone, appears likely to be associated with an increased mitotic rate in the secretory cells, respectively of the trachea, bronchi, and bronchioles. The secretory cells continue to show mitotic activity when proliferating in suprabasal position and even at the luminal surface of hyperplastic epithelia.

In a current long-term study we are investigating the effects of intratracheal wounding, dosing with saline alone, with Fe_2O_3 in saline, and with BP/Fe_2O_3 in saline, on hamster respiratory epithelium treated at five weeks of age with a subcarcinogenic, single dose of MNU. We are using such young hamsters because age is another variable factor in respiratory epithelial proliferation. In the five week-old juvenile hamster trachea, the mitotic rate was much higher than in the adult hamster, and most mitotic activity was in secretory cells (70).

The results of these experiments should help clarify the respective roles of carcinogens, mechanical wounding, Fe_2O_3 particulates, and saline, as proliferative stimuli and enhancing factors in respiratory tract carcinogenesis.

Recovery of BP from hamster lungs after instillation of a fine particle size suspension of BP/Fe_2O_3 in saline, lasted up to 7 to 10 days (96,99). The frequency of intratracheal treatment is an important determinant of the carcinogenic response, high for weekly treatments and much lower for treatments every two weeks (77). The higher response to weekly treatments can be explained by the maintenance throughout the treatment period of a high level of BP in target tissues as well as of a high mitotic rate, while treatments at 2-week intervals allow partial recovery in the second week.

DIFFERENTIATION OF THE RESPIRATORY EPITHELIUM AND CELLS OF ORIGIN OF RESPIRATORY TRACT TUMORS

Tumor Phenotypes

Lung tumors show a range of histologies because they express multiple and complex phenotypes (72). In fact, the majority of human tumors show two or more histologic patterns when multiple sections are examined (89,92). It is very common for carcinomas which are predominantly epidermoid (squamous), to show foci of glandular specialization and *vice versa* (21,26). There are, however, regional differences in the expression of the predominant phenotype; in humans, carcinomas which are predominantly epidermoid usually arise in larger bronchi, while tumors that are predominantly glandular, i.e., adenocarcinomas, arise most commonly from small bronchi at the periphery of the lung (17).

Glandular tumors are characterized by the nature of the products which are packaged in granules for export, such as mucosubstances (mucus-secreting adenocarcinomas), and peptide hormones (small cell carcinomas and carcinoid tumors). Epidermoid tumors are characterized by the accumulation of large amounts of intermediate-sized (57 and 59 kd) cytoplasmic keratin proteins, and by the presence of the cross-linked envelope protein, involucrin (7,106). Furthermore, epidermoid specialization is associated with a more complex cytokeratin pattern than the glandular phenotype (15).

The phenotypic mosaics expressed by lung tumors are reflected in the numerous schemes of lung tumor classification, including the World Health Organization (WHO) classification (134) and one which relies more heavily on the phenotype(s) of the tumor cells (69). The WHO classification is descriptively based on the light microscopic histological growth patterns. Using WHO criteria only, tumors with overt keratinization are classified as epidermoid carcinomas. Moreover, tumors with dense-cored endocrine granules, but which do not show light microscopic morphologies characteristic of either small cell carcinomas or carcinoid tumors, will inevitably be placed into another tumor category.

The use of electron microscopy and light microscopic immunocytochemistry is rapidly increasing in tumor diagnosis and there is little doubt that the increasing use of more sophisticated methods, compared with the WHO classification, will result in a different diagnostic pattern of tumor phenotypes, since light microscopic diagnosis may change upon ultrastructural and/or immunocytochemical examination.

The tumors induced in hamsters by BP/Fe_2O_3 resemble the human tumors not only in their morphology, distribution and histogenesis, as noted above, but also in their mixed phenotypic expression. The exception is represented by the endocrine type tumors, including small cell carcinomas and carcinoid tumors, which are rare in the hamster model.

Cell Kinetics of the Adult Tracheobronchial Epithelium

Studies of adult human (41) and animal respiratory epithelia (16,55) show that the normal epithelium has very low mitotic and labeling indices. Secretory cells and basal cells divide but until recently the mitotic potential of secretory cells had received very little attention. The notion that basal cells are responsible for maintenance of the tracheobronchial epithelium has been a commonly held belief, together with the supposition that basal cells are the "stem" cells which give rise to other cell types during normal development and maintenance, during regeneration following injury, and during tumorigenesis resulting in neoplastic cells. However, evidence against this premise is rapidly mounting and several reports have described considerable mitotic activity in columnar secretory cells in rodents, primates and humans in normal and abnormal states (16,41,53,55,58,60,70,71,133). In the hamster tracheal epithelium, secretory cells outnumber basal cells 6:1 (58), and the cell cycle time of the secretory cells is considerably shorter than that of basal cells (16).

Fetal and Neonatal Development

Characterization of normal development of any epithelium helps us understand the histogenesis and morphogenesis of non-neoplastic and neoplastic lesions in the mature tissue. It is important that the origin of the various cell types, their proliferative potentials, and their range of phenotypic expression be defined because understanding the fluctuations in cellular composition and the cytodifferentiation patterns during development yields insight into the pathological mechanisms. Regenerating epithelia in adults display structures and properties essentially similar to those of the corresponding immature tissues of the fetus (132). The tracheobronchial epithelium is no exception and there are some striking similarities between the modulations which normally occur in the developing tracheal epithelium and those which occur in hamster tracheal epithelium regenerating following mechanical injury (62), or vitamin A deficiency (70,71), and during the genesis of neoplastic states in several species (73).

Studies on the development of the tracheal epithelium in fetal and neonatal Syrian golden hamsters are presently underway (McDowell et al., unpublished). The gestation period is 16 days. The following developmental sequence was demonstrated by light microscopy, histochemistry, and electron microscopy. Up to fetal day 11 the primordial trachea was lined by a single layer of primitive columnar cells and many of the cells were replicating. All cells reached the lumen and none of the cells were short. On day 12 the epithelium remained simple columnar but groups of endocrine cells had become specialized to form discrete neuroepithelial bodies which were most obvious in the dorsal epithelium. On day 13 the epithelium was pseudostratified, i.e., a few cells were short. At this time, some preciliated and ciliated cells were present, but of all the cells in mitotic division, 92% were columnar and only 8% were short.

The proliferating cells, both short (prebasal) and columnar (presecretory), appeared to be poorly-differentiated until day 14. On this day primitive hemidesmosomes were seen. As these structures are unique to basal cells (55,125), we conclude that the short cells had specialized to become basal cells by day 14. Moreover, rough endoplasmic reticulum developed in the columnar cells heralding the specialization of secretory cells. These cells were mucus-producing by day 15.

It is clear from these studies that poorly-differentiated columnar cells were the primordial "stem cells" capable of division and giving rise to the specialized cells. Proliferative activity in columnar cells (at first poorly-differentiated and later secretory cells) dominated numerically over that in basal cells during all stages of fetal development. On the day of birth (day 16), about 80% of all mitotic activity was in columnar secretory cells, yet the basal cells were well established at this time. During the first postnatal week, the mitotic index was low (about 1%) and the cellular proportions remained similar to those of fetal days 15 and 16. This indicates that most of the cells of the early neonatal period were formed *in utero*. Mitotic activity in secretory cells predominated (over 60% of the total), proportionate with the greater number of secretory cells compared to basal cells in the tracheal epithelium. Based on the results, a hypothetical model (McDowell, unpublished) is being proposed for the formation of the pseudostratified mucociliary epithelium. The model proposes that basal cells, secretory cells, and ciliated cells are established *in utero* from poorly-differentiated columnar cells. Thereafter, basal cells replicate to produce basal cells, whereas secretory cells replicate to produce secretory cells and ciliated cells. This model is being tested in further studies.

Regeneration Following Focal Lethal Injury

Studies of epithelial regeneration following mechanical, chemical, and nutritional (vitamin A deficiency) injury have been helpful in clarifying the histogenesis of stratification and epidermoid metaplasia, and the restoration of the mucociliary state.

The various stages of regeneration of adult hamster tracheal epithelium following mechanical injury were characterized morphologically and quantified by cell type (58-60). In this experimental model, the cells were scraped from the epithelium at a focal area by intratracheal cannulation. Within a few hours columnar secretory cells and basal cells, which were adjacent to the wound, changed shape, flattened and migrated to cover the wound site. Most of the flattened cells were altered secretory cells (62). Twenty-four hr following wounding about 30% of the cells in the wound were in mitosis. Thereafter, they piled up and formed a typical multilayered epidermoid (keratin producing) metaplastic epithelium. The keratinizing metaplastic cells also contained mucous granules, indicative of their secretory nature and consistent with their origin from secretory cells. Within three days, some of the metaplastic cells desquamated from the epithelium while division of metaplastic and columnar secretory cells gave rise to presecretory and preciliated cells. A nearly normal mucociliary epithelium was restored within 5 to 6 days following wounding. The preciliated cells had an electron-lucent cytoplasm and bore long slender apical microvilli. Ciliogenesis was evident as fibrogranular areas and/or basal bodies at the cell apices. Cell quantitation and labeling experiments with tritiated thymidine indicated that presecretory and preciliated cells were the progeny of division of secretory cells, both normal columnar and polygonal keratinizing metaplastic secretory cells. Many preciliated cells contained mucous granules in their apical cytoplasm, but they lacked well-developed endoplasmic reticulum and Golgi apparatus, indicating that the mucous granules had been carried over from the parent secretory cell (58-60,62).

Essentially similar processes occurred during regeneration of the tracheal epithelium of bonnet monkeys following exposure to ozone (133). Foci of stratification and transient metaplasia were generated, associated with proliferation of secretory cells. Thereafter, cilia formed from cells which contained secretory granules, and the mucociliary state was restored. Preciliated cells with a few mucous granules (formerly called "indifferent cells") are also seen in human bronchial epithelium (72).

Vitamin A Deficiency

Vitamin A is a growth factor essential for maintaining the mucociliary state. The effect of vitamin A in the inhibition of hamster respiratory tract carcinogenesis was first reported by Saffiotti et al. (103). Subsequent studies examined the histogenesis of squamous metaplasia *in vivo* (46). Organ culture studies reported the effects of retinoids on BP binding to DNA and on the reversion of keratinizing epidermoid metaplasia induced by vitamin A deficiency (19,33,112,113). In recent detailed studies of the tracheal epithelium in the vitamin A deficient hamster, a continuum of change was observed ranging from minimal morphologic change, through hyperplasia and stratification of secretory cells, to non-cornifying and cornifying epidermoid metaplasia (70). Mitotic activity was reduced to near zero in the minimally changed epithelium but was increased in foci of stratification and metaplasia. Epidermoid metaplastic cells were characterized by well-developed tonofilament bundles and desmosomes, yet they retained many features of secretory cells, i.e., abundant cytoplasm, well-developed RER and Golgi apparatus and mucous granules, suggesting that the metaplastic cells were altered secretory cells. Epidermoid metaplasia also occurs in the tracheal glands during vitamin A deficiency (18). Since basal cells are absent from the glandular epithelium, this observation further supports the premise that the metaplastic cells are altered secretory cells, not basal cells.

The reversal of the epithelium to the normal mucociliary state following restoration of dietary vitamin A was studied quantitatively in hamster trachea (71). In the deficient epithelium, preciliated cells were virtually absent and mitotic activity of secretory cells was reduced 14-fold. The number of ciliated cells was also reduced. The basal cell mitotic rate, which was very low even in control hamsters, was reduced 3-fold by deficiency of vitamin A. Within two days of restoring vitamin A, mitotic activity began to increase in columnar secretory cells and was maintained at near normal over the next five days. Mitotic activity of basal cells remained below control level throughout the restorative period. Preciliated cells reappeared in the epithelium following increased proliferation of secretory cells. The preciliated cells, many of which contained secretory granules, rapidly developed cilia and matured into ciliated cells. The normal mucociliary epithelium was restored over 7 days.

Cells of Origin of Preneoplastic and Neoplastic Lesions

Only cells that have the potential to divide are capable of hyperplastic, metaplastic, and neoplastic change. In the tracheobronchial epithelium the candidate cells of origin are secretory (mucous) cells and basal cells, both of which divide in the adult, and possibly also endocrine cells which divide in the fetal airways but rarely if ever divide in the normal adult epithelium (25). It has been conventionally assumed that epidermoid carcinomas arise from basal cells, adenocarcinomas from mucous cells (especially those in the mucosal glands), and small cell carcinomas and carcinoid tumors from endocrine cells, but there are many reasons that make this generalization simplistic. Data presented here and elsewhere (10,32,73,74,111,136) indicate that lung cancers derive from endodermal pluripotent cells that display a continuum of phenotypic expression. This premise is now widely accepted although there are still disagreements between investigators regarding the nature of the progenitor cell(s). Tumors grown in rats from clones derived from single cells of combined epidermoid and adenocarcinomas showed differentiative instability and the nascent tumors expressed different degrees of epidermoid and mucus-secreting specializations in an apparently uncontrolled manner (114). Similarly, when a transplantable adenocarcinoma of the colon (an organ also derived from endoderm) comprised of mucous, endocrine, columnar and undifferentiated cells was cloned, each of the nascent tumors derived from a single cell was composed of mucous, endocrine, columnar and undifferentiated elements (22).

In the tracheobronchial epithelium the true origin of the pluripotential progenitor cell(s) remains unclear but one hypothesis proposes that neoplastic changes in secretory cells are responsible for most bronchogenic neoplasms in humans and animals (73).

ACKNOWLEDGEMENTS

Work at the University of Maryland was supported in part by Contract N01-CP-15738 from the National Cancer Institute and Grant HL-24722 from the National Heart, Lung and Blood Institute, National Institutes of Health.

REFERENCES

1. Althoff, J., Cardesa, A., Pour, P., and Mohr, U. (1973): *J. Natl. Cancer Inst.*, 50:323-329.
2. Althoff, J., Eagen, M., and Grandjean, C. (1975): *J. Natl. Cancer Inst.*, 55:1209-1211.
3. Argyris, T. S. (1980): *J. Invest. Dermatol.*, 75:360-362.
4. Autrup, H., Harris, C. C., Stoner, G., Selkirk, J., Schafer, P., and Trump, B. F. (1978): *Lab. Invest.*, 38:217-223.
5. Autrup, H., Harris, C. C., Trump, B. F., Stoner, G. D., and Hsu, I.-C. (1979): *Proc. Soc. Exp. Biol. Med.*, 161:280-284.
6. Autrup, H., Wefald, F. C., Jeffrey, A. M., Tate, H., Schwartz, R. D., Trump, B. F., and Harris, C. C. (1980): *Int. J. Cancer*, 25:293-300.
7. Banks-Schlegel, S. P., McDowell, E. M., Wilson, T. S., Trump, B. F., and Harris, C. C. (1984): *Am. J. Pathol.*, 114:273-286.
8. Banks-Schlegel, S. P., Schlegel, R., and Pinkus, G. S. (1981): *Exp. Cell Res.*, 136:465-469.
9. Barrett, L. A., McDowell, E. M., Frank, A. L., Harris, C. C., and Trump, B. F. (1976): *Cancer Res.*, 36:1003-1010.
10. Baylin, S. B., and Mendelsohn, G. (1980): *Endocr. Rev.*, 1:45-77.
11. Becci, P. J., McDowell, E. M., and Trump, B. F. (1978): *J. Natl. Cancer Inst.*, 61:551-561.

12.   Becci, P. J., McDowell, E. M., and Trump, B. F. (1978): *J. Natl. Cancer Inst.*, 61:577-586.
13.   Becci, P. J., McDowell, E. M., and Trump, B. F. (1978): *J. Natl. Cancer Inst.*, 61:607-618.
14.   Bertolero, F., Kaighn, M. E., Gonda, M. A., and Saffiotti, U. (1984): *Exp. Cell Res.*, 155:64-80.
15.   Blobel, G. A., Moll, R., Franke, W. W., and Vogt-Moykopf, I. (1984): *Virchows Arch. (Cell Pathol.)*, 45:407-429.
16.   Boren, H. G., and Paradise, L. J. (1978): In: *Pathogenesis and Therapy of Lung Cancer*, edited by C. C. Harris, pp. 369-418. Marcel Dekker, New York.
17.   Carter, D., and Eggleston, J. C. (1980): *Tumors of the Lower Respiratory Tract. Atlas of Tumor Pathology*. Armed Forces Institute of Pathology, Washington, D.C.
18.   Chopra, D. P., and Cooney, R. A. (1983): *Carcinogenesis*, 4:1345-1347.
19.   Clamon, G. H., Sporn, M. B., Smith, J. M., and Saffiotti, U. (1974): *Nature*, 250:64-66.
20.   Clark-Lewis, I., and Murray, A. W. (1978): *Cancer Res.*, 38:494-497.
21.   Corson, J. M., and Pinkus, G. S. (1982): *Am. J. Pathol.*, 108:80-87.
22.   Cox, W. F., and Pierce, G. B. (1982): *Cancer*, 50:1530-1538.
23.   Craddock, V. M. (1976): In: *Liver Cell Cancer*, edited by H. M. Cameron, D. S. Linsell, and G. P. Warwick, pp. 153-201. Elsevier, Amsterdam.
24.   Dagle, G. E., Wehner, A. P., Clark, M. L., and Buschbom, R. L. (1985): In: *Silica, Silicosis and Cancer: Controversy in Occupational Medicine*, edited by D. F. Goldsmith, D. M. Winn, and C. M. Shy, in press. Praeger Publ., Philadelphia.
25.   Di Augustine, R. P., and Sonstegard, K. S. (1984): *Environ. Health Perspect.*, 55:271-295.
26.   Dingemans, K. P., and Mooi, W. J. (1984): *Pathol. Annual*, 19:289-273.
27.   Evans, M. J. (1982): In: *Mechanisms in Respiratory Toxicology*, edited by H. Witschi and P. Nettesheim, pp. 189-218. CRC Press, Boca Raton, FL.
28.   Farber, E. (1982): *Am. J. Pathol.*, 106:271-296.
29.   Feron, V. J., van den Heuvel, P. D., Koëter, H. B. W. M., and Beems, R. B. (1980): *Int. J. Cancer*, 25:301-307.
30.   Frei, J. V., and Harsomo, T. (1967): *Cancer Res.*, 27:1481-1484.
31.   Friedewald, W. F., and Rous, P. (1944): *J. Exp. Med.*, 80:101-125.
32.   Gazdar, A. F., Carney, D. N., Guccion, J. G., and Baylin, S. B. (1981): In: *Small Cell Lung Cancer*, edited by F. A. Greco, R. K. Oldham, and P. A. Bunn, pp. 145-175. Grune and Stratton, New York.
33.   Genta, V. M., Kaufman, D. G., Harris, C. C., Smith, J. M., Sporn, M. B., and Saffiotti, U. (1974): *Nature*, 247:48-49.
34.   Goldsmith, D. F., Winn, D. M., and Shy, C. M., editors (1985): *Silica, Silicosis and Cancer: Controversy in Occupational Medicine*, in press. Praeger Publ., Philadelphia.
35.   Groth, D. H., Stettler, L. E., Platek, S. F., Lal, J. B., and Burg, J. R. (1985): In: *Silica, Silicosis and Cancer: Controversy in Occupational Medicine*, edited by D. F. Goldsmith, D. M. Winn, and C. M. Shy, in press. Praeger Publ., Philadelphia.
36.   Harris, C. C. (1983): In: *Lung Cancer. Clinical Diagnosis and Treatment*, edited by M. J. Straus, pp. 1-20. Grune and Stratton, New York.
37.   Harris, C. C., and Autrup, H., editors (1983): *Human Carcinogenesis*. Academic Press, New York.

38. Harris, C. C., Autrup, H., Connor, R., Barrett, L. A., McDowell, E. M., and Trump, B. F. (1976): *Science*, 194:1067-1069.
39. Harris, C. C., Autrup, H., Stoner, G. D., McDowell, E. M., Trump, B. F., and Schafer, P. (1977): *Cancer Res.*, 37:2309-2311.
40. Harris, C. C., Autrup, H., Stoner, G. D., McDowell, E. M., Trump, B. F., and Schafer, P. (1977): *J. Natl. Cancer Inst.*, 59:1401-1406.
41. Harris, C. C., Frank, A., Barrett, L. A., McDowell, E. M., Trump, B. F., Paradise, L. J., and Boren, H. (1975): *J. Cell Biol.*, 67:158a.
42. Harris, C. C., Frank, A. L., Van Haaften, C., Kaufman, D. G, Connor, R., Jackson, F., Barrett, L. A., McDowell, E. M., and Trump, B. F. (1976): *Cancer Res.*, 36:1011-1018.
43. Harris, C. C., Hsu, I.-C., Stoner, G. D., Trump, B. F., and Selkirk, J. K. (1978): *Nature*, 272:633-634.
44. Harris, C. C., Kaufman, D. G., Sporn, M. B., and Saffiotti, U. (1973): *Cancer Chemother. Rep.*, 4:43-54.
45. Harris, C. C., Kaufman, D. G., Sporn, M. B., Smith, J. M., Jackson, F., and Saffiotti, U. (1973): *Int. J. Cancer*, 12:259-269.
46. Harris, C. C., Sporn, M. B., Kaufman, D. G., Smith, J. M., Jackson, F. E., and Saffiotti, U. (1972): *J. Natl. Cancer Inst.*, 48:743-761.
47. Hennings, H., and Boutwell, R. K. (1970): *Cancer Res.*, 30:312-320.
48. Henry, M. C., and Kaufman, D. G. (1973): *J. Natl. Cancer Inst.*, 51:1961-1964.
49. Henry, M. C., Port, C. D., and Kaufman, D. G. (1974): In: *Experimental Lung Cancer Carcinogenesis and Bioassays*, edited by E. Karbe and J. F. Park, pp. 173-185. New York.
50. Herrold, K. M. (1970): *Int. J. Cancer*, 6:217-222.
51. Holland, L. M., Wilson, J. S., Tillery, M. I., and Smith, D. M. (1985): In: *Silica, Silicosis and Cancer: Controversy in Occupational Medicine*, edited by D. F. Goldsmith, D. M. Winn, and C. M. Shy, in press. Praeger Publ., Philadelphia.
52. Hsu, I.-C., Harris, C. C., Yamaguchi, M., Trump, B. F., and Schafer, P. W. (1979): *J. Clin. Invest.*, 64:1245-1252.
53. Jeffery, P. K., Ayers, M., and Rogers, D. (1982): In: *Mucus in Health and Disease*, edited by E. N. Chantler, J. B. Elder, and M. Elstein, Vol. II, pp. 399-409. Plenum Press, New York.
54. Jones, R., Bertolero, F., Kaighn, M. E., and Saffiotti, U. (1984): *In Vitro*, 20:115a.
55. Kaufman, D. G., Baker, M. S., Harris, C. C., Smith, J. M., Boren, H., Sporn, M. B., and Saffiotti, U. (1972): *J. Natl. Cancer Inst.*, 49:783-792.
56. Kaufman, D. G., and Madison, R. M. (1974): In: *Experimental Lung Cancer: Carcinogenesis and Bioassays*, edited by E. Karbe, and J. F. Park, pp. 207-218. Springer-Verlag, New York.
57. Kawanami, O., Ferrans, V. J., and Crystal, R. G. (1979): *Am. Rev. Resp. Dis.*, 120:595-611.
58. Keenan, K. P., Combs, J. W., and McDowell, E. M. (1982): *Virchows Arch. (Cell Pathol.)*, 41:193-214.
59. Keenan, K. P., Combs, J. W., and McDowell, E. M. (1982): *Virchows Arch. (Cell Pathol.)*, 41:215-229.
60. Keenan, K. P., Combs, J. W., and McDowell, E. M. (1982): *Virchows Arch. (Cell Pathol.)*, 41:231-252.
61. Keenan, K. P., Stinson, S. F., Saffiotti, U., and McDowell, E. M. (1984): *Fed. Proc.*, 43:700.

62. Keenan, K. P., Wilson, T. S., and McDowell, E. M. (1983): *Virchows Arch. (Cell Pathol.)*, 43:213-240.
63. Lechner, J. F., Haugen, A., Autrup, H., McClendon, I. A., Trump, B. F., and Harris, C. C. (1981): *Cancer Res.*, 41:2294-2304.
64. Lechner, J. F., Haugen, A., McClendon, I. A., and Pettis, E. W. (1982): *In Vitro*, 18:633-642.
65. Lechner, J. F., Haugen, A., McClendon, I. A., and Shamsuddin, A. M. (1984): *Differentiation*, 25:229-237.
66. Lee, T.-C., Wu, R., Brody, A. R., Barrett, J. C., and Nettesheim, P. (1984): *Exp. Lung Res.*, 6:27-45.
67. Little, J. B., McGandy, R. B., and Kennedy, A. R. (1978): *Cancer Res.*, 38:1929-1935.
68. McDowell, E. M., Barrett, L. A., Galvin, F., Harris, C. C., and Trump, B. F. (1978): *J. Natl. Cancer Inst.*, 61:539-549.
69. McDowell, E. M., Harris, C. C., and Trump, B. F. (1982): In: *Morphogenesis of Lung Cancer*, edited by Y. Shimosato, M. R. Melamed, and P. Nettesheim, pp. 1-36. CRC Press, Boca Raton, FL.
70. McDowell, E. M., Keenan, K. P., and Huang, M. (1984): *Virchows Arch. (Cell Pathol.)*, 45:197-219.
71. McDowell, E. M., Keenan, K. P., and Huang, M. (1984): *Virchows Arch. (Cell Pathol.)*, 45:221-240.
72. McDowell, E. M., McLaughlin, J. S., Merenyi, D. K., Kieffer, R. F., Harris, C. C., and Trump, B. F. (1978): *J. Natl. Cancer Inst.*, 61:587-606.
73. McDowell, E. M., and Trump, B. F. (1983): *Surv. Synth. Path. Res.*, 2:235-279.
74. McDowell, E. M., Wilson, T. S., and Trump, B. F. (1981): *Arch. Pathol. Lab. Med.*, 105:20-28.
75. Montesano, R., and Saffiotti, U. (1968): *Cancer Res.*, 28:2197-2210.
76. Montesano, R., Saffiotti, U., Ferrero, A., and Kaufman, D. G. (1974): *J. Natl. Cancer Inst.*, 53:1395-1397.
77. Montesano, R., Saffiotti, U., and Shubik, P. (1970): In: *Inhalation Carcinogenesis*, edited by M. G. Hanna, Jr., P. Nettesheim, and J. R. Gilbert, pp. 353-371. U.S. Atomic Energy Commission Symposium Series No. 18, Oak Ridge, TN.
78. Mossman, B. T., Ezerman, E. B., Adler, K. B., and Craighead, J. E. (1980): *Cancer Res.*, 40:4403-4409.
79. Nettesheim, P., and Barrett, J. C. (1984): *CRC Crit. Rev. Toxicol.*, 12:215-239.
80. Nettesheim, P., and Griesemer, R. A. (1978): In: *Pathogenesis and Therapy of Lung Cancer*, edited by C. C. Harris, pp. 75-78. Marcel Dekker, New York.
81. Nettesheim, P., Klein-Szanto, A. J. P., Marchok, A. C., Steele, V. E., Terzaghi, M., and Topping, D. C. (1981): *Arch. Pathol. Lab. Med.*, 105:1-10.
82. Niemeier, R. W., Mulligan, L. T., and Rowland, J. (1985): In: *Silica, Silicosis and Cancer: Controversy in Occupational Medicine*, edited by D. F. Goldsmith, D. M. Winn, and C. M. Shy, in press. Praeger Publ., Philadelphia.
83. Pai, S. B., Steele, V. E., and Nettesheim, P. (1983): *Carcinogenesis*, 4:369-374.
84. Pershagen, G., Nordberg, G., and Björklund, N.-E.: *Environ. Res.*, in press.
85. Pour, P., Althoff, J., Cardesa, A., Krüger, F. W., and Mohr, U. (1974): *J. Natl. Cancer Inst.*, 52:1869-1874.
86. Pour, P., Krüger, F. W., Althoff, J., Cardesa, A., and Mohr, U. (1975): *J. Natl. Cancer Inst.*, 54:141-146.
87. Pour, P., Krüger, F. W., Cardesa, A., Althoff, J., and Mohr, U. (1973): *J. Natl. Cancer Inst.*, 51:1019-1027.

88. Pour, P., Krüger, F. W., Cardesa, A., Althoff, J., and Mohr, U. (1974): *J. Natl. Cancer Inst.*, 52:457-462.

89. Reid, J. D., and Carr, A. H. (1961): *Cancer*, 14:673-698.

90. Reznik-Schüller, H. M. (1983): In: *Comparative Respiratory Carcinogenesis, Vol. II, Experimental Respiratory Tract Carcinogenesis*, edited by H. M. Reznik-Schüller, pp. 109-134. CRC Press, Boca Raton, FL.

91. Reznik, G., Mohr, U., and Lijinski, W. (1978): *J. Natl. Cancer Inst.*, 60:371-378.

92. Roggli, V. I., Vollmer, R. T., McGavran, M. H., Greenberg, S. D., Spjut, H. T., and Yesner, R. (1984); *Lab. Invest.*, 50:50a.

93. Saffiotti, U. (1960): *Med. Lavoro*, 51:10-17.

94. Saffiotti, U. (1962): *Med. Lavoro*, 53:5-18.

95. Saffiotti, U. (1969): In: *Progress in Experimental Tumor Research*, edited by F. Homburger, Vol. 11, pp. 302-333. Karger, New York.

96. Saffiotti, U. (1970): In: *Inhalation Carcinogenesis*, edited by M. G. Hanna, Jr., P. Nettesheim, and J. R. Gilbert, pp. 27-54. U.S. Atomic Energy Commission Symposium Series No. 18, Oak Ridge, TN.

97. Saffiotti, U. (1970): In: *Morphology of Experimental Respiratory Carcinogenesis*, edited by P. Nettesheim, M. G. Hanna, Jr., and J. W. Deatherage, Jr., pp. 245-254. U.S. Atomic Energy Commission Symposium Series No. 21, Oak Ridge, TN.

98. Saffiotti, U. (1985): In: *Silica, Silicosis and Cancer: Controversy in Occupational Medicine*, edited by D. F. Goldsmith, D. M. Winn, and C. M. Shy, in press. Praeger Publ., Philadelphia.

99. Saffiotti, U., Borg, S. A., Grote, M. I., and Karp, D. B. (1964): *Chicago Med. Sch. Quart.*, 24:10-17.

100. Saffiotti, U., Cefis, F., and Kolb, L. H. (1968): *Cancer Res.*, 28:104-124.

101. Saffiotti, U., Cefis, F., and Shubik, P. (1966): In: *Lung Tumors in Animals*, edited by L. Severi, pp. 537-546. University of Perugia, Perugia.

102. Saffiotti, U., and Harris, C. C. (1979): In: *Carcinogens: Identification and Mechanisms of Action*, edited by A. C. Griffin, and C. R. Shaw, pp. 65-82. Raven Press, New York.

103. Saffiotti, U., Montesano, R., Sellakumar, A. R., and Borg, S. A. (1967): *Cancer*, 20:857-864.

104. Saffiotti, U., Tommasini Degna, A., and Mayer, L. (1960): *Med. Lavoro*, 51:518-552.

105. Said, J. W., Nash, G., Banks-Schlegel, S, Sassoon, A. F., Murakami, S., and Shintaku, I. P. (1983): *Am. J. Pathol.*, 113:27-32.

106. Said, J. W., Nash, G., Sassoon, A. F., Shintaku, I. P., and Banks-Schlegel, S. P. (1983): *Lab. Invest.*, 49:563-568.

107. Schreiber, H., Martin, D. H., and Pazmiño, N. (1975): *Cancer Res.*, 35:1654-1661.

108. Schreiber, H., Schreiber, K., and Martin, D. H. (1975): *J. Natl. Cancer Inst.*, 54:187-197.

109. Sellakumar, A. R., Montesano, R., Saffiotti, U., and Kaufman, D. G. (1973): *J. Natl. Cancer Inst.*, 50:507-510.

110. Shami, S. G., Thibodeau, L. A., Kennedy, A. R., and Little, J. B. (1982): *Cancer Res.*, 42:1405-1411.

111. Sidhu, G. S. (1979): *Am. J. Pathol.*, 96:5-20.

112. Sporn, M. B., Clamon, G. H., Dunlop, N. M., Newton, D. L., Smith, J. M., and Saffiotti, U. (1975): *Nature*, 253:47-50.

113. Sporn, M. B., Clamon, G. H., Smith, J. M., Dunlop, N. M., Newton, D. L., and Saffiotti, U. (1974): In: *Experimental Lung Cancer. Carcinogenesis and Bioassays*, edited by E. Karbe and J. F. Park, pp. 575-582. Springer-Verlag, New York.
114. Steele, V. E., and Nettesheim, P. (1981): *J. Natl. Cancer Inst.*, 67:149-154.
115. Stenbäck, F. G., Ferrero, A., and Shubik, P. (1973): *Cancer Res.*, 33:2209-2214.
116. Stenbäck, F. G., and Rowland, J. (1977): *Experientia*, 34:1065-1066.
117. Stenbäck, F. G., and Rowland, J. (1978): *Eur. J. Cancer*, 14:321-326.
119. Stenbäck, F. G., Rowland, J., and Sellakumar, A. (1976): *Oncology*, 33:29-34.
120. Stenbäck, F. G., Sellakumar, A., and Shubik, P. (1975): *J. Natl. Cancer Inst.*, 54:861-867.
121. Stinson, S. F., and Lilga, J. C. (1980): *Cancer Res.*, 40:609-613.
122. Stinson, S. F., Reznik-Schüller, H. M., Reznik, G., and Donahoe, R. (1983): *Am. J. Pathol.*, 111:21-26.
123. Stinson, S. F., and Saffiotti, U. (1983): In: *Comparative Respiratory Carcinogenesis, Vol. II, Experimental Respiratory Tract Carcinogenesis*, edited by H. M. Reznik-Schüller, pp. 75-93. CRC Press, Boca Raton, FL.
124. Stoner, G. D., Katoh, Y., Foidart, J. M., Myers, G. A., and Harris, C. C. (1980): In: *Methods in Cell Biology: Respiratory, Cardiovascular, and Integumentary Systems*, edited by C. C. Harris, B. F. Trump, and G. D. Stoner, pp. 15-35. Academic Press, New York.
125. Tandler, B., Sherman, J., and Boat, T. F. (1981): *Am. Rev. Resp. Dis.*, 124:469-475.
126. Thomas, P., Said, J. W., Nash, G., and Banks-Schlegel, S. (1984): *Lab. Invest.*, 50:36-41.
127. Thomassen, D. G., Gray, T. E., Mass, M. J., and Barrett, J. C. (1983): *Cancer Res.*, 43:5956-5963.
128. Thyssen, J., Althoff, J., Kimmerle, G., and Mohr, U. (1981): *J. Natl. Cancer Inst.*, 66:575-577.
129. Trump, B. F., McDowell, E. M., Glavin, F., Barrett, L. A., Becci, P. J., Schürch, W., Kaiser, H. E., and Harris, C. C (1978): *J. Natl. Cancer Inst.*, 61:563-575.
130. Valerio, M. G., Fineman, E. L., Bowman, R. L., Harris, C. C., Stoner, G. D., Autrup, H., Trump, B. F., McDowell, E. M., and Jones, R. T. (1981): *J. Natl. Cancer Inst.*, 66:849-859.
131. Warwick, G. P. (1971): *Fed. Proc.*, 30:1760-1765.
132. Willis, R. A. (1962): *The Borderland of Embryology and Pathology*, pp. 495-518. Butterworths, Washingon.
133. Wilson, D. W., Plopper, C. G., and Dungworth, D. L. (1984): *Am. J. Pathol.*, 116:193-206.
134. World Health Organization (1981): *Histological Typing of Lung Tumors*, 2nd Edition, International Histological Classification of Tumors, No. 1, World Health Organization, Geneva.
135. Wu, R., Groelke, J. W., Chang, L. Y., Porter, M. E., Smith, D., and Nettesheim, P. (1982): In: *Growth of Cells in Hormonally Defined Media*, Cold Spring Harbor Conferences on Cell Proliferation, Vol. 9, pp. 641-656. Cold Spring Harbor Laboratory, Cold Spring Harbor, NY.
136. Yesner, R. (1978): *Pathol. Annual*, 13(Part 1):217-240.

Carcinogenesis, Vol. 8, edited by M. J. Mass et al.
Raven Press, New York © 1985.

Glass Fibers and Vapor Phase Components of Cigarette Smoke as Cofactors in Experimental Respiratory Tract Carcinogenesis

V. J. Feron, C. F. Kuper, B. J. Spit, P. G. J. Reuzel,
and R. A. Woutersen

Institute CIVO—Toxicology and Nutrition TNO, 3700 AJ Zeist, The Netherlands

Sarcomas and mesotheliomas have been found in rats after intrapleural or intraperitoneal administration of glass fibers (28,33,34,36). Physical factors such as length and diameter of the fibers have been shown to be related to their carcinogenic potential (28,34). However, other factors such as chemical composition of mineral fibers (16) and compounds adsorbed on the fibers (7,9,32) are thought to also play a role in the carcinogenicity of fibers. Asbestos enhances the induction of lung cancer by cigarette smoke (22,30,31). In mice, inhaled glass fibers appeared able to enhance the adverse effect of styrene vapor on the bronchiolar epithelium (23). Within the scope of a research program on the significance of nonspecific injury to the respiratory tract for the formation of tumors at the site of damage, intratracheal administration of glass fibers to Syrian golden hamsters was used as one of the methods to induce damage to the pulmonary tissue. The clearance of glass fibers from the lungs and their acute and chronic effects on the lung tissue after a single intratracheal instillation have recently been described in detail (35). The present paper describes preliminary results of a long-term study in hamsters given multiple intratracheal instillations of glass fibers with or without benzo(a)pyrene (BP).

It is conceivable that the carcinogenicity of cigarette smoke is the result of initiating, promoting and inhibiting factors present in this complex mixture of many hundreds of gaseous and liquid or solid components. The carcinogen BP and the comutagen norharman are known to occur in the particulate phase of cigarette smoke (13,27). Components occurring in the vapor phase of cigarette smoke at relatively high or even very high concentrations and possibly significant for the induction of lung cancer are isoprene, methyl chloride, methyl nitrite and acetaldehyde (13). Against this background, a 23-month study was carried out in which Syrian golden hamsters were exposed by inhalation to a mixture of the four vapor phase components. A proportion of the animals were also given multiple intratracheal instillations of BP or norharman in saline solution. In addition, a 28-month inhalation carcinogenicity study of acetaldehyde in rats was performed using exposure levels of 0, 750, 1500 and 3000 → 1000 ppm (concentration reduced from 3000 ppm to 1000 ppm after 52 weeks). Preliminary results of these studies in hamsters and rats are presented in the present paper.

MATERIALS AND METHODS

Glass Fiber Study

Glass and Asbestos Fibers

Glass microfibers (code 104, Johns-Manville, Denver, CO) were obtained commercially. After milling of the glass wool, fibers of the following size distribution by number were obtained: length, 95% < 20 μm, 89% < 12 μm, 58% < 5 μm and 25% < 2 μm; diameter, 88% < 1.0 μm, 60% < 0.5 μm and 31% < 0.25 μm. The asbestos fibers used, an UICC standard reference sample of crocidolite, were a generous gift from Dr. V. Timbrell, Medical Research Council, Pneumoconiosis Unit, Llandough Hospital, Penarth, UK. The size distribution of the crocidolite fibers by number was: length, 90% < 20 μm, 78% < 12 μm, 42% < 5 μm and 21% < 2 μm; diameter, 91% < 1.0 μm, 67% < 0.5 μm and 37% < 0.25 μm. (The distribution measurements of the glass and crocidolite fibers were carried out by M. J. van Noord and Mrs. Ing. C. J. G. Blok-van Hoek, Centre for Analytical Electron Microscopy TNO, Leiden, The Netherlands.)

Animals

Syrian golden hamsters were obtained from the randomly-bred colony of the Central Institute for the Breeding of Laboratory Animals TNO, Zeist, The Netherlands.

Experimental Design and Procedures

Six groups of hamsters (12 weeks old), each consisting of 35 males and 35 females, were given the following intratracheal instillations once every two weeks for a period of 52 weeks: group 1 (control), 0.2 ml 0.005% gelatin solution in saline; group 2, 1 mg BP in 0.2 ml 0.005% gelatin solution in saline; group 3, 1 mg glass fibers in 0.2 ml 0.005% gelatin solution in saline; group 4, 1 mg glass fibers + 1 mg BP in 0.2 ml 0.005% gelatin solution in saline; group 5, 1 mg crocidolite in 0.2 ml 0.005% gelatin solution in saline; group 6, 1 mg crocidolite + 1 mg BP in 0.2 ml 0.005% gelatin solution in saline. The groups treated with asbestos were included in the study to be able to compare the results found after glass fiber-treatment to those obtained with asbestos under the same experimental conditions. The experiment was terminated at week 85; at that week all survivors were killed. All animals not lost by cannibalism or severe autolysis were autopsied and thoroughly examined for gross pathological changes. Histopathological examination was done on the respiratory tract, tumors and gross changes suspected of being tumors.

Studies with Vapor Phase Components of Cigarette Smoke

Twenty-Three-Month Inhalation/Intratracheal Instillation Study with Six Cigarette Smoke Components in Hamsters

Four vapor phase components viz. isoprene, methyl chloride, methyl nitrite and acetaldehyde, and two components of the particulate phase viz. BP and norharman were examined. The vapor phase compounds were administered as a mixture by inhalation for 6 hours/day, 5 days/week during 23 months, at the end of which the survivors were killed. The concentrations of the various compounds in the mixture were: 800 → 700 ppm (concentration reduced from 800 ppm to 700 ppm after 12 weeks) isoprene, 1000 → 900 ppm (concentration reduced from 1000 ppm to 900 ppm after 12 weeks) methyl chloride, 200 → 190 ppm (concentration reduced from 200 ppm to 190 ppm after 12 weeks) methyl nitrite and 1400 → 1200 ppm (concentration reduced from 1400 ppm to 1200 ppm after 12 weeks) acetaldehyde. BP and norharman were administered separately by intratracheal instillation. The animals treated with BP received 6 instillations, each consisting of 15 mg BP suspended in 0.2 ml 0.02% gelatin solution in saline (total dose: 90 mg BP per hamster). The instillations were given on days 29,

32, 36, 113, 116 and 120 of the experimental period. The animals treated with norharman were given 2 mg norharman dissolved in 0.2 ml saline once every two weeks during the first 52 weeks of the study (total dose: 52 mg norharman per hamster). Inhalation of the vapor mixture was also combined with intratracheal instillation of BP or norharman.

Seven groups of hamsters (the same strain as used in the glass fiber study; 6 weeks old), each consisting of 35 males and 35 females, were treated as follows: group 1 (controls), no treatment; group 2, inhalation of the vapor mixture; group 3, inhalation of the vapor mixture + intratracheal instillation of BP; group 4, inhalation of the vapor mixture + intratracheal instillation of norharman; group 5, intratracheal instillation of BP; group 6, intratracheal instillation of norharman; group 7, intratracheal instillation of BP + norharman. At autopsy all hamsters were thoroughly examined for gross pathological changes. Histopathological examination was carried out on the respiratory tract, tumors and gross lesions suspected of being tumors.

Twenty-Eight-Month Inhalation Study with Acetaldehyde in Rats

Four groups of rats (Cpb:WU; Wistar Random; 5 weeks old), each consisting of 55 males and 55 females, were exposed to acetaldehyde vapor at concentrations of 0 (controls), 750, 1500 and 3000 → 1000 ppm, respectively, during 6 hr/day, 5 days/week, for a period of at most 28 months, after which the survivors were killed. All animals were autopsied and subjected to a thorough gross examination. Extensive histopathological examinations are currently being performed with special attention to the various segments of the respiratory tract, tumors and gross lesions suspected of being tumors. To date, all noses have been examined microscopically for the presence of tumors.

RESULTS

Glass Fiber Study

Body Weights and Mortality

Body weights were not affected by any of the treatments. There were no relevant differences in mortality between any of the treatment groups and the control group (Table 1).

TABLE 1. Cumulative mortality of hamsters given intratracheal instillations of saline, BP, glass fibers, glass fibers + BP, crocidolite, or crocidolite + BP[a]

| | Number of deaths at end of week | | | | | | | | | | | |
| | Males | | | | | | Females | | | | | |
Treatments[b]	13	26	52	65	78	85	13	26	52	65	78	85
Saline	2	4	8	12	16	17	2	4	13	20	26	29
BP	1	3	5	8	12	14	2	5	13	20	30	34
Glass fibers	3	5	7	15	18	20	1	9	18	27	29	33
Glass fibers + BP	0	2	6	8	8	12	0	3	10	21	26	31
Crocidolite	1	1	5	8	9	13	2	10	14	23	25	30
Crocidolite + BP	0	4	9	14	14	18	3	7	21	23	27	32

[a]Initial number of animals per group: 35 males and 35 females.
[b]For details for the treatments see text.

Pathology

Tumors of the respiratory tract were found only in hamsters treated with BP, either with BP alone or with BP + glass fibers or BP + crocidolite (Table 2). The incidences of respiratory tract tumors were low and amounted to 7/63 (11%), 4/66 (6%) and 4/52 (8%) in the groups given BP alone, BP + glass fibers and BP + crocidolite fibers, respectively. Two peripheral lung tumors were found; both were adeno-squamous carcinomas and both occurred in the group of hamsters treated with crocidolite + BP.

In addition to neoplasms of the respiratory tract, slight to moderate hyperplasia and metaplasia with or without atypia of the laryngeal and tracheal epithelium were seen in hamsters receiving BP with or without glass fibers or crocidolite. The degree and incidence of these non-neoplastic epithelial alterations were similar in each of the BP-groups.

"Silicotic granulomas" (Fig. 1) were the predominant pulmonary lesions in animals given glass fibers. The granulomas consisted of clusters of tightly packed, iron-positive macrophages filled with glass fibers and surrounded by a layer of alveolar epithelial cells (Fig. 2 and 3). Free glass fibers, free macrophages with glass fibers and multinucleated giant cells containing glass fibers were occasionally

TABLE 2. Type and incidence of respiratory tract tumors in hamsters given intratracheal instillations of saline, BP, glass fibers, glass fibers + BP, crocidolite or crocidolite + BP[a]

Site and type of tumors	Incidence of tumors					
	Saline	BP	Glass fibers	Glass fibers + BP	Croci-dolite	Croci-dolite + BP
Males						
Number of animals examined	31	34	34	35	34	27
Trachea						
Papilloma	0	3	0	2	0	0
Squamous cell carcinoma	0	1	0	0	0	0
Sarcoma	0	1	0	1	0	0
Bronchi						
Papilloma	0	1	0	0	0	0
Lungs						
Adeno-squamous carcinoma	0	0	0	0	0	1
Females						
Number of animals examined	28	29	30	31	26	25
Larynx						
Carcinoma *in situ*	0	1	0	0	0	0
Trachea						
Papilloma	0	0	0	0	0	1
Sarcoma	0	0	0	1	0	1
Lungs						
Adeno-squamous carcinoma	0	0	0	0	0	1

[a]Initial number of animals: 35 males and 35 females per group. For details of the treatments see text.

seen. Coated glass fibers were found only sporadically. Areas not containing "silicotic nodules" or glass fibers were indistinguishable from pulmonary tissue of controls.

Hamsters treated with crocidolite often contained massive amounts of asbestos fibers either lying free in alveolar or bronchiolar lumens, or present in or surrounded by macrophages or multinucleated giant cells. Many asbestos fibers were coated and the characteristic

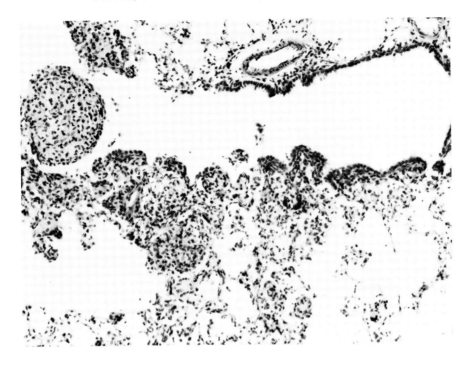

FIG. 1. "Silicotic granuloma" in the lung of a female hamster treated with glass fibers (H.E., × 160).

asbestos bodies occurred very frequently. Focal pulmonary fibrosis and calcified foci within asbestos granulomas were common findings (Fig. 4). Mesotheliomas were not observed.

Randomly distributed tumors in organs outside the respiratory tract unrelated to treatment included 8 adrenocortical tumors, 2 thyroid adenomas, 2 leukemias, 2 melanosarcomas, 2 subcutaneous sarcomas, 1 pheochromocytoma, 1 cholangioma, 1 renal carcinoma, 1 hepatocellular carcinoma and 1 adenocarcinoma of the large intestine.

Study with Six Cigarette Smoke Components

Body Weights and Mortality

Body weights were significantly lower in each of the groups exposed to the mixture of vapor phase components than in the control group.

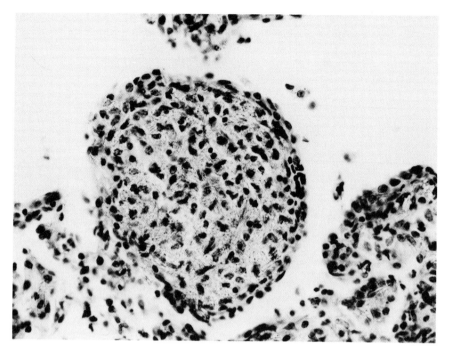

FIG. 2. Higher magnification of the "silicotic granuloma" depicted in Fig. 1. The granuloma consists of tightly packed macrophages filled with glass fibers and surrounded by a layer of epithelial cells (H.E., × 400).

After an experimental period of 26 weeks, mortality increased less rapidly in male control animals and in males only exposed to the vapor mixture than in the other groups. The death rate was highest in males treated with BP alone (Table 3). In females no differences in mortality occurred between groups; death rates were rather similar in the various groups.

Pathology

Pathological changes attributable to treatment were found in the nose, larynx and forestomach.

Hyperplasia and stratified squamous metaplasia with or without keratinization of the nasal respiratory epithelium (Fig. 5) were seen to be more severe and more extensive and occurred more frequently in hamsters exposed to the vapor mixture than in the other groups (Table 4). There was no evidence that intratracheal instillation of BP or

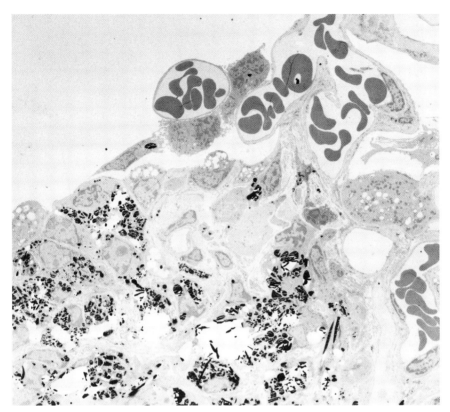

FIG. 3. Part of a "silicotic nodule" lined by alveolar epithelial cells and continuous with the adjacent pulmonary tissue of a male hamster treated with glass fibers (uranyl acetate and lead citrate, × 1700).

norharman influenced the effects of the vapor mixture on the nasal mucosa. A total of three squamous cell carcinomas (Fig. 5 and 6) were observed in the nose, one in a male and one in a female exposed to the vapor mixture only, and one in a female exposed to the vapor mixture and treated with BP. The olfactory epithelium was not affected by exposure to the vapor phase components. Three adenocarcinomas derived from the olfactory epithelium were found, one in a female control animal, one in a male exposed to the vapor phase mixture only, and one in a female treated with norharman. These tumors are considered fortuitous findings unrelated to treatment.

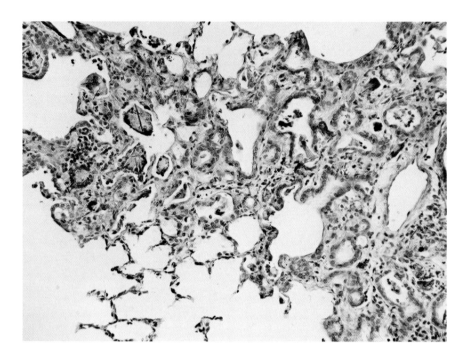

FIG. 4. Focal pulmonary fibrosis, adenomatous proliferation of epithelial cells and several multinucleated giant cells containing asbestos fibers in a male hamster treated with crocidolite (H.E., × 375).

Inhalation exposure to the mixture of vapor phase components resulted in exophytic and inverted (pseudoepitheliomatous) hyperplastic and metaplastic changes of the laryngeal epithelium (Fig. 7). Severe changes invariably exhibited nuclear and cellular atypia. A considerable number of hamsters in each of the three groups exposed to the vapor mixture had a squamous cell carcinoma of the larynx (Fig. 8) viz. 12 out of 63 (19%) animals exposed to the vapor mixture alone, 8 out of 61 (13%) animals exposed to the vapors + BP, and 8 out of 64 (13%) exposed to the vapors and treated with norharman. These figures and those of the non-neoplastic epithelial changes of the larynx (Table 4) clearly demonstrate that intratracheal administration of BP or norharman did not aggravate the adverse effects of the vapor mixture on the larynx.

TABLE 3. Cumulative mortality of hamsters exposed to air or vapor phase components of cigarette smoke and treated or not treated intratracheally with BP or norharman, or treated intratracheally with BP + norharman alone[a]

| | Number of deaths at end of week | | | | | | | | | | | |
| | Males | | | | | | Females | | | | | |
Treatments[b]	13	26	52	65	78	100	13	26	52	65	78	100
Air	0	0	0	2	4	20	0	1	5	11	17	21
VPCCS[c]	0	0	0	2	7	18	0	0	1	6	12	18
VPCCS + BP	0	1	3	6	7	26	0	0	6	11	16	22
VPCCS + norharman	1	1	3	6	8	22	2	2	5	6	10	14
BP	2	2	4	9	18	33	0	0	3	9	15	21
Norharman	0	1	3	6	9	26	0	1	4	8	12	22
BP + norharman	1	1	1	8	11	29	0	0	6	14	21	28

[a]Initial number of animals per group: 35 males and 35 females.
[b]For details for the treatments see text.
[c]VPCCS = vapor phase components of cigarette smoke (isoprene, methyl chloride, methyl nitrite and acetaldehyde).

The incidence of exophytic and inverted hyperplasia and metaplasia of the laryngeal epithelium was somewhat higher in the groups treated with norharman alone or with norharman + BP than in the group treated with BP alone or in the control group (Table 4), indicating a slight effect of norharman on the larynx. In this context it is interesting to note that in the group treated with norharman alone 3 out of 30 (10%) males, but 0 out of 24 females, had developed a laryngeal tumor, viz. one papilloma and two squamous cell carcinomas. However, in the group treated with norharman + BP no laryngeal tumor was observed.

In each of the three groups given intratracheal instillations of BP squamous cell carcinomas of the forestomach were found. Their incidences varied from 6 to 10%. No forestomach carcinomas were encountered in any of the other groups.

TABLE 4. Type and incidence of non-neoplastic and neoplastic changes in the nose and larynx of hamsters exposed to air or vapor phase components of cigarette smoke and treated or not treated intratracheally with BP or norharman, or treated intratracheally with BP + norharman alone[a]

Site and type of lesions	Incidence of lesions						
	Air	VPCCS[b]	VPCCS + BP	VPCCS + norharman	BP	Norharman	BP + norharman
Males							
Nose							
Respiratory epithelium:	(29)	(29)	(28)	(29)	(27)	(29)	(22)
1. disarrangement	0	0	2	1	0	0	0
2. hyperplasia	0	3	5	1	0	0	0
3. squamous metaplasia	3	13	12	9	3	1	3
4. squamous cell carcinoma	0	1	0	0	0	0	0
Olfactory epithelium:							
1 disarrangement	0	0	0	0	0	1	0
2. adenocarcinoma	0	1	0	0	0	0	0
Larynx	(26)	(31)	(27)	(29)	(24)	(30)	(23)
1. exophytic hyper/metaplasia							
a. slight	0	4	0	4	0	2	3
b. moderate	0	2	4	4	1	1	1
c. severe (with atypia)	0	2	0	2	0	1	0
2. inverted hyper/metaplasia							
a. slight	1	6	3	0	1	2	4
b. moderate	0	2	4	6	1	2	1
c. severe (with atypia)	0	1	2	2	0	0	0
3. papilloma	0	1	0	0	0	1	0
4. squamous cell carcinoma	0	6	6	5	0	2	0
5. sarcoma	0	0	1	0	0	0	0

Females

Nose	(25)	(28)	(25)	(32)	(25)	(29)	(27)
Respiratory epitehlium:							
1. disarrangement	0	1	0	1	0	0	0
2. hyperplasia	0	0	3	3	0	0	0
3. squamous metaplasia	0	12	12	12	0	0	0
4. squamous cell carcinoma	0	1	1	0	0	0	0
Olfactory epithelium:							
1. replacement by respiratory epithelium	0	1	1	1	3	2	5
2. adenocarcinoma	1	0	0	0	0	1	0
Sarcoma	0	0	0	0	0	1	0

Larynx	(25)	(32)	(34)	(35)	(31)	(34)	(33)
1. exophytic hyper/metaplasia							
a. slight	0	2	2	7	0	0	0
b. moderate	1	6	0	3	0	2	0
c. severe (with atypia)	0	2	3	1	0	1	0
2. inverted hyper/metaplasia							
a. slight	0	1	2	1	0	0	0
b. moderate	0	3	1	1	0	1	0
c. severe (with atypia)	0	2	0	0	0	0	0
3. papilloma	0	0	0	0	1	0	0
4. squamous cell carcinoma	0	6	2	3	0	0	0

[a] Initial number of animals per group: 35 males and 35 females. For details of the treatments see text. The number of organs examined is given in parentheses.

[b] VPCCS = vapor phase components of cigarette smoke (isoprene, methyl chloride, methyl nitrite and acetaldehyde).

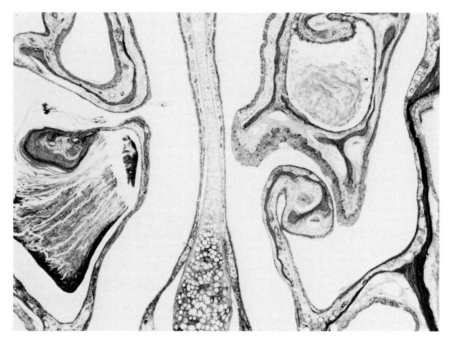

FIG. 5. Nose of hamster exposed to a mixture of isoprene, methyl chloride, methyl nitrite and acetaldehyde. Maxillary turbinate lined by metaplastic keratinized stratified squamous epithelium (left side). Accumulation mainly of poly-morphonuclear leucocytes and cellular debris (left side). Carcinoma *in situ* of the nasal turbinate (right side) (H.E., × 90).

Long-Term Inhalation Study with Acetaldehyde in Rats

Body Weights and Mortality

Reduced weight gain was seen in males of each of the test groups and in females of the intermediate- and high-dose groups; there was a clear dose-response relationship.

Mortality was low during the first six months of the experimental period (Table 5). Thereafter a sharp increase in mortality occurred in the high-dose group. The mean survival time decreased with increasing dose levels (Table 5).

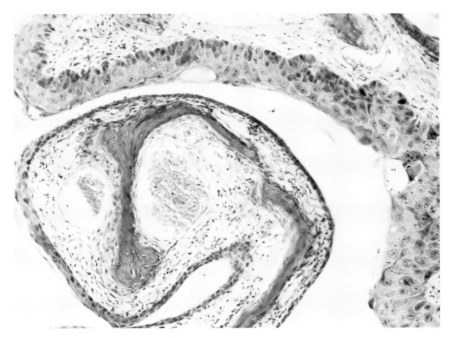

FIG. 6. Higher magnification of the carcinoma *in situ* depicted in Fig. 5 (H.E., × 375).

Pathology

Pathological changes attributable to the inhalation of acetaldehyde vapor occurred in the nose and larynx. A detailed description of the gross and microscopic pathology observed during the first 15 months of the study has recently been published (37). The changes found in the nose can be summarized as follows: (a) degeneration and focal basal cell hyperplasia of the olfactory epithelium and thickening of its submucosa along with loss of Bowman's glands and nerve bundles in all dose groups, (b) stratified squamous metaplasia with or without keratinization and with or without atypia of the respiratory epithelium in the high-dose group, and (c) carcinomas in all dose groups. The laryngeal changes comprised hyperplasia and keratinized stratified squamous metaplasia of the epithelium in the intermediate- and high-dose groups.

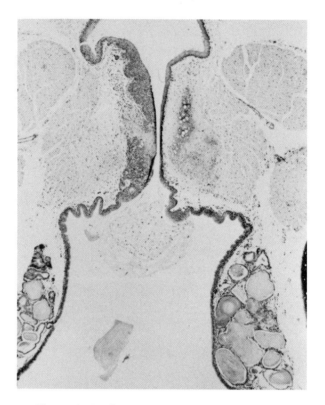

FIG. 7. Inverted hyperplasia of the laryngeal epithelium of a male hamster exposed to a mixture of isoprene, methyl chloride, methyl nitrite and acetaldehyde (H.E., × 75).

Type and incidence of nasal tumors in the various groups are presented in Table 6. The table shows that squamous cell carcinomas (Fig. 9) occurred in all dose groups and that their incidence increased with increasing dose level. Adenocarcinomas of the olfactory epithelium (Fig. 10) were also found in all dose groups, their incidence being highest at the intermediate-dose level in both males and females. The absence of a dose-response relationship, which is also true for the total number of males bearing a nasal tumor, is almost surely due to the much shorter mean survival time of high-dose animals as compared to that of animals in the other groups (Table 5). It is noteworthy that the ratio of squamous cell carcinomas/adenocarcinomas shifted from about 1/1 in the high-dose group to about 1/3 in the intermediate-dose group to about 1/6 in the low-dose group.

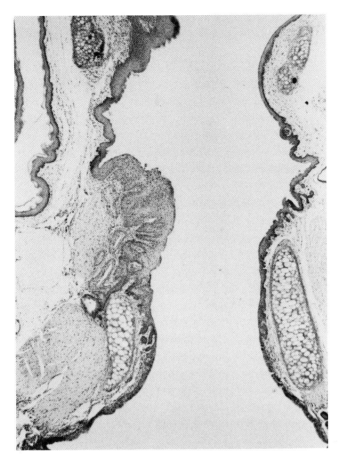

FIG. 8. Carcinoma *in situ* of the larynx of a female hamster exposed to a mixture of isoprene, methyl chloride, methyl nitrite and acetaldehyde (H.E., × 120).

DISCUSSION

In the present study hamsters given repeated intratracheal instillations of glass fibers developed chronic focal non-neoplastic pulmonary lesions characteristic for exposure of experimental animals to high concentrations of glass fibers (5,6,14,20,21). Bronchogenic carcinomas or mesotheliomas were not found, which is in agreement with the absence of treatment-related lung tumors in Fischer rats exposed to atmospheres containing 10 mg/m^3 of different kinds of man-made mineral fibers for 6 to 7 hr/day, 5 days/week during one year (18). In addition, it appeared that glass fibers did not enhance the development of BP-induced respiratory tract tumors. An obvious

TABLE 5. Cumulative mortality and mean survival time of rats exposed to various concentrations of acetaldehyde vapor[a]

Acetaldehyde concentration (ppm)	Males							Females						
	4	26	52	80	104	122	Mean survival time (days)	4	26	52	80	104	122	Mean survival time (days)
0	0	0	0	3	22	33	747 ± 16[b]	0	0	0	1	9	29	782 ± 14
750	1	1	4	6	27	44	704 ± 18	0	1	1	5	21	44	739 ± 19
1500	0	0	1	12	27	46	683 ± 20	0	0	0	6	27	48	729 ± 15
3000 → 1000	0	4	15	38	55	55	434 ± 23	0	3	7	31	55	55	502 ± 19

[a] Initial number of animals per group: 55 males and 55 females.
[b] Standard error of the mean.

TABLE 6. Type and incidence of nasal tumors in rats exposed to various concentrations of acetaldehyde vapor for 28 months[a]

	Incidence of tumors							
	Males				Females			
Type of tumors	Acetaldehyde concentration (ppm)				Acetaldehyde concentration (ppm)			
	0	750	1500	3000 → 1000	0	750	1500	3000 → 1000
Number of animals examined	52	51	50	49	52	52	52	51
Number of tumor-bearing animals	1	16	34	28	0	7	33	37
Carcinoma *in situ*	0	0	0	1	0	0	3	3
Squamous cell carcinoma	1	2	9	15	0	1	5	16
Adeno-squamous carcinoma	0	0	0	0	0	0	0	1
Adenocarcinoma of olfactory epithelium	0	14	25	17	0	6	26	17
Carcinoma (unclassified)	0	0	0	0	0	0	0	2

[a] Initial number of animals per group: 55 males and 55 females.

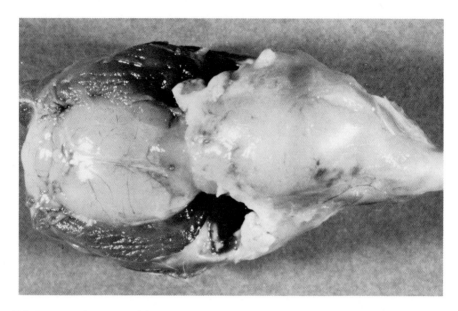

FIG. 9. Large tissue mass lying over the premaxilla and extending into the brain; it was diagnosed microscopically as an osteolytic squamous cell carcinoma derived from the nasal epithelium. Male rat exposed to 3000 → 1000 ppm acetaldehyde for 15 months.

conclusion, therefore, is that under the conditions of the present experiment the glass fibers used did not exert carcinogenic or co-carcinogenic activity. However, this conclusion also holds for the crocidolite fibers examined. Since intratracheal instillation of asbestos fibers mixed with BP has been shown by several investigators to produce a markedly increased incidence of lung tumors in hamsters or rats as compared to treatment with the separate materials (24), the hamster model used in the present study might not be sensitive enough to detect possible carcinogenic or co-carcinogenic properties of glass fibers.

A long-term inhalation study in Syrian hamsters showed that exposure to 1500 ppm acetaldehyde vapor for 7 hr/day, 5 days/week during 52 weeks followed by an observation period of 29 weeks caused severe hyperplasia and metaplasia of the nasal respiratory epithelium and of the laryngeal epithelium (10). However, no tumors were found in

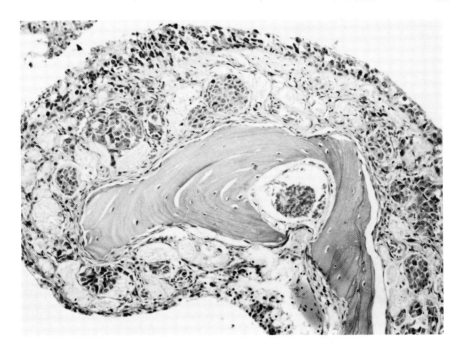

FIG. 10. Adenocarcinoma of the nasal olfactory epithelium of a male rat exposed to 3000 → 1000 ppm acetaldehyde for 15 months (H.E., × 200).

the nose or larynx. In a subsequent study of very similar design but using a higher exposure concentration of acetaldehyde vapor (2500 → 1650 ppm; concentration reduced from 2500 ppm to 1650 ppm after 45 weeks), again hyperplasia and metaplasia of the nasal and laryngeal epithelium of hamsters were observed, but now also a few nasal tumors and a considerable number of laryngeal carcinomas occurred (11). Because the main difference between the former and the latter study was a difference in exposure level, it seems justified to assume that the higher exposure concentration in the latter study was responsible for the induction of nasal and laryngeal tumors. In the present study the nasal and laryngeal changes observed in the three groups of hamsters exposed to the vapor mixture were very similar in type and incidence to those occurring in the second acetaldehyde experiment. Because of these striking similarities the possibility was considered that the effects of the vapor mixture on the nose and larynx have to be ascribed to acetaldehyde alone. The exposure level of acetaldehyde in the present study was, however, relatively low

(1400 → 1200 ppm), even lower than that (1500 ppm) used in the first acetaldehyde study. On the other hand the exposure period (100 weeks) was almost twice as long as in the previous studies (52 weeks). Moreover, in the present study the total exposure to acetaldehyde expressed in ppm·hr was 3.9×10^6, which is very close to the total exposure of 3.7×10^6 ppm·hr in the second acetaldehyde study (11) and much higher than the exposure of 2.7×10^6 ppm·hr in the first acetaldehyde study (10). It is, therefore, concluded that the nasal and laryngeal effects observed in hamsters exposed to the vapor mixture were most probably caused by acetaldehyde alone. This conclusion is further supported by the fact that in 4-week inhalation studies with the other compounds of the mixture, no histopathological changes of the nasal or laryngeal epithelium were observed at any of the exposure levels tested, which were comparable to (methyl nitrite) or much higher (isoprene, methyl chloride) than the concentrations in the mixture (Personal communication, P. G. J. Reuzel, CIVO-Toxicology and Nutrition TNO, Zeist, The Netherlands).

The feeding of norharman to male rats at a dietary level of 500 ppm either alone or in combination with various levels of aniline for 80 weeks did not produce evidence for carcinogenicity or co-carcinogenicity of this compound (15). In the present study there was some evidence of norharman adversely affecting the laryngeal epithelium in hamsters; however, in view of the way of administering the compound and the relatively slight effect on the larynx the evidence is considered insufficient to allow any conclusion as to irritating or carcinogenic properties of norharman.

The long-term inhalation study with acetaldehyde in rats clearly showed that this aldehyde is capable of inducing squamous cell carcinomas and adenocarcinomas in the nose of rats at exposure levels of 750 ppm and above. In the top-dose group (3000 → 1000 ppm) the incidences of squamous cell carcinomas and adenocarcinomas were about equal; in the lower dose groups (750 and 1500 ppm) the large majority of the nasal tumors were adenocarcinomas. Squamous cell carcinomas originated mainly, if not exclusively, from metaplastic respiratory epithelium, and adenocarcinomas from damaged olfactory epithelium. As has been reported previously (37) the olfactory epithelium was injured by acetaldehyde at each exposure level, the severity of the injuries increasing with increasing dose level. The respiratory epithelium was severely damaged at the top-dose level, slightly affected at the intermediate-dose level, and not damaged at all at the low-dose level. These findings suggest that the tumors in the nose arise from epithelium which is injured by acetaldehyde, viz. mainly the olfactory epithelium in the low- and mid-dose groups and both the respiratory and the olfactory epithelium in the top-dose group. This indicates that the cytotoxic effects of acetaldehyde have played a significant role in the development of nasal tumors (37).

Recent studies have shown that acetaldehyde induced sister chromatid exchanges (4,17,29) and chromosomal aberrations (26) in human peripheral lymphocytes *in vitro*. Acetaldehyde also induced sister chromatid exchanges in cultured ovary cells of Chinese hamsters (8,25) and in the bone marrow of mice (26) and Chinese hamsters (19). Moreover, acetaldehyde has been found to induce cell transformations in C3H10T½ cells (1) and micronuclei, chromosomal aberrations and aneuploidies in rat fibroblasts (2,3). It is, therefore, obvious to assume that acetaldehyde possesses initiating activity which played a role in the induction of nasal tumors in rats and laryngeal tumors in hamsters (11,37). The full results of the long-term study in rats should be available before the relative importance can be judged of the cytotoxic and initiating activity of acetaldehyde for its carcinogenicity. For the time being, however, it seems justified, thinking in terms of cytotoxic concentrations, to consider acetaldehyde a complete carcinogen. It would be of interest to investigate whether chronic exposure of rats to subcytotoxic concentrations of acetaldehyde leads to nasal tumors.

Since acetaldehyde is known to occur in cigarette smoke at levels up to 2000 ppm (13), this and several other aldehydes, e.g., formaldehyde (12) may significantly contribute to the induction of bronchogenic cancer by cigarette smoke in man. Particularly, a smoker who actively inhales may expose his larynx and bronchi to high concentrations of acetaldehyde. The preliminary results of the present studies did not produce evidence that isoprene, methyl chloride or methyl nitrite, all major components of the vapor phase of cigarette smoke (13), or norharman occurring in the particulate phase of smoke, are of significance for the induction of lung cancer by cigarette smoke.

SUMMARY

Syrian golden hamsters were given intratracheal instillations of glass fibers with or without BP suspended in saline, once a fortnight for 52 weeks; the experiment was terminated at week 85. No tumors of the respiratory tract were observed in hamsters treated with glass fibers alone. There was no indication that glass fibers enhanced the development of respiratory tract tumors induced by BP.

In another study Syrian golden hamsters were exposed to fresh air or to a mixture of 4 major vapor phase components of cigarette smoke, viz. isoprene (800 → 700 ppm), methyl chloride (1000 → 900 ppm), methyl nitrite (200 → 190 ppm) and acetaldehyde (1400 → 1200 ppm) for a period of at most 23 months. Some of the animals were also given repeated intratracheal instillations of BP or norharman in saline. Laryngeal tumors were found in 7/31 male and 6/32 female hamsters exposed only to the vapor mixture, whereas no laryngeal tumors occurred in controls. The tumor response of the larynx most probably has to be ascribed entirely to the action of acetaldehyde. Simultaneous treatment with norharman or BP did not affect the tumor response of the larynx.

Acetaldehyde may occur in the vapor phase of cigarette smoke at levels up to 2000 ppm. Chronic inhalation exposure of rats to acetaldehyde at levels of 0 (controls), 750, 1500 or 3000 → 1000 ppm resulted in a high incidence of nasal carcinomas, both squamous cell carcinomas of the respiratory epithelium and adenocarcinomas of the olfactory epithelium.

It was discussed that acetaldehyde may significantly contribute to the induction of bronchogenic cancer by cigarette smoke in man. No evidence was obtained for a role of isoprene, methyl chloride or methyl nitrite in the induction of lung cancer by cigarette smoke.

ACKNOWLEDGEMENTS

The studies were supported by grants from the Stichting Koningin Wilhelmina Fonds (Netherlands Cancer Foundation), Amsterdam, and the Ministery of Housing, Physical Planning and Environmental Protection, Leidschendam.

REFERENCES

1. Abernethy, D. J., Frazelle, J. H., and Boreiko, C. J. (1982): *Environ. Mutagen.*, 4:331 (abstract).
2. Bird, R. P., and Draper, H. H. (1980): *J. Toxicol. Environ. Health*, 6:811-833.
3. Bird, R. P., Draper, H. H., and Basrur, P. K. (1982): *Mutat. Res.*, 101:237-246.
4. Böhlke, J. U., Singh, S., and Goedde, H. W. (1983): *Human Genet.*, 63:285-289.
5. Botham, S. K., and Holt, P. F. (1971): *J. Pathol.*, 103:149-156.
6. Botham, S. K., and Holt, P. F. (1973): *Brit. J. Indust. Med.*, 30:232-236.
7. Cralley, L. J., and Lainhart, W. S. (1973): *J. Occup. Med.*, 15:262-266.
8. DeRaat, W. K., Davis, P. B., and Bakker, G. L. (1983): *Mutat. Res.*, 124:85-90.
9. Dixon, J. R., Lowe, D. B., Richards, E. E., Cralley, L. J., and Stokinger, H. E. (1970): *Cancer Res.*, 30:1068-1074.
10. Feron, V. J. (1979): *Prog. Exp. Tumor Res.*, 24:162-176.

11. Feron, V. J., Kruysse, A., and Woutersen, R. A. (1982): *Eur. J. Cancer Clin. Oncol.*, 18:13-31.
12. Feron, V. J., Woutersen, R. A., and Appelman, L. M. (1985): In: *Zur Problematik von Inhalationstoxizitäts-Untersuchungen.* Proceedings of a Symposium, BGA, 2-4 April 1984, Berlin, in press.
13. Groenen, P. J. (1978): *Bestanddelen van Tabaksrook: Aard en Hoeveelheid; Potentiële Invloed op de Gezondheid*, 30 pp. Rapport No. R 5787. Centraal Instituut voor Voedingsonderzoek TNO: Zeist.
14. Gross, P., Kaschak, M., Tolker, E. E., Babyak, M. A., and DeTreville, R. T.P. (1970): *Arch. Environ. Health*, 20:696-704.
15. Hagiwara, A., Arai, M., Hirose, M., Nakanowatari, J., Tsuda, H., and Ito, N. (1980): *Toxicol. Lett.*, 6:71-75.
16. Harington, J. S., Allison, A. C., and Badami, D. V. (1975): *Adv. Pharmacol. Chemother.*, 12:291-402.
17. Jansson, T. (1982): *Hereditas*, 97:301-303.
18. Kolk, J. J. (1982): *T. Soc. Geneesk.*, 60:770-772.
19. Korte, A., Obe, G., Ingwersen, I., and Rückert, G. (1981): *Mutat. Res.*, 88:389-395.
20. Lee, K. P., Barras, C. E., Griffith, F. D., and Waritz, R. S. (1979): *Lab. Invest.*, 40:123-133.
21. Lee, K. P., Barras, C. E., Griffith, F. D., Waritz, R. S., and Lapin, C. A. (1981): *Environ. Res.*, 24:167-191.
22. Meurman, L. O., Kiviluoto, R., and Hakama, M. (1979): *Ann. N.Y. Acad. Sci.*, 330:491-496.
23. Morisset, Y., P'an, A., and Jegier, Z. (1979): *J. Toxicol. Environ. Health*, 5:943-956.
24. Mossman, B., Light, W., and Wei, E. (1983): *Ann. Rev. Pharmacol. Toxicol.*, 23:595-615.
25. Obe, G., and Beek, B. (1979): *Drug Alcohol Depend.*, 4:91-94.
26. Obe, G., Natarajan, A. T., Meyers, M., and Den Hertog, A. (1979): *Mutat. Res.*, 68:291-294.
27. Poindexter, E. H., and Carpenter, R. D. (1962): *Phytochemistry*, 1:215-221.
28. Pott, F., Huth, F., and Friedrichs, K. H. (1976): In: *Occupational Exposure to Fibrous Glass*, pp. 183-191. Proceedings of a Symposium, College Park, MD, 26-27 June 1974, HEW Publications No. (NIOSH) 76-151, U.S. Department of Health, Education and Welfare, Washington, DC.
29. Ristow, H., and Obe, G. (1978): *Mutat. Res.*, 58:115-119.
30. Saracci, R. (1977): *Int. J. Cancer*, 20:323-331.
31. Selikoff, I. J., Seidman, H., and Hammond, E. C. (1980): *J. Natl. Cancer Inst.*, 65:507-513.
32. Shabad, L. M., Pylev, L. N., Krivosheeva, L. V., Kulagina, L. F., and Nemenko, B. A. (1974): *J. Natl. Cancer Inst.*, 52:1175-1187.
33. Stanton, M. F., Layard, M., Tegeris, A., Miller, E., May, M., and Kent, E. (1977): *J. Natl. Cancer Inst.*, 58:587-603.
34. Stanton, M. F., and Wrench, C. (1972): *J. Natl. Cancer Inst.*, 48:797-821.
35. Van Graft, M., Spit, B. J., Immel, H. R., and Feron, V. J. (1984): *Pulmonary Response of Syrian Golden Hamsters to Fibrous Glass Following Intratracheal Instillation. I. Clearance and Morphological Changes After a Single Administration*, 28 pp. Report No. V 84.094, Institute CIVO-Toxicology and Nutrition TNO: Zeist.

36.   Wagner, J. C., Berry, G., and Skidmore, J. W. (1976): In: *Occupational Exposure to Fibrous Glass*, pp. 193-197. Proceedings of a Symposium, College Park, MD, 26-27 June 1974, HEW Publications No. (NIOSH) 76-151, U.S. Department of Health, Education and Welfare, Washington, DC.
37.   Woutersen, R. A., Appelman, L. M., Feron, V. J., and Van Der Heijden, C. A. (1984): *Toxicology*, 31:123-133.

Carcinogenesis, Vol. 8, edited by M. J. Mass et al.
Raven Press, New York © 1985.

In Vivo Studies on Enhancement and Promotion of Respiratory Tract Carcinogenesis: Studies with Heterotopic Tracheal Transplants

A. J. P. Klein-Szanto, *A. C. Marchok,
and *M. Terzaghi

*Science Park—Research Division, The University of Texas System Cancer Center,
Smithville, Texas 78957; *Biology Division, Oak Ridge National Laboratory,
Oak Ridge, Tennessee 37831*

Several chemical and nonchemical agents are able to enhance the development and incidence of experimentally induced squamous cell carcinomas of the respiratory tract *in vivo*. This review will deal more extensively with the promoting effects of exogenous chemicals which seem to qualify as true promoters of tumors in the respiratory tract epithelium (although some of these agents have characteristics of weak carcinogens). Several other factors that enhance the development of airway neoplasia have been recently reviewed (16) and will be mentioned succinctly. Among these factors, the most important are immunosuppression and chronic infection.

Although the inverse relationship between immunocompetence and development of malignancy has been studied profusely in several animal models (2,10,24), few studies have employed *in vivo* lung models in order to analyze this phenomenon (18,22). Only one of these models was used to study the influence of immunosuppression on the process of carcinogenesis leading to squamous cell carcinomas of the respiratory tract epithelium. Using syngeneic heterotopic tracheal transplants treated with 7,12-dimethylbenz(a)anthracene (DMBA), Nettesheim et al. (16) demonstrated an almost two-fold enhancement of tumor incidence in immunosuppressed animals. In addition, the latency period was also shortened in the immunodeficient animals.

In another study, Schreiber et al. (19) showed that conventional animals with clear histologic signs of chronic murine pneumonia had a higher incidence of nitrosamine-induced squamous cell carcinomas than specific pathogen free (SPF) and germ free rats of the same parental stock. The mechanism of tumor enhancement in infected mice is not yet resolved but several possible factors have been suggested on the basis of experimental data, i.e., decreased local immunocompetence (17), alterations in carcinogen metabolism (4), and impaired clearance of carcinogen or carcinogen carrying particles when the lungs are subjected to inhalation exposure (5).

A nutritional factor, namely the lack of adequate levels of vitamin A, has also been implicated in the enhancement of 3-methyl-cholanthrene-induced lung cancer in rats (15). Several possible mechanisms by which hypovitaminosis A could enhance squamous cell carcinoma induction in the respiratory tract epithelium have been proposed. Genta et al. (7) have demonstrated an increase in binding of benzo(a)pyrene (BP) to DNA in tracheal cells maintained under conditions of vitamin A deficiency. On the other hand, on the basis of studies indicating that retinoids inhibit metabolic activation of polycyclic hydrocarbons (9), it could be expected that vitamin A deficiency would enhance the production of ultimate carcinogens. Recently, it has been suggested that vitamin A deficiency may act by establishing biological autarchy of initiated cell populations (6), a phenomenon which would be equivalent to promotion.

PROMOTION OR PROMOTION-LIKE ENHANCEMENT STUDIES IN TRACHEAL TRANSPLANTS

Chemical enhancement of respiratory tract tumor induction includes syncarcinogenesis and cocarcinogenesis, utilizing several administration modalities of two or more known or putative complete carcinogens, and will be described in detail in other chapters of this volume. In this section, we will describe the most relevant data on *in vivo* lung tumor induction which adhere to, or approximate, the basic definition of two-stage carcinogenesis as originally described by Berenblum (1).

These experiments used the induction of squamous carcinomas in heterotopic tracheal transplants as the endpoint to evaluate the ability of 12-O-tetradecanoylphorbol-13-acetate (TPA) and asbestos to promote tumors in respiratory tract epithelium. In this model, which has been extensively described previously (8,11,12) tracheas from donor rats are transplanted into the subcutaneous tissue of syngeneic Fischer 344 rats. The mucociliary epithelium, after initial suffering and partial cell shedding, is reestablished in 3-4 weeks after transplantation and survives for the duration of the transplant without noticeable differences from homotopic tracheal epithelium. Under these conditions, the tracheal transplants can be exposed to precisely quantifiable amounts of carcinogens and/or promoters (18). Based on the extensive experience acquired by the Oak Ridge National Laboratory group, the tracheal transplants could be exposed to a very low initiating dose of DMBA (35 and 100 µg) followed by the protracted exposure to 100 µg of TPA (25,30). TPA embedded in a beeswax matrix was released at a rate of 1-2 µg per day during the first 30 days. Thereafter, the release rate dropped to 0.2-0.5 µg/day. The data showed in Table 1 summarizes the results of this experiment. Although the doses of DMBA utilized were not subcarcinogenic, a marked enhancement of tumor production and a notable decrease in the latency period could be demonstrated. Using the same experimental model, Topping and Nettesheim (29) showed an asbestos-induced enhancement of respiratory tract carcinogenesis by sequentially treating the tracheal transplants with DMBA and 200 µg of chrysotile asbestos (Table 2). In both experiments, these authors utilized initiating doses which proved to be complete carcinogenic doses in some of the experimental groups. This complication did not prevent the clear demonstration of tumor enhancement produced both by TPA and asbestos. Furthermore, these experiments represent the only *in vivo* attempts to reproduce the classical sequential administration of an initiator and a promoter, thus representing the most reliable evidence that promoters play an important role in the pathogenesis of carcinogenesis in respiratory epithelium.

TABLE 1. Percentage of carcinoma incidence in tracheal transplants initiated with DMBA and promoted with TPA[a]

DMBA initiation (µg)	TPA promotion (µg)	Weeks of treatment		
		75	90	100
188	100	47	55	73
188	0	0	10	20
35	100	10	40	ND[b]
35	0	0	5	ND

[a] Modified from ref. 25 and ref. 30.
[b] Not determined.

TABLE 2. Percentage of carcinoma incidence in tracheal transplants
initiated with DMBA and promoted with asbestos[a]

DMBA initiation (μg)	Asbestos promotion (μg)	Percentage squamous carcinoma
50	200	15
50	0	0
25	200	23
25	0	0
12.5	200	3
12.5	0	3
0	200	0

[a] Modified from ref. 29.

This argument is further supported by an additional set of experiments in which the effects of TPA on tracheal epithelium initiated by DMBA *in vivo* were investigated using an *in vitro* growth assay. This study was based on previous experience in which the same epithelial focus assay (EF assay) (26) was used for the quantitative evaluation of the emergence of carcinogen-altered and neoplastic cells.

Briefly, the EF assay consists of the following sequential phases. Heterotopic tracheal transplants are exposed to DMBA followed by TPA in beeswax or by beeswax pellets alone. At various time intervals after initiation of exposure, prior to the development of frank neoplastic lesions, or even before the appearance of preneoplastic lesions, tracheal transplants are removed from host animals. Luminal epithelial cells are dispersed enzymatically and seeded into tissue culture dishes in order to establish primary cultures, and the number of EFs per dish are scored. When isolated, each EF contains roughly 5×10^4 cells. They are removed from the primary dish enzymatically and each EF seeded into a separate secondary culture dish. The fraction of foci which can be subcultured two or more times is noted. All subcultured EFs (EF_s) are tested for the capacity to grow in soft agarose. In this system, the capacity to grow in soft agarose has been found to correlate with the capacity of a cell population to yield tumors when inoculated i.m. into immunosuppressed rats (14,28).

The EF assay has made it possible to monitor the development *in vivo* of cell compartments endowed with different proliferative and neoplastic potentials *in vitro*. Epithelia from normal noncarcinogen-exposed tracheas yield few EFs in primary culture. Epithelia from carcinogen-exposed tracheas (without TPA promotion) yield 10 to 100 times more EFs than control cultures. The capacity of EFs to be subcultured (EF_s) and the capacity of EF_s to grow in soft agarose ($EF_{s,ag+}$) appear to reflect the severity of carcinogen-induced changes in tracheal epithelium. The frequency of EF_s and $EF_{s,ag+}$ populations increase both with carcinogen dose and time after exposure (27).

When the DMBA exposure was followed with TPA treatment, there was no increase in the yield of EFs. In a similar fashion, the number of EFs were not affected by subsequent TPA exposure. On the other hand, there was a marked effect of promoter treatment on the maintenance and size of the cell pool giving rise to $EF_{s,ag+}$. Although this effect is already evident 3 months after TPA exposure, it becomes extremely clear after 12 and 18 months of promotion (Table 3). This increase in the anchorage independent cell population correlates very well with the late appearance of tumors in the *in vivo* experiments using the same doses of initiator and promoter (23, 25) and indicates that TPA permits the persistence of carcinogen-altered cells which otherwise might revert to normal or disappear. Furthermore, these TPA-dependent populations not only persist but are most probably amplified and some could finally develop into neoplastic cells.

TABLE 3. Percentage of subculturable anchorage-independent epithelial foci detected during tumor promotion in heterotopic tracheal transplants[a]

Duration of exposure to TPA (wk)	Exposure regimen		
	Beeswax-cholesterol followed by TPA[b]	DMBA followed by beeswax-cholesterol[b]	DMBA followed by TPA[b]
0	0	32	32
3	0	29	38
12	0	4	82
18	0	12	70

[a] Modified from ref. 25.
[b] Percentage of subculturable epithelial foci that grew in soft agarose.

FORMALDEHYDE AS A SECOND STAGE PROMOTER IN TRACHEAL TRANSPLANTS

A recent improvement in the use of tracheal transplants has permitted the investigation of the effects of chemicals in solution or in gaseous form. It consists of regular s.c. tracheal transplants that are connected, four weeks after implantation, to the outside by way of two terminal tracheostomies. This model, called open-ended rat tracheal implant (OERTI), has been successfully used to evaluate the toxic effects of formadelhyde solutions and formaldehyde gas (20,21) (Fig. 1).

Recently, we have evaluated the effect of 0.1% formaldehyde in phosphate-buffered saline (PBS) as a promoter. Briefly, the tracheal transplants were treated with beeswax pellets containing 800 μg of BP for one month, at this time the pellets were removed and the ends of the transplants were fixed to the skin producing two terminal tracheostomies. Rats with OERTI were treated twice a week for 30 weeks. Each treatment consisted of an intratracheal injection of approximately 60 μl of formaldehyde or PBS for 3 hr. After 30 weeks the animals were pulse labeled with [3H]thymidine and sacrificed (Fig. 2). Table 4 shows the marked increase in the labeling index on the BP/formaldehyde-treated OERTI; in addition large numbers of squamous metaplasias, some of them with moderate atypias, were seen in this group. The other OERTI groups, formaldehyde control groups, as well as the animals treated only with BP showed variable degrees of hyperplasia, and only occasionally regular squamous metaplasia. It is worthwhile to mention that OERTI treated only with PBS exhibited normal mucociliary epithelium with occassional areas of hyperplasia, especially near the tracheostomies (Fig. 3).

Although it is premature to conclude that these changes elicited by formaldehyde constitute an integral part of a tumor promotion process, the production of squamous metaplasia and moderate dysplastic lesions is compatible with the hypothesis that this compound enhances and/or promotes BP-initiated carcinogenesis of the respiratory tract.

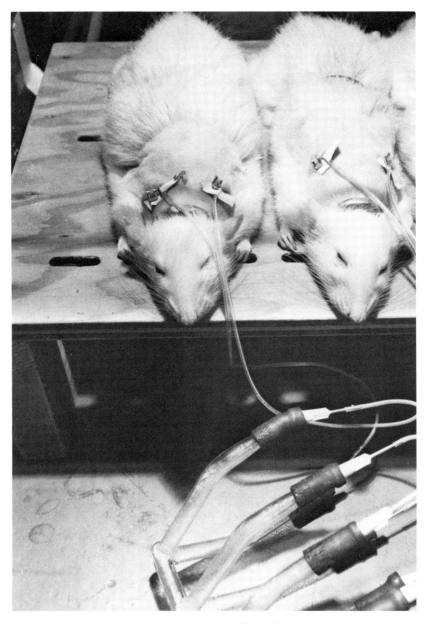

FIG. 1. Two rats undergoing treatment with formaldehyde gas. Each animal has two open ended tracheal implants (OERTI) connected to a formaldehyde exposure system. The proximal tracheostomy of the OERTI is connected to a tubing and divider system (lower part), the distal tracheostomy remains open.

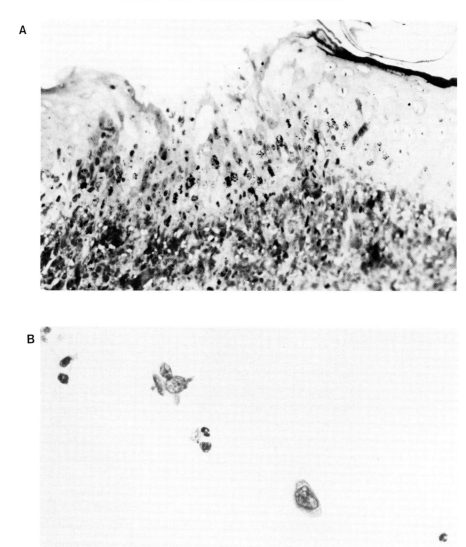

FIG. 2. (A) Squamous metaplasia of an OERTI epithelium initiated with BP and promoted with a formaldehyde solution for 30 weeks. Note the moderate degree of atypia and a high thymidine labeling index. (B) Exfoliative cytology of similarly treated OERTI shows desquamated epithelial cells with moderate atypia.

TABLE 4. Labeling indices of respiratory tract epithelia exposed to formaldehyde

Exposure regimen	Labeling index[a]
Beeswax pellets followed by PBS (phosphate buffered saline)	1.5 ± 0.8
Beeswax pellets followed by formaldehyde in PBS	4.2 ± 1.3
Benzo(a)pyrene in beeswax followed by formaldehyde in PBS	7.9 ± 4.0
Benzo(a)pyrene in beeswax pellets	0.4 ± 0.2

[a] Percentage of cells labeled by [^{3}H]thymidine ± standard deviation.

EFFECTS OF CARCINOGENS AND PROMOTERS ON TRACHEAL TRANSPLANTS CONTAINING HUMAN EPITHELIUM

Recently, we have developed a method permitting the repopulation of rat tracheal transplants stripped of their epithelium and replaced with human respiratory tract epithelium derived from immediate autopsies (13). In brief, epithelial cells from the respiratory tract of premature and full-term human fetuses were enzymatically removed and inoculated into rat tracheas devoid of native epithelium. These were sealed at both ends and transplanted subcutaneously into nude mice. After 3-4 weeks, a normal mucociliary epithelium covered the tracheal lumen. At this stage, the human epithelial cells could be isolated again and transplanted into other denuded rat tracheas. This passaging could be repeated up to six times, each permitting an amplification factor of approximately 3-fold. Tracheal transplants containing cells of human origin (*in vivo* passages 2-4) were treated with beeswax pellets containing either 100-200 μg of DMBA or 100 μg of TPA. Treatment of the human respiratory tract epithelium with the polycyclic hydrocarbon produced after 4-8 weeks squamous metaplasias without atypia as well as some mild to moderate dysplastic lesions. The promoter TPA produced hyperplasias and stratified metaplasias without atypias after 4 weeks of treatment. Although these experiments are now in progress, it is reasonable to conclude that these responses in xenotransplanted human tissue are very similar to those described previously in rodent respiratory tract epithelium.

A

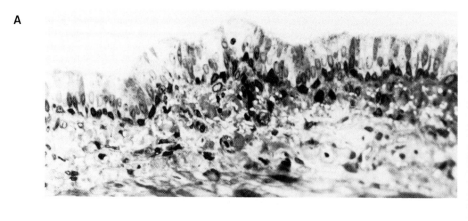

B

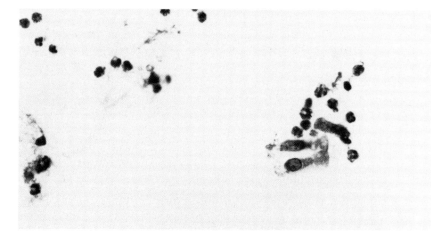

FIG. 3. (A) Slightly hyperplastic epithelium of OERTI 30 weeks after twice weekly injection of phosphate buffered saline solution. (B) Exfoliative cytology of similarly treated OERTI shows normal ciliated cells.

CONCLUSION

Although most of the *in vivo* work on tumor promotion in the respiratory tract does not fulfill the most strict and dogmatic requirements of the two-stage carcinogenesis model (probably because the initiating doses utilized have not been low enough), the available data do show an important enhancement of tumor production, which is still compatible with a promoting effect. The tracheal transplant system seems to be an adequate tool for continuing these investigations. New methodological advances permitting a combined *in vivo-in vitro* evaluation of the effects of known amounts of carcinogens and/or promoters, flow-through tracheal-implants, and the xenotransplanted human epithelia offer an ideal set of conditions under which to study the effects of promoters and suspected promoters of probable importance in the development of cancer in humans.

ACKNOWLEDGEMENTS

This investigation was supported by PHS grants CA 35552 and CA 34137 awarded by the National Cancer Istitute, NIH, DHHS.

REFERENCES

1. Berenblum, I. (1954): *Cancer Res.*, 14:471-477.
2. Cohen, S. M., Headley, D. B., and Bryan, G. T. (1973): *Cancer Res.*, 33:637-641.
3. Cone, M. V., and Nettesheim, P. (1973): *J. Natl. Cancer Inst.*, 50:1599-1606.
4. Corbett, T. H., and Nettesheim, P. (1973): *J. Natl. Cancer Inst.*, 50:778-782.
5. Creasia, D. A., Nettesheim, P., and Hammons, A. S. (1973): *Arch. Environ. Health*, 26:197-201.
6. DeLuca, L. M. (1983): *J. Natl. Cancer Inst.*, 70:405-407.
7. Genta, V. M., Kaufman, D. G., Harris, C. C., Smith, J. M., Sporn, M. B., and Saffiotti, U. (1974): *Nature*, 247:48-49.
8. Griesemer, R. A., Nettesheim, P., Martin, D., and Caton, J. E., Jr. (1977): *Cancer Res.*, 37:1266-1271.
9. Hill, D. L., and Shih, T. W. (1974): *Cancer Res.*, 34:564-570.
10. Johnson, S. (1968): *Brit. J. Cancer*, 22:755-760.
11. Kendrick, J., Nettesheim, P., and Hammons, A. S. (1974): *J. Natl. Cancer Inst.*, 52:1317-1325.
12. Klein-Szanto, A. J. P., Pal, B., Terzaghi, M., and Marchok, A. C. (1984): *Environ. Health Perspect.*, in press.
13. Klein-Szanto, A. J. P., Terzaghi, M., Mirkin, L. D., Martin, D., and Shiba, M. (1982): *Am. J. Pathol.*, 108:231-239.
14. Marchok, A. C., Rhoton, J. C., and Nettesheim, P. (1978): *Cancer Res.*, 38:2030-2037.
15. Nettesheim, P., Snyder, C., and Kim, J. C. (1979): *Environ., Health Perspect.* 29:89-93.
16. Nettesheim, P., Topping, D. C., and Jamasbi, R. (1981): *Ann. Rev. Pharmacol. Toxicol.*, 21:133-163.
17. Nettesheim, P., and Williams, M. L. (1974): *Ann. N.Y. Acad. Sci.*, 221:220-233.
18. Pal, B. D., Topping, D. C., Griesemer, R. A., Nelson, F. R., and Nettesheim, P. (1978): *Cancer Res.*, 38:1376-1383.

19. Schreiber, H., Nettesheim, P., Lijinsky, W., Richter, C. B., and Walburg, H. E., Jr. (1972): *J. Natl. Cancer Inst.*, 49:1107-1114.
20. Shiba, M., Marchok, A. C., and Klein-Szanto, A. J. P. (1983): *Toxicol. Lett.*, 16:241-248.
21. Shiba, M., Marchok, A. C., and Klein-Szanto, A. J. P. (1984): *Toxicol. Lett.*, in press.
22. Shimkin, M. B., and Stoner, G. D. (1975): *Adv. Cancer Res.*, 21:1-58.
23. Steele, V. E., and Nettesheim, P. (1983): In: *Mechanism of Tumor Promotion, Vol. 1*, edited by T. J. Slaga, pp. 91-105. CRC Press, Boca Raton, FL.
24. Stutman, O. (1969): *Science*, 166:620-621.
25. Terzaghi, M., Klein-Szanto, A. J. P., and Nettesheim, P. (1983): *Cancer Res.*, 43:1461-1466.
26. Terzaghi, M., and Nettesheim, P. (1979): *Cancer Res.*, 39:4003-4010.
27. Terzaghi, M., Nettesheim, P., and Riester (1980): *Cancer Res.*, 42:4511-4518.
28. Terzaghi, M., Nettesheim, P., and Williams, M. L. (1978): *Cancer Res.*, 38:4546-4553.
29. Topping, D. C., and Nettesheim, P. (1980): *J. Natl. Cancer Inst.*, 65:627-630.
30. Topping, D. C., and Nettesheim, P. (1980): *Cancer Res.*, 40:4352-4355.

Carcinogenesis, Vol. 8, edited by M. J. Mass et al.
Raven Press, New York © 1985.

Experimental Methods for the Detection of the Carcinogenicity and/or Cocarcinogenicity of Inhaled Polycyclic-Aromatic-Hydrocarbon-Containing Emissions

Uwe Heinrich, *Friedrich Pott, †Ulrich Mohr,
and Werner Stöber

*Fraunhofer-Institut für Toxikologie und Aerosolforschung, 3000 Hannover 61; *Medizinisches
Institut für Umwelthygiene, 4000 Düsseldorf; †Institut für Experimentelle Pathologie,
Medizinische Hochschule Hannover, 3000 Hannover 61, Federal Republic of Germany*

The aim of our investigations is to develop a sensitive method for testing all aspects of the total carcinogenic potential of various inhaled emissions from incomplete combustion processes on the respiratory tract of experimental animals, and to quantify the carcinogenic or cocarcinogenic effects detected.

There is no doubt that the greater part of all human lung cancer cases is caused by the inhalation of cigarette smoke. This special type of effluent from incomplete combustion contains several carcinogens and promoters or cocarcinogens which are held responsible for the tumor induction; some of these compounds are also discharged with emissions of incomplete combustion processes of other organic materials, e.g., fossil fuels. So far, however, it has not been possible to find an experimental inhalation mode sensitive enough to detect carcinogen dose-response relationships for emissions containing polycyclic aromatic hydrocarbons (PAH) by utilizing relatively small numbers of animals (50 to 100 per group).

Besides carcinogens and promoters there are several other factors whose impact on the induction of lung cancer is known or may be anticipated. These factors may promote as well as inhibit the development of tumors in different ways. The concepts of promoter, cocarcinogen, and enhancer do not yet have a generally accepted, standardized definition by which they can be distiguished according to biochemical events and/or operational processes. Therefore, this presentation defines all compounds and interferences which enhance tumor induction to be cocarcinogens. This comprehensive definition of cocarcinogenicity also comprises, for example, the potential enhancement of lung tumor incidence rates by irritant gases; such an influence on the development of lung cancer has been assumed for a long time but has not yet been proven conclusively. Many scientists are engaged in elucidating various mechanisms of carcinogenicity. If this aim were achieved, and a complete exhaust analysis were available, then it might be possible to assess the carcinogenic potential of various emissions without further testing. However, it would take a long time before the existing gaps in our knowledge could be filled. Thus, we are looking for alternative ways of establishing a basis for assessing carcinogenic risk by measuring the effect of all initiating, promoting, enhancing, and inhibiting factors involved in the development of lung cancer by exhaust inhalation in experimental animals. It is assumed that the ranking of carcinogenic potency of the various exhaust gases tested can be extrapolated to the human situation (18). Perhaps, it may not be feasible to establish an experimental model allowing a quantitative comparison of the total carcinogenic potential of various kinds of emissions. However, since research on inhaled source emissions is important to preventive medicine and public health policies, in that it may enable a more reliable assessment of cancer risk to both the general public and the occupationally exposed, the efforts of such work appear to be justified.

A review of published inhalation experiments using exhaust gases revealed that most investigations were conducted with cigarette smoke (1,3,4,5,9) and automobile exhaust (7,11,12,16,17); only one study examined the effects of another PAH-containing emission (14). Reasons for this may include scarcity of adequately equipped inhalation laboratories and the relatively low content of carcinogenic substances in many exhaust emissions as compared to some acutely toxic components. These toxic compounds often require a high dilution of the exhaust gas before they can be used in long term inhalation experiments.

Emissions from diesel and gasoline engines have a very low content of PAH (6). Even if the irritant gases would considerably enhance tumor induction, there is only a remote chance of detecting a carcinogenic effect after chronic inhalation of the diluted exhaust. Likewise, distinguishing between the carcinogenic potential of diesel and gasoline emissions would be next to impossible. Thus, it would be improper to interpret negative observations of this kind as evidence for no risk to the exposed population.

RATIONALE

Except for cigarette smoking and certain occupational exposures, there is no epidemiological or experimental evidence from inhalation studies of the anticipated weak carcinogenicity of emissions from several forms of incomplete combustion, like exhaust from furnaces or combustion engines. In view of this, the question was tabled as to whether a treatment of animals with a known carcinogen, generating a significant base tumor incidence rate, would provide a means for producing a superimposed and quantitatively detectable dose-response relationship of tumor incidence rates by chronic exposure to the emissions under investigation. Combinations of known carcinogens with cigarette smoke were already used for this purpose by several authors. Recently, Hoffmann et al. summarized such investigations (10).

This Institute is concerned with four emission sources involving PAH as exhaust constituents under the experimental arrangement discussed. As sources with low PAH concentration, we make use of:

- a Daimler-Benz diesel engine running at constant load
- a Volkswagen diesel engine running on a driving cycle
- a Volkswagen gasoline engine running on a driving cycle.

As an emission source with extremely high PAH concentration we use:

- a domestic coal furnance, the exhaust of which is enriched with PAH by adding pyrolized pitch effluents.

Some groups of the animals exclusively inhaled the exhaust emissions whereas other groups were additionally treated with one of the carcinogens listed in Table 1. Most of the experiments, which are presently still in progress, are conducted with three animal species: rats, hamsters and mice.

Of all these studies, only the investigation with the Daimler-Benz diesel engine was completed at the time of this report. All other experiments are at various stages of progress.

The animals were exposed to the exhaust gases for a maximum of $2\frac{1}{2}$ years and, as far as possible, for 19 hr/day and 5 days/week. The additional carcinogens were usually applied intratracheally once a week for at least 15 weeks during exhaust exposure; the substances used were two PAH, four metal compounds and two fiber dusts. In case of two nitrosamines, subcutaneous injection replaced the intratracheal instillation; diethylnitrosamine (DEN) was applied to hamsters and dipentylnitrosamine to rats. Finally, newborn mice received a

TABLE 1. Various carcinogens and mode of administration used for the additional treatment of laboratory rodents exposed to exhaust gases

Treatment	Animal species
i.tr. instillation	
- benzo(a)pyrene	hamster, mouse
- dibenz(a,h)anthracene	rat
- calcium arsenate	hamster
- cadmium chloride	hamster
- cadmium oxide	hamster
- nickel oxide	hamster
- crocidolite asbestos	rat, hamster
- glass fibers	hamster
s.c. injection	
- diethylnitrosamine	hamster
- dipentylnitrosamine	rat
- dibenz(a,h)anthracene	mouse (newborn)
i.p. injection	
- urethane	mouse

subcutaneous injection of dibenz(a,h)anthracene (DBahA), and mice about 10 weeks old were treated intraperitoneally with urethane. The experimental details will be described below.

The carcinogenic substances were administered at the beginning of the experiment along with the exhaust exposures. After that, the exhaust exposures continued for between $1\frac{1}{2}$ and $2\frac{1}{2}$ years depending on the average life-span of the species used. Some of the additionally applied caricnogens are believed to persist and may have an effect lasting beyond the treatment period. Therefore, the exhaust exposure and the simultaneously administered carcinogens were considered as two phases taken in separately but interfering in the respiratory tract and modifying the basic carcinogenic effect. A quantitative evaluation appeared to be possible, and was to be examined. This long known experimental arrangement was previously named the "two phase model" (8,18,19) and should not be confused with the "two-stage model" which refers to the action of an initiator and promoter. The changes of the base tumor incidence rates as effected by a mixture with multiple constituents like exhaust emission gases does not permit a distinction between initiators, promoters, or enhancers which may all be contained in the exhaust. Instead, the reported investigations focus on the influence of the exhaust on the base tumor incidence rate induced by the known carcinogen. However, since the mechanisms of action are mostly unknown, no assessment is intended as to which of the primary inducing substances or class of substances used in our experiments are best suited for a subsequent alteration of the tumor induction by the exhaust exposure. An enhancement as well as an inhibition is envisioned.

THE EXHAUST GENERATION SYSTEM

Motor vehicle engines are typical exhaust generators. If fuel consumption remains the same, the mixture of pollutants in the exhaust emission of an individual engine can be reproduced easily by controlling the operating conditions, and the composition of exhaust components may be maintained constantly during a chronic 1-2 year study. The reproducible generation of exhausts from coal combustion is far more difficult. This is not only because the collective term "coal" covers many and varied coal blends, but also because the combustion process in stoves, furnaces, or ovens is far more difficult to regulate and to standardize than that of motor vehicle engines. A particular disadvantage of generating exhaust from coal ovens is that, during the initial burning phase, the concentrations of different pollutants vary considerably and can attain extremely high values. Although an environmentally obnoxious emission develops during this phase, it cannot be used for inhalation experiments because of the considerable variations including acute toxicity levels despite standard dilution. This is partiuclarly unfortunate for carcinogenicity studies because the largest portion of PAH is produced during the initial burning phase but must be discarded. The concentration of benzo(a)pyrene (BP) in the exhaust emitted after a 2-3 hr initial burning phase in a domestic coal oven is very low and can be compared with the BP concentration of clean air in the normal environment.

Against this background, it was decided to mix the coal oven emissions with the effluent generated by pyrolizing pitch at about 700° in a nitrogen atmosphere. As already mentioned, the coal oven emission contains only small amounts of PAH when the coal is glowing after the initial burning phase. Coal pitch contains approximately 1% BP and is still used outside West Germany as a binding medium in the production of hard coal briquets.

Under such experimental conditions, the BP concentration in the exposure chambers increased from less than 1 ng/m^3 to about 120 μg/m^3, i.e., an increase by a factor of 10^5 (Table 2). Some other PAH measured in the exposure chambers have been determined in correspondingly high concentrations. Similar and even higher BP concentrations can be found at some work places, e.g., in coking plants.

TABLE 2. Concentration of some components in coal oven exhaust (COE) diluted 1:10 with clean air (average of 19 hr of exposure)

Components	COE	COE + Pitch[a]
BP (ng/m^3)	0.2	120.000
Particles (mg/m^3)	0.3	6
CnHm (ppm)	3	4
CO (ppm)	110	110
CO$_2$ (vol %)	0.3	0.3
SO$_2$ (ppm)	3	3
NO$_2$ (ppm)	0.4	0.1

[a]   COE mixed with PAH-rich exhaust from pyrolized pitch

Fortunately, the concentrations of other gaseous exhaust components like CO, CO$_2$, SO$_2$, NO$_2$, and total hydrocarbons were, on average, not clearly increased by the addition of a pyrolized pitch exhaust (Table 2). Thus, it was possible to achieve a strong and almost selective increase of the PAH content of an exhaust by pyrolized pitch. There is a chance that this model atmosphere may directly induce tumors in the respiratory tract of experimental animals.

THE EXPOSURE FACILITIES

Figure 1 shows one of the Institute's inhalation laboratories with the generating unit for the domestic coal oven exhaust. The animal rooms into which the chambers open are part of the animal barrier system. The technical measuring area with the equipment for adjusting, controlling and characterizing the exposure atmosphere in the chambers is hermetically sealed from the animal rooms and located between the rear sides of two rows of chambers. The advantage of this arrangement is that the technical staff responsible for the control and maintainance of the exposure facilities and the analytical instruments for the chamber atmosphere need not enter the animal quarters. The exhaust gas and the clean air pipes as well as the mixing boxes for the individual chambers are located on an accessible air distribution floor above the inhalation laboratories. The exhaust diluted in the mixing boxes flows from the upper left hand side into a space behind the perforated wall of the exposure chamber and from there through the perforation horizontally across the chamber and via another perforated wall on the opposite side to an exhauster pipeline (Fig. 2). The horizontal airflow caused by the perforated walls provides an even particle distribution in the chamber and, thus, a uniform burden on the animals. Several exhaust components, such as CO, CO_2, SO_2, NO, NO_2, methane, and total hydrocarbons can be measured simultaneously and continuously by means of a computer-operated, compact measuring cabinet; filter samples are taken for determining the concentrations of particles and PAH.

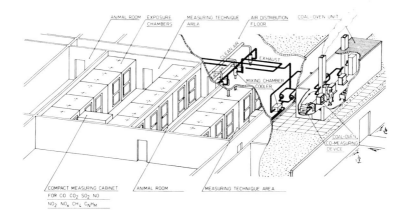

FIG. 1. Exposure facilities of the Fraunhofer-Institute, Hannover with inhalation chambers and the coal oven exhaust generating unit.

Figure 3 shows measured data for various emissions. The concentrations of CO, CO_2, SO_2, and NO_2 in 4 exhaust experiments are given in columns relating to the German maximum allowable concentration at workplaces (MAK). Mass concentrations of particulate matter (dust) are also given; these cannot be related to the general MAK value of 6 mg/m³ for particulate matter because the particles contain numerous toxic and carcinogenic substances. The abbreviations D1 and D2 refer to two experiments with diesel exhaust, G signifies exhaust from a gasoline engine, and CP designates domestic coal oven exhaust with pyrolized pitch. The only figures clearly exceeding the MAK values are those for the CO content of the gasoline engine and the coal oven exhaust. Furthermore, leaded gasoline as fuel

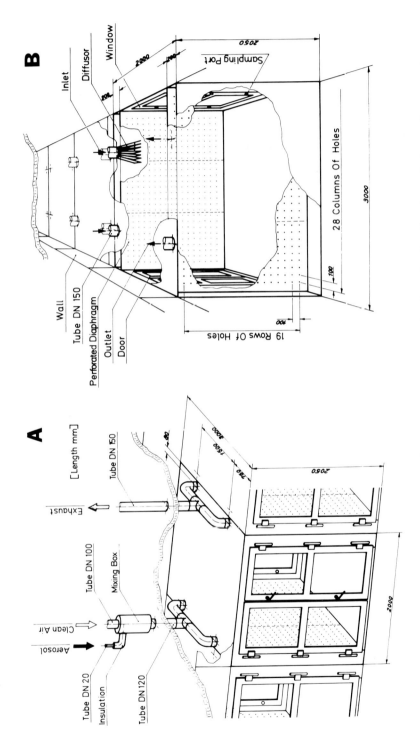

FIG. 2. Horizontal air flow exposure chamber (12 m³). Exterior view (A) and view into the chamber through the partly removed walls (B). (The total area of the holes/diaphragm amount to 417 cm² = 0.7% of the whole diaphragm; the diameter of the holes is 10 mm).

results in concentrations of approximately 40 μg/m³ of lead in the exposure chamber. Regarding the burden on the animals, it should be noted that, except for the first diesel experiment (D1), the exposures per week were as great as 5 exposures for about 19 hr instead of 5 exposures for 8 hr, which is the exposure time at the workplace (15). The particularly high BP content of the domestic coal oven exhaust due to additional effluents of pyrolized pitch has already been explained.

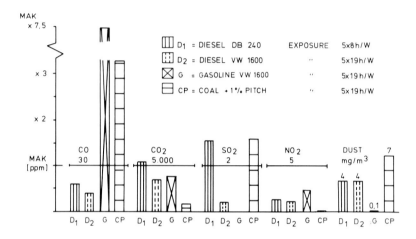

FIG. 3. Concentrations of some exhaust components in the exposure chambers in comparison to the MAK-values (MAK = German maximum allowable concentration at workplaces).

SOME RESULTS AND CONCLUSIONS

At the earliest, results of long term inhalation experiments of the kind reported here are available 2 to 3 years after the beginning of exposure. Since the capacity of our inhalation laboratories is limited, we cannot conduct all of the exposures to various emissions side by side, so we do not yet have enough results to draw firm conclusions.

As expected, no exposure-related tumors could be detected in rats, hamsters, and mice merely exposed to diluted diesel and gasoline engine exhaust for about 2 years. The amount of particle-bound BP deposited in the rodent lung after a 2 year exhaust exposure may amount to less than 1 μg; similar values were estimated for other PAH. This clearly demonstrates that, at least with regard to particle-bound

PAH, exposure-related tumor development within a latency period of about 2-2½ years is most unlikely. Figure 4 shows that all hamster groups exposed to the total diesel exhaust developed a higher percentage of animals with proliferative alterations in the lungs than did the groups that were exposed to the particle-free exhaust or that inhaled clean air (7).

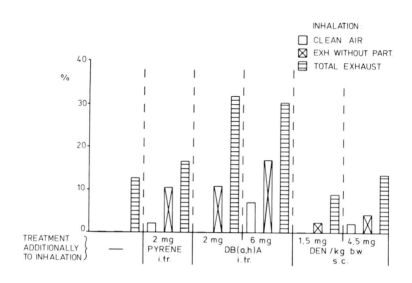

FIG. 4. Hamster with focal proliferations in the lung (in % per group).

Furthermore, by comparing the various experimental groups treated additionally with different known carcinogens, the intratracheally instilled DBahA facilitated the most pronounced influence of the inhaled exhaust on the base incidence rate of proliferative lesions. The percentage of animals with proliferative alterations in the lung was highest in both of these groups.

The experiments using coal oven exhaust enriched with PAH by adding pyrolized pitch are not yet finished. An exposure related tumorigenic effect is expected in these experiments. The investigation by Mestizova and Kossey in 1961 (14) clearly shows a definite increase in the lung tumor incidence rate of mice exposed to the exhaust of heated coal tar. Also, the inhalation of cigarette smoke, mainly in hamsters, demonostrates the possibility of inducing tumors in the respiratory tract of experimental animals by the inhalation of PAH-containing exhaust gases, although the nitrosamine content of the cigarette smoke is higher than that of other exhaust gases from incomplete combustion processes.

From our experiments, the following preliminary results concerning cocarcinogenicity and the "two-phase model" may be mentioned.

The initial experiment combining diesel engine exhaust with DEN seems to demonstrate a tumor induction enhancing effect of the exhaust. After inhalation of diesel engine exhaust, the 45% base tumor incidence rate induced in the larynx/trachea of Syrian golden hamsters by s.c. injections of 4.5 mg DEN/kg was significantly incresed to 70% (Fig. 5) (7). As this effect was observed for both the total exhaust and the exhaust without particles, this may indicate that there is no specific action of the PAH absorbed onto diesel soot. Similar cocarcinogenic effects obtained as an enhancement of the tumor incidence rate by DEN have already been described by Dontenwill (5), and by Hoffmann (10) following exposure to cigarette smoke, and by Dalbey (2) after inhalation of formaldehyde. However, we were not yet able to confirm our findings in additional experiments. So far, our investigations showed that a cocarcinogenic effect is not detected when the induced base tumor incidence rate is low. In both investigations, the diesel exhaust study and the gasoline engine inhalation experiments in Syrian hamsters, a cocarcinogenic effect could not be ascertained when the base tumor incidence rate by DEN was as low as 10-15% (Fig. 5). With gasoline exhaust, no statistically significant influence on DEN-induced tumor incidence was observed (Table 3) (8). On the other hand, whatever the effect on tumor induction, the percentage of animals with hyperplastic alterations in the exposed groups was higher than in the control group.

Apparently, the intratracheally instilled dose of DBahA used in the diesel experiment was also too low to induce tumors in the lungs of hamsters irrespective of exposure to diesel exhaust or clean air. This experiment was already mentioned in conection with the DBahA-dependent increase in exposure-related proliferative alterations in the lung of the experimental animals.

Furthermore, some experiments were carried out with the adenoma test in mice. The advantage of this test is that multiple lung adenomas can be seen macroscopically by 6 months after subcutaneous injection of newborn mice with, for example, 10 μg of DBahA. In an initial experiment by Pott et al. (20), the inhalation of a mixture of SO_2 and NO_2, and the inhalation of ozone seemed to enhance the base tumor

% Hamsters with papillomas in larynx and/or trachea

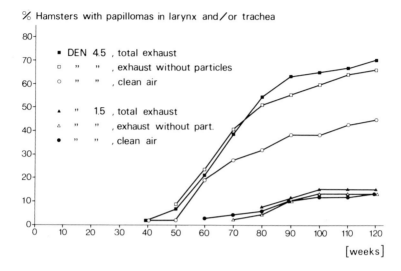

FIG. 5. Tumor (papilloma) incidence in the respiratory tract of hamsters exposed to diesel exhaust and additionally treated (s.c.) with 4.5 or 1.5 mg/kg DEN.

TABLE 3. Hamsters with papillomas and hyperplasia in larynx and/or trachea after s.c. injection of 4.5 mg/kg diethylnitrosamine and inhalation of diluted gasoline exhaust

	Animals (%) with papillomas	Animals (%) with hyperplasia
Clean Air (n = 79)	13.9	13.9
Exhaust diluted with air 1:61 (n = 80)	12.5[a]	18.8
Exhaust diluted with air 1:27 (n = 78)	6.4	27.0

[a] Included are 2 animals with papillomas in the nasal cavity.

incidence rate induced by 10 µg DBahA. The base tumor rate of the group kept in clean air for 7 months was about 65% (Fig. 6). Nearly 100% of the animals that inhaled a mixture of 30 mg SO_2/m^3 and 18 mg NO_2/m^3 for 100 hr per week developed lung adenomas. After inhalation of 0.5 mg ozone/m^3, a tumor incidence of 90% was observed. Correspondingly, differences in the average number of tumors per lung were assessed. But, so far, these results could not be confirmed to the same extent in subsequent experiments. However, an effect of enhancing tumor induction by SO_2 was observed earlier by Peacock and Spencer in 1967 (15). The lung tumor incidence rate of SO_2-exposed mice was about 50% higher than the tumor incidence of the control animals. Laskin et al. (13) found more tumors in rats and hamsters after inhalation of SO_2 and BP than after exposure to BP only. However, it should be noted that up to now all of these studies lack confirmation, and it is premature to take them as proof of a cocarcinogenic effect of the irritant gases investigated.

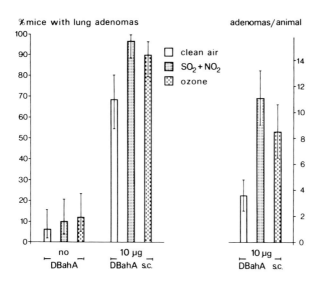

FIG. 6. NMRI-mice with lung adenomas (% per group with 95% confidence limits) and number of adenomas per lung (average per group) after s.c. injection of dibenz(a,h)anthracene and inhalation of clean air or SO_2 + NO_2 or O_3 (20).

The adenoma test in mice was further used to investigate the influence of diesel and gasoline engine exhaust on the base tumor incidence rate. Table 4 shows the results of the experiment with diesel engine exhaust. Comparing the clean air group with the group exposed to total exhaust, both treated with 10 µg DBahA, a statistically significant lower tumor incidence rate and lower average number of adenomas per lung could be detected in the exhaust group.

Although these results should be interpreted with caution, it is remarkable that similar results with diesel exhaust were recently

TABLE 4. Number of lung adenomas/animal ($\bar{x}$) and adenoma bearing animals (%) 6 months after s.c. injection of newborn mice exposed to diesel exhaust (n = 96 female mice per group; confidence limit 95%)

	Total exhaust		Exhaust without particles		Clean air	
s.c. injection	Tumors/ animal ($\bar{x}$)	%	Tumors/ animal ($\bar{x}$)	%	Tumors/ animals ($\bar{x}$)	%
10 µg DBahA	4.16 ± 1.15[a]	62.8[a]	7.33 ± 1.86	71.6	7.8 ± 1.74	81.3
5 µg DBahA	1.17 ± 0.40	51.1	1.71 ± 0.52[a]	53.2	0.97 ± 0.42	45.7
------	------	----	------	----	0.075 ± 0.054	7.5

[a] $p < 0.05$ related to the corresponding group exposed to clean air.

reported by Pepelko (16) as well as by the Southwest Research Institute (12). The tumor incidences of the clean air group and the total exhaust group treated with 5 µg DBahA showed no significant difference. However, the average number of tumors per animal of the group exposed to diesel exhaust devoid of particles was higher than the average number of the control group (the error probability was 4.6% using the U-test). Finally, the newborn mice model did not indicate any influence of gasoline engine exhaust exposure on the incidence of adenomas. Thus, at the present time, it is the prevailing impression that the influence of automobile engine exhaust on the induction of adenomas in mice may, rather, be an inhibitory one.

Although, to date, the results are not very conclusive, they may become consistent by the time all our various experiments are finished.

ACKNOWLEDGEMENTS

The inhalation experiments with diesel and gasoline engine emissions as well as with coal oven exhaust were partially supported by the German governmental agencies and German industries: Umweltbundesamt, Bundesministerium für Forschung und Technologie, Forschungsvereinigung Automobiltechnik, e.V., Volkswagenwerk AG, Daimler Benz AG.

REFERENCES

1.   Bernfeld, P., Homburger, F., Soto, E., and Pai, K. (1979): *J. Natl. Cancer Inst.*, 63:675-689.
2.   Dalbey, W. E. (1982): *Toxicology*, 24:9-14.
3.   Dalbey, W. E., Nettesheim, P., Griesemer, R., Caton, J. E., and Guerin, M. R. (1980): *J. Natl. Cancer Inst.*, 64:383-390.
4.   Dontenwill, W. P. (1974): In: *Experimental Lung Cancer: Carcinogenesis and Bioassays*, edited by E. Karbe and J. F. Park, pp. 331-382. Springer Verlag, New York.
5.   Dontenwill, W., Chevalier, H. J., Harke, H.P., Lafrenz, U., Reckzeh, G., and Schneider, B. (1973): *J. Natl. Cancer Inst.*, 51:1781-1832
6.   Grimmer, G. (1983): In: *Handboook of Polycyclic Aromatic Hydrocarbons*, edited by A. Bjorseth, pp. 150-181. Marcel Dekker, Inc., New York.
7.   Heinrich, U., Peters, L., Funcke, W., Pott, F., Mohr, U., and Stöber, W. (1982): In: *Toxicological Effects of Emissions from Diesel Engines*, edited by J.Lewtas, pp. 225-242. Elsevier Biomedical Press, New York.
8.   Heinrich, U., Stöber, W., and Klingenberg, H. (1984): Society of Automotive Engineers, Inc., Warrendale, PA, USA (Hrsg.), XX FISITA Congress, Wien, 6.-11. Mai 1984, The Automotive Future, SAE P-143,3, S. 3.132/3.141.
9.   Hoffman, D., Rivenson, A., Hecht, S. S., Hilfrich, J., Kobayaschi, N., and Wynder, E. L. (1979): *Prog. Exp. Tumor Res.*, 24:370-390.

10. Hoffmann, D., Hecht, S. S., and Wynder, E. L. (1983): *Environ. Health Perspect.*, 50:247-257.
11. Hyde, D., Orthoefer, J., Dungworth, D., Tyler, W., Carter, R., and Lum, H. (1978): *Lab. Invest.*, 38:455-469.
12. Kaplan, H. L., Springer, K. L., and MacKenzie, W. F. (1983): *Final Report (SWRI Project No. 01-0750-103, and SFRE Project No. 1239)*, 58 pp. Southwest Research Institute, San Antonio, TX.
13. Laskin, S., Kuschner, M., and Drew, R. T. (1970): In: *Inhalation Carcinogenesis*, edited by M. G. Hanna, P. Nettesheim, and J. R Gilbert, pp. 321-350. U.S. Atomic Energy Commission, Oak Ridge, TN.
14. Mestizova, M., and Kossey, P. (1961): *Neoplasma*, 8:27-39.
15. Peacock, P. R., and Spence, J. B. (1967): *Brit. J. Cancer*, 21:696-698.
16. Pepelko, W. E., and Peirano, W. B. (1983): *J. Am. Coll. Toxicol.* 2:253-305.
17. Plopper, C. G., Hyde, D. M., and Weir, A. J. (1983): *Lab. Invest.*, 49:391-399.
18. Pott, F., and Heinrich, U. (1983): In: *Jahresbericht 1982 d. Med. Inst. f. Umwelthygiene, Düsseldorf, FRG*, 15: 86-97.
19. Pott,F., and Stöber, W. (1983): *Environ. Health Perspect.*, 47:293-303.
20. Pott, F., Ziem, U., and Brockhaus, A. (1983): *Zur Frage der krebsfördernden Wirkung von Reizgasen in Verbindung mit polyzyklischen aromatischen Kohlenwasserstoffen.* Stellungnahme zu Frage 10 des Fragenkatalogs zur öffentlichen Anhörung über Säuredepositionen der Europäischen Gemeinschaft vom 20.01.1983.

Carcinogenesis, Vol. 8, edited by M. J. Mass et al.
Raven Press, New York © 1985.

Enhancement of Lung Tumor Formation in Mice

H. P. Witschi

*Biology Division, Oak Ridge National Laboratory,
Oak Ridge, Tennessee 37831*

A substantial body of evidence is now available to document that the development of lung tumors in mice can be enhanced by certain chemicals. The subject has recently been reviewed in detail (34). Experiments in several laboratories have shown that lung tumor formation can be enhanced by phorbol, by saccharin and by the antioxidant butylated hydroxytoluene (BHT). It is perhaps no coincidence that the same agents also have been found to promote or to enhance skin, bladder, or liver tumors. While data on the enhancing effects of phorbol or saccharin in mouse lung remain rather limited, a considerable body of information on the effects of BHT has accumulated over the last ten years (34-41).

The present symposium addresses topics related to promotion or enhancement of respiratory tract cancer in both humans and in experimental systems. Any discussion of how mouse lung tumor formation may be influenced by a common food additive needs therefore to address four fundamental questions: how do lung tumors in mice relate to human respiratory tract cancer; does BHT fulfill all criteria of a promoting agent, as usually defined in mouse skin; how do findings of the effects of BHT on lung tumors relate eventually to the continued use of BHT as a food additive; and what is the mechanism of action of BHT.

EPITHELIAL LUNG TUMORS IN MICE

Certain mouse strains develop with age a high incidence of spontaneous lung tumors (19). In 2-year-old male A/Jax mice we found that 80% of all surviving animals had tumors and that approximately half of the tumor-bearing animals had more than one tumor per lung (25). The Swiss Webster mouse strain also develops a high incidence of spontaneous tumors, whereas in such strains as C57 black or C3H, only very few animals ever develop spontaneous lung tumors. If mice with high spontaneous lung tumor incidence are exposed to a variety of carcinogens, invariably both tumor incidence (number of tumor-carrying animals) and tumor multiplicity (average number of tumors found per lung) increase (19). Both the multiplicity and the incidence of tumors induced by chemical carcinogens in susceptible strains is dependent upon dose. It now seems to be established that two genes are responsible for tumor susceptibility in mice (3,9,15).

Macroscopically, lung tumors appear as pearly-white nodules on the surface of the lung. As the tumors grow they compress the surrounding lung parenchyma, although they seldom show aggressive infiltration associated with malignancy. In animals six months of age treated with the carcinogen urethan, all tumors are clearly separated from each other and on the average have a diameter of 0.8 to 1.4 mm (39). After one year, tumors become 3 to 8 mm large, begin to become confluent, and are no longer easily distinguishable from each other.

It is possible to recognize two major types of tumors by light microscopy. One tumor type consists of continuous bands of uniform cuboidal cells which line the alveolar septa and fill alveolar spaces. On occasion the cells are arranged in tubular patterns which resemble fetal lung tissue. When visualized by scanning electron microscopy the tumors have a smooth surface. Transmission electron microscopy has shown that the tumors are most likely derived from type II alveolar cells. The second form of tumor consists of columnar epithelial cells arranged in a tubular or capillary pattern. The scanning electron microscope shows a rough surface with many microvilli, and on transmission electron microscopy it was found that the cells forming such tumors were derived most likely from nonciliated bronchiolar, or so called Clara cells (12, 18).

Some observations made recently have revealed that not all mouse strains show the same proportion of alveolar type II cell tumors and Clara cell tumors (37). In A/J mice we found that most tumors produced by urethan, when classified by light microscopy, were type II alveolar cell tumors (70 to 80% of all tumors counted) (32). On the other hand, in Swiss Webster mice, BALB/c, or Sencar mice, 70 to 100% of all tumors when identified by light microscopy were Clara cell tumors (Table 1). It will be important in future experiments to confirm these findings by electron microscopy. It also needs to be established whether the spontaneously occurring tumors in different mouse strains follow a similar distribution pattern and whether it may be influenced by various chemical carcinogens.

The commonly seen epithelial lung tumors in mice are therefore derived from type II alveolar epithelial cells or from the Clara cells of

TABLE 1. Classification of lung tumors in different mouse strains[a]

Strain or stock	Type II cell tumors	Clara cell tumors
A/J	118 (72%)	46 (28%)
A/J	22 (61%)	14 (39%)
Ha:1 CR	5 (28%)	13 (72%)
Sencar	0 (0%)	11 (100%)
BALB/c	0 (0%)	16 (100%)
Swiss Webster	22 (27%)	59 (73%)

[a] Tumors induced by urethan and classified under the light microscope 4-12 months later; data from ref. 36 and unpublished observations.

the small airways. Obviously, such tumors may not be directly comparable to the most common forms of human bronchogenic carcinoma. However, they may have a counterpart in a comparatively small group of human lung tumors, the so called bronchiolo-alveolar carcinoma. Ultrastructural data show that such tumors are derived from alveolar type II epithelial cells or from Clara cells (6,11,20-22). Originally, the incidence of these tumors was estimated to be between 4 and 5% in man. It has been remarked that this figure probably underestimates the current incidence, particularly if the incidence of peripheral lung scar adenocarcinomas was included in this group of lung cancers (26). Other authors list a much lower incidence for human bronchiolo-alveolar carcinoma (1 to 2%) (16). The common lung tumors in mice and the rare human bronchiolo-alveolar carcinoma thus seem to have the same cell of origin. For this reason alone we probably should not consider that the biological behavior of mouse lung tumors is irrelevant to man. On the other hand, it must be remembered that tumors in experimental animals are model systems which allow study of mechanisms and principles of tumor generation and tumor biology. To conclude from anatomical location, or from observations made on histogenesis, that some tumors are relevant to man whereas others are not, is probably not warranted.

TWO-STAGE CARCINOGENESIS IN MOUSE LUNG

Two-stage carcinogenesis was first described in experiments on tumor development in mouse skin (4). The terms initiation-promotion were coined early and have by now assumed some very specific meanings. Initiators and promoters were originally defined in operational terms; initiators as agents capable of producing tumors, and promoters as agents capable of furthering tumor development. In order to be considered a promoter, a chemical would have to fulfill several criteria. These can be summarized as follows: promoters are effective, i.e., enhance development of tumors, only if they are administered after a carcinogen. However, the interval between exposure to the initiator and to the first application of the promoter may last from several weeks to several months. If the sequence of exposure is reversed and a promoter is given before a carcinogen, it is without any effect. Promoters are also effective in inducing tumors in tissues which have been exposed to a dose of initiating agent small enough to be without tumorigenic effect if there is no subsequent exposure to a promoting agent. Finally, it is generally assumed that promoters do not have any tumorigenic activity *per se* (23).

The above criteria were developed from observations made in mouse skin tumorigenesis. In recent years it has become obvious that there are several agents which enhance tumor formation in the epithelial tissues of internal organs such as the liver, the gastrointestinal tract, the lung, and the bladder, although none of these agents has been shown to fulfill rigorously all the criteria developed for promoters in mouse skin (24). The most likely reason for this is that not all necessary experiments have been done, or are impossible or impractical to perform. For example, longitudinal studies can be carried out most easily and certainly economically by observing the development of papillomas on mouse skin, where tumor development can be followed and quantitated repeatedly without killing the animals. In the lung and other internal organs data can only be gathered after the animal is sacrificed. This makes longitudinal studies expensive.

One of the most complete data bases on tumor enhancement in an internal organ has been developed by studying the enhancement of lung tumors in mice by BHT (32,36,39). In animals treated with a single dose of a carcinogen such as urethan, diethylnitrosamine, dimethyl-nitrosamine, benzo(a)pyrene, or 3-methylcholanthrene, BHT given after the carcinogen will invariably increase the number of lung tumors which develop over the next 4 to 9 months, regardless of whether BHT is introduced by injection, by gavage, or in the diet. The first dose of BHT can be given as late as 5 months after urethan and it will still enhance lung tumor formation during the next 4 months. However, if BHT is given before a carcinogen, tumor development is not enhanced and may actually be decreased. Given by itself, BHT does not usually increase tumor incidence or tumor multiplicity; in the few experiments where these parameters were increased, the effects were marginal (e.g. see Table 2).

TABLE 2. Effect of BHT on lung tumor development in A/J mice treated with 3-methylcholanthrene (3-MC) or benzo(a)pyrene (BP)

Treatment, dose (mg/kg)[a]	Tumor multiplicity[b]		Tumor incidence[c]	
	BHT	Controls	BHT	Controls
3-MC, 5 (i.p.)	10.2 ± 1.0^{d}	2.8 ± 0.5	24/24	27/29
3-MC, 2.5 (i.p.)	2.3 ± 0.5^{d}	0.6 ± 0.2	$17/20^{d}$	12/28
3-MC, 1.5 (i.p.)	0.8 ± 0.2^{d}	0.3 ± 0.1	$13/24^{d}$	8/29
3-MC, 0.5 (i.p.)	0.5 ± 0.1^{d}	0.2 ± 0.1	$10/26^{d}$	4/30
BP, 150 (p.o.)	30.8 ± 2.4^{d}	4.9 ± 0.6	30/30	29/29
BP, 30 (p.o.)	1.0 ± 0.3	0.6 ± 0.2	15/27	11/30
BP, 15 (p.o.)	0.3 ± 0.1	0.3 ± 0.1	8/28	8/30
Untreated[e]	0.5 ± 0.2	0.2 ± 0.1	$8/19^{d}$	6/35

[a] Male A/J mice treated with 3-MC (i.p.) or BP (p.o.) and then fed 0.5% BHT in diet for 6-8 weeks; all animals were killed 4 months after the carcinogen.
[b] Number of tumors per lung ± standard error.
[c] Number of tumor bearing animals/total number of animals per group.
[d] $p < 0.05$ compared to corresponding controls by t-test (tumor multiplicity) or x^2-test (tumor incidence).
[e] Controls: animals injected with 0.9% NaCl and fed 0.75% BHT for 8 weeks (data from ref. 40). In other studies (e.g., ref. 32, 38, 39) the differences between BHT-treated and control animals was found not to be statistically significant.

It must be noted that at one time it was thought that BHT did not meet all the criteria of a promoting agent because it did not enhance tumor formation in animals treated with subcarcinogenic doses of urethan (34). More recent data obtained by using 3-methylcholanthrene or benzo(a)pyrene as the initiating agents tended to confirm this conclusion (Table 2). Therefore, we must conclude that BHT fails to increase significantly lung tumor incidence or multiplicity in animals treated with a carcinogen dose which by itself yields only a minimal response. It might therefore be appropriate to state that BHT enhances lung tumor formation rather than to insist that it is a promoting agent in mouse lung. This proper use of the terminology restricts the use of the terms promotion and promoter exclusively to compounds which show a certain operational behavior in mouse skin. While this is in the interest of using precise terminology, it tends to diminish the biological significance of the term promotion; terminology derived from and defined by a single system will by necessity be irrelevant to any other system. On the other hand, the term initiation-promotion also has come to denote a broad and important concept in toxicology: adverse interactions between two chemical agents can occur even if exposure to the two agents is separated in time, provided the sequential exposure occurs in a defined manner (33). Therefore, the biological implications derived from the mouse lung tumor model should not be dismissed, although it might be necessary to adopt, for the sake of precision, some different terminology.

THE CONTINUED USE OF BHT AS A FOOD ADDITIVE

BHT is used widely as a direct food additive and as such was considered to be generally recognized as safe (GRAS). However, in 1973 it was removed from the GRAS list and at present is under interim regulation (2). Its effects on lung tumor development in mice have given rise to little, if any, concern. This has mostly been rationalized by the fact that lung tumors occur only in certain mouse strains and that the tumors do not seem to have any, or have only limited counterparts in human pathology. Moreover, it was also thought that BHT cannot be called a promoting agent in the classical sense, since it did not fulfill all criteria applicable to a mouse skin promoter. We have discussed these two problems earlier. To further complicate the picture it must be remembered that in certain experiments BHT did the opposite of enhancing tumor formation: it was found to protect animals against chemical carcinogenesis (2). At one point BHT was even considered to be an effective antipromoting agent (31), although the experimental observations leading to this conclusion were made in an *in vitro* system only.

It must be mentioned at this point that among the agents which in the last decade have acquired some notoriety for being tumor promoters in internal organs (saccharin, fatty acids, bile salts, DDT, phenobarbital), BHT has been shown to have the broadest range of biological activity. BHT enhances tumor development in two different species, the mouse and the rat, and in several organ systems such as the liver (14,17), bladder (10,13), lung (15,39), and possibly the gastro-intestinal tract (30). In two *in vitro* systems BHT has been found to act like 12-O-tetradecanoylphorbol-13-acetate (TPA) (7,29). Several of the findings, such as the enhancement of lung tumors in mice, and enhancement of bladder or liver tumors in rats have been confirmed independently in more than one laboratory.

It also has become obvious by now that the lowest cumulative dose of BHT that has biological activity in the mouse lung tumor system is quite low. We found that a total of 6 intraperitoneal injections of 50 mg/kg BHT (39) or feeding 7,500 ppm of BHT in the diet for two weeks (40) enhanced the development of lung tumors. Recently, we found that in strain A mice treated with a single dose of 3-methyl-cholanthrene and exposed for 2-4 weeks to a concentration of 500 or 1000 ppm BHT in the diet, the number of lung tumors observed 4 months later is increased (Table 3). The total dose of BHT ingested during the shortest (2 week) exposure to 500 ppm was on the average of 470 mg/kg corresponding to a total cumulative intake of 35 mg/kg/day. This is about 70 times higher than the unconditional acceptable daily intake for BHT for man, set presently at 0.5 mg/kg body weight. This daily acceptable intake occurs at an approximate concentration of 30 ppm BHT in the total diet (2). While the concentration of dietary BHT in our experiment (500 ppm) exceeded the BHT concentration in the human diet by a factor of almost 20, and the cumulative daily intake of 35 mg/kg/day was about 75-fold higher than the acceptable daily intake, it must not be overlooked that the enhancing effects on tumor occurrence was obtained by only a 2 week exposure. This corresponds to about 1/75th of the normal life span of a mouse. The minimal exposure conditions found to enhance tumor formation should be compared to the proposed levels of BHT required and claimed to have some protective action against certain chemical carcinogens (5,27). Such a comparison makes it obvious that in animals pre-exposed to a carcinogen, the amounts of BHT required to enhance tumor formation are lower by several orders of magnitude than are the amounts of BHT needed in the food to allow for a marginal beneficial effect.

THE MECHANISM OF ACTION OF BHT

In the early 1970's it had become obvious that most if not all agents capable of promoting skin tumors in mice were agents which produced hyperplasia (4). At about the same time it was discovered that BHT injected i.p. in mice would produce a profuse proliferation of type II alveolar epithelial cells (1). Since type II alveolar cells were thought to be the cells of origin of lung tumors in mice it was logical to see whether repeated BHT injection followed by repeated proliferation of type II alveolar cells would enhance lung tumor formation.

TABLE 3. Lung tumor enchancement by BHT in the diet

BHT in diet (ppm)[a]	Exposure to diet (days)[b]	Number of tumors/lung (mean ± SEM)	Cumulative intake of BHT (g/kg)[c]
0 (no BHT)	14	5.7 ± 0.9	-
	21	9.6 ± 1.2	-
	28	8.7 ± 1.0	-
500	14	10.6 ± 1.2[d]	0.47
	21	17.4 ± 1.5[d]	0.86
	28	20.2 ± 2.2[d]	1.11
1000	14	19.5 ± 1.7[d]	0.99
	21	24.7 ± 2.2[d]	1.65
	28	25.1 ± 1.9[d]	2.22
5000	14	26.7 ± 2.7[d]	2.77
	28	24.7 ± 2.3[d]	9.58

[a] Male A/J mice treated initially with a single dose of 10 mg/kg of 3-methyl-cholanthrene i.p. and killed 4 months later; composition of BHT-containing diet described in ref. 40.

[b] All animals placed on BHT diet immediately after 3-MC and returned to lab chow 2, 3 or 4 weeks later.

[c] Estimated by measuring amount of food consumed.

[d] $p < 0.05$ compared to animals fed a BHT-free control diet for the same length of time.

The first few experiments seemed to bear out this prediction. However, some evidence has become available which suggests that overall and diffuse cell proliferation in lung is not necessarily a prerequisite for enhancement of lung tumor development. Several lines of evidence are available to support such a conclusion. Some time ago we found that lung tumor development could be enhanced by BHT in animals treated with SKF525A prior to each BHT injection to the same extent that it was in animals injected with BHT alone (38). Since SKF525A pretreatment has been found to abolish BHT induced cell proliferation in lung, the observation was interpreted to mean that cell proliferation was not a prerequisite for enhancement of lung tumor development. Additional support for this hypothesis was obtained in an experiment where we injected male A/J mice with urethan and then gave them 4 weekly intraperitoneal injections of BHT. When we measured the cumulative labeling index of alveolar cells we found a significant increase in proliferation of cells in the alveolar zone occurred only after the first 2 injections of BHT. Two injections of BHT only would not be enough to influence tumor development (39). Taken together these observations led us to conclude that enhancement of tumor development can be separated from overall cell hyperplasia in lung. This conclusion was reinforced although indirectly by the observation that methylcyclopentadienyl manganese tricarbonyl or oxygen do not enhance lung tumor formation although they both stimulate cell proliferation in mouse lung (36,38). However, final evidence on whether to accept or to refute our hypothesis is still missing.

We also examined the effects of oxygen on tumor development in mouse lung. Male A/J mice, given a single injection of 1000 mg/kg of urethan, were placed into a plastic chamber ventilated continuously with a mixture of air and oxygen so as to give a chamber concentration of 70% oxygen. Groups of 20 animals were removed from the oxygen after 1, 2, 4, 8 or 16 weeks. All animals were killed 4 months after the urethan injection (Lindenschmidt, R. C., unpublished observations).

The data presented in Fig. 1 show that animals which were kept for 4, 8 or 16 weeks in 70% oxygen had significantly fewer tumors than did the animals exposed for 1 or 2 weeks, or animals kept in room air throughout. At first this finding seemed surprising. Oxygen free radicals seem to enhance development of mouse skin tumors (28). It was thought possible that in a continuous atmosphere of 70% oxygen more oxygen free radicals might be generated than in room air and therefore lung tumor development might be enhanced. However, 70% oxygen also inhibits cell proliferation in the lung, particularly proliferation of alveolar type II epithelial cells (8). This observation may account for the decrease in lung tumors.

BHT is an effective antioxidant and an excellent inducer of microsomal mixed function oxidases. However, it does not seem likely that the antioxidant properties of BHT are instrumental in promoting lung tumors. Several other antioxidants, among them the structurally closely related butylated hydroxyanisole (BHA) do not enhance lung tumor development in mice (35). Induction of mixed function oxidases by BHT could account for several observations showing that prefeeding or pretreatment with BHT may sometimes convey some protection against the carcinogenic effect of agents such as benzo(a)pyrene. It also has been found that rats fed simultaneously BHT and N-2-fluorenylacetamide (FAA) are protected against liver carcinogenesis while urinary bladder carcinogenesis is enhanced (13). Shifting pathways in the metabolism of the carcinogen as a consequence of mixed function oxidase induction could explain this phenomenon.

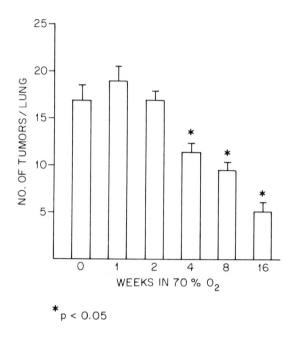

FIG. 1. Influence of 70% oxygen on lung tumor development in A/J mice. Male A/J mice were injected with 1000 mg/kg of urethan and then exposed to 70% oxygen for 1, 2, 4, 8 or 16 weeks. All animals were killed 16 weeks after urethan. *$p < 0.05$ compared to animals kept in room air throughout. (Lindenschmidt, R. C., and Witschi, H. P. unpublished observation.)

SUMMARY AND CONCLUSION

There is now a great deal of data available that show that BHT enhances the development of lung tumors in mice (15,34). In many ways BHT behaves like a promoting agent. Interestingly, it also has tumor enhancing or promoting properties in other organs than mouse lung, such as rat liver (14,17), rat bladder (10, 13), possibly rat GI tract (30), and in *in vitro* systems (7,29). The development of lung tumors by BHT may be influenced by comparatively low exposure regimens; the minimum dose found so far to be effective is 6 intraperitoneal injections of 50 mg/kg of BHT (39) or feeding a diet containing 500 ppm of BHT for 2 weeks (Table 2). While these findings seem to require that the continued use of BHT as a food additive needs to be reevaluated, it should be mentioned that other considerations have led to the conclusion that the use of BHT probably has a large margin of safety (14).

This makes it important to establish the mechanism of action of BHT which at this time remains unknown.

ACKNOWLEDGEMENTS

Research sponsored by the Office of Health and Environmental Research, U.S. Department of Energy under contract DE-AC05-840R21400 with the Martin Marietta Energy Systems, Inc. By acceptance of this article, the publisher or recipient acknowledges the U.S. Government's right to retain a non-exclusive, royalty-free license in and to any copyright covering the article.

REFERENCES

1.   Adamson, I. Y. R., Bowden, D. H., Côté, M. G., and Witschi, H. P. (1974): *Lab. Invest.*, 36:26-32.
2.   Babich, H. (1982): *Environ. Res.*, 29:1-29.
3.   Bloom, J. L., and Falconcer, D. S. (1964): *J. Natl. Cancer Inst.*, 33:607-618.
4.   Boutwell, R. K. (1974): *CRC Crit. Rev. Toxicol.*, 2:419-447.
5.   Cohen, L. A., Polanski, M., Faraya, K., Reddy, M., Beke, H., and Weisburger, J. H. (1984): *J. Natl. Cancer Inst.*, 72:165-174.
6.   Dermer, G. D. (1982): *Cancer*, 49:881-887.
7.   Djurhuus, R., and Lillehaug, J. R. (1982): *Bull. Environ. Contam. Toxicol.*, 29:115-120.
8.   Haschek, W. M., Reiser, K. M., Klein-Szanto, A. J. P., Kehrer, J. P., Smith, L. H., Last, J. A., and Witschi, H. P. (1983): *Am. Rev. Respir. Dis.*, 127:28-34.
9.   Heston, W. E. (1942): *J. Natl. Cancer Inst.*, 3:69-78.
10. Imaida, K., Fukushima, S., Shirai, T., Ohtani, M., Nakanishi, K., and Ito, H. (1983): *Carcinogenesis*, 4:895-899.
11. Jacques, J., and Currie, W. (1977): *Cancer*, 40:2171-2180.
12. Kauffman, S. L., Alexander, L., and Sass, L. (1979): *Lab. Invest.*, 40:708-718.
13. Maeura, Y., Weisburger, J. H., and Williams, G. M. (1984): *Cancer Res.*, 44:1604-1610.
14. Maeura, Y., and Williams, G. M. (1984): *Food Chem. Toxicol.*, 22:191-198.
15. Malkinson, A. M., and Beer, D. S. (1983): *J. Natl. Cancer Inst.*, 70:931-936.
16. Muller, K. M. (1983): In: *Comparative Respiratory Tract Carcinogenesis, Vol. I: Spontaneous Respiratory Tract Carcinogenesis*, edited by H. M. Reznik-Schuller, pp. 55-78. CRC Press, Boca Raton, FL.
17. Peraino, C., Fry, R. J., Staffeldt, E., and Christopher, P. (1977): *Food Cosmet. Toxicol.*, 15:93-96.
18. Sato, K., and Kauffman, S. L. (1982): *Lab. Invest.*, 43:28-36.
19. Shimkin, M. B., and Stoner, G. D. (1975): *Adv. Cancer Res.*, 21:1-58.
20. Sidler, G. S., and Forrester, E. M. (1977): *Cancer*, 40:2209-2215.
21. Singh, G., Katyal, S. L., Ordoney, N. G., Dail, D. H., Negishi, Y., Weeden, V. W, Marcus, P. B., Weldon-Linue, C. M., Axiotis, C. A., Alvarez-Fernandez, E., and Smith, W. I. (1984): *Arch. Pathol. Lab. Med.*, 108:44-48.
22. Singh, G., Katyal, S. L., and Torikata, C. (1982): *Cancer*, 50:946-948.

23.   Slaga, T. J., Fisher, S. M., Weeks, C. E., and Klein-Szanto, A. J. P. (1981): *Rev. Biochem. Toxicol.*, 3:231-282.
24.   Slaga, T. J., Sivak, A., and Boutwell, R. (1978): In: *Carcinogenesis - A Comprehensive Survey, Vol. 2: Mechanisms of Tumor Promotion and Carcinogenesis.* Raven Press, New York.
25.   Smith, L. H., and Witschi, H. P. (1983): Oak Ridge National Laboratory, Technical Report ORNL-5961.
26.   Spencer, W. (1977): *Pathology of the Lung.* Pergamon Press, London.
27.   Tatsuta, M., Mikuni, T., and Taniguchi, H. (1983): *Int. J. Cancer*, 32:253-254.
28.   Troll, W., Witz, G., Goldstein, B., Stone, D., and Sugimura, T. (1982): In: *Carcinogenesis - A Comprehensive Survey, Vol. 7: Cocarcinogenesis and Biological Effects of Tumor Promoters*, edited by E. Hecker, N. E. Fusenig, W. Kunz, F. Marks, and H. W. Thielmann, pp. 583-597. Raven Press, New York.
29.   Trosko, J. E., Yotti, L. P., Warren, P., Tushimoto, G., and Chang, C. C. (1982): In: *Carcinogenesis - A Comprehensive Survey, Vol. 7: Cocarcinogenesis and Biological Effects of Tumor Promoters*, edited by E. Hecker, N. E. Fusenig, W. Kunz, F. Marks, and H. W. Thielmann, pp. 565-585. Raven Press, New York.
30.   Weisburger, E. K., Evarts, R. P., and Wenk, M. L. (1977): *Food Cosmet. Toxicol.*, 15:139-141.
31.   Weiss, J. A., and Archer, D. C. (1982): *Proc. Soc. Exp. Biol. Med.*, 170:427-430.
32.   Witschi, H. P. (1981): *Toxicology*, 21:95-104.
33.   Witschi, H. P. (1982): In: *Assessment of Multichemical Contamination. Proceedings of an International Workshop*, Milan, Italy. April 28-30, 1981, pp. 263-288. National Academy Press, Washington, DC.
34.   Witschi, H. P. (1983): In: *Mechanisms of Tumor Promotion, Vol. I: Tumor Promotion in Internal Organs*, edited by T. J. Slaga, pp. 71-89. CRC Press, Boca Raton, FL.
35.   Witschi, H. P., and Doherty, D. G. (1984): *Toxicologist*, 4:104.
36.   Witschi, H. P., Hakkinen, P. J., and Kehrer, J. P. (1981): *Toxicology*, 21:37-45.
37.   Witschi, H. P., and Haschek, W. M. (1982): *J. Natl. Cancer Inst.*, 70:991-992.
38.   Witschi, H. P., and Kehrer, J. P. (1982): *J. Am. Coll. Toxicol.*, 1:171-184.
39.   Witschi, H. P., and Lock, S. (1979): *Toxicol. Appl. Pharmacol.*, 50:391-400.
40.   Witschi, H. P., and Morse, C. C. (1983): *J. Natl. Cancer Inst.*, 71:859-866.

Carcinogenesis, Vol. 8, edited by M. J. Mass et al.
Raven Press, New York © 1985.

Effects of Tumor Promoters, Aldehydes, Peroxides, and Tobacco Smoke Condensate on Growth and Differentiation of Cultured Normal and Transformed Human Bronchial Cells

Curtis C. Harris, James C. Willey, *Andrew J. Saladino, and
†Roland C. Grafstrom

*Laboratory of Human Carcinogenesis, Division of Cancer Etiology, National Cancer Institute,
Bethesda, Maryland 20205; *Baltimore Veterans Administration Medical Center,
Baltimore, Maryland 21218; †Department of Toxicology, Karolinska Institutet,
S-104 01 Stockholm, Sweden*

Carcinogenesis is clearly a multistage process (Fig. 1) in which the stage of tumor promotion can be an important determinant of tumor incidence and latency period. The central tenet of tumor promotion is selective clonal expansion of initiated (preneoplastic) cells. Therefore, we propose several mechanisms of tumor promotion that can be considered as *selective clonal expansion advantages* of preneoplastic and neoplastic cells (Table 1). This brief report will focus on one of these mechanisms, resistance of preneoplastic and neoplastic cells to inducers of terminal differentiation. The effects of known and putative cocarcinogens and tumor promoters on growth and differentiation of normal and transformed human bronchial cells will be described and used to exemplify data supportive of this hypothetical mechanism.

Because tumor promoters exhibit a relative tissue specificity and their potency varies among animal species (21), we have initiated systematic studies of the pathobiological effects of these agents using cultured normal human bronchial epithelial cells (NHBE). We have selected agents from several different chemical classes (Fig. 2) that have promoting activity in the mouse skin carcinogenesis model. Because epidemiological studies suggest that tobacco smoke has promoting activity in human lung carcinogenesis (2), and cigarette smoke condensate (CSC) contains both tumor initiators and promoters (see Hoffmann et al., this volume), we have also chosen to investigate the effects of CSC and its fractions. The aldehydes formaldehyde, acrolein, and acetaldehyde are found in the gaseous phase of tobacco

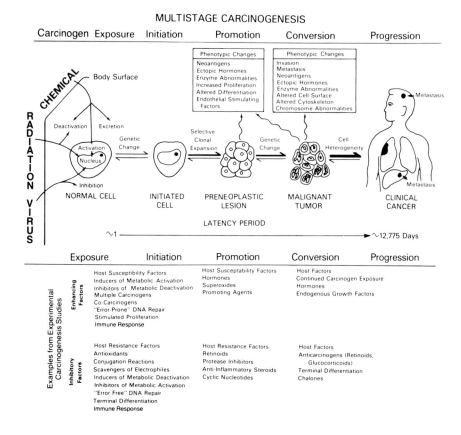

FIG. 1. Multistage process of carcinogenesis.

TABLE 1. Selective clonal expansion advantages[a]

1. Resistance to inducers of terminal differentiation
   a. endogenous agents
   b. exogenous agents
2. Resistance to cytotoxicity of viral gene products
3. Increased sensitivity to growth factors
4. Autocrine production of growth factors
5. Cell surface modifications

[a] Properties of preneoplastic and neoplastic cells that provide them with a survival advantage over normal cells.

smoke. These aldehydes are also of interest because of their potential carcinogenicity in the human respiratory tract and the fact that they are metabolites of xenobiotics such as N-nitrosodimethylamine, cyclophosphamide, and ethanol, and are also formed endogenously as products of normal intermediary metabolism (8,9,19).

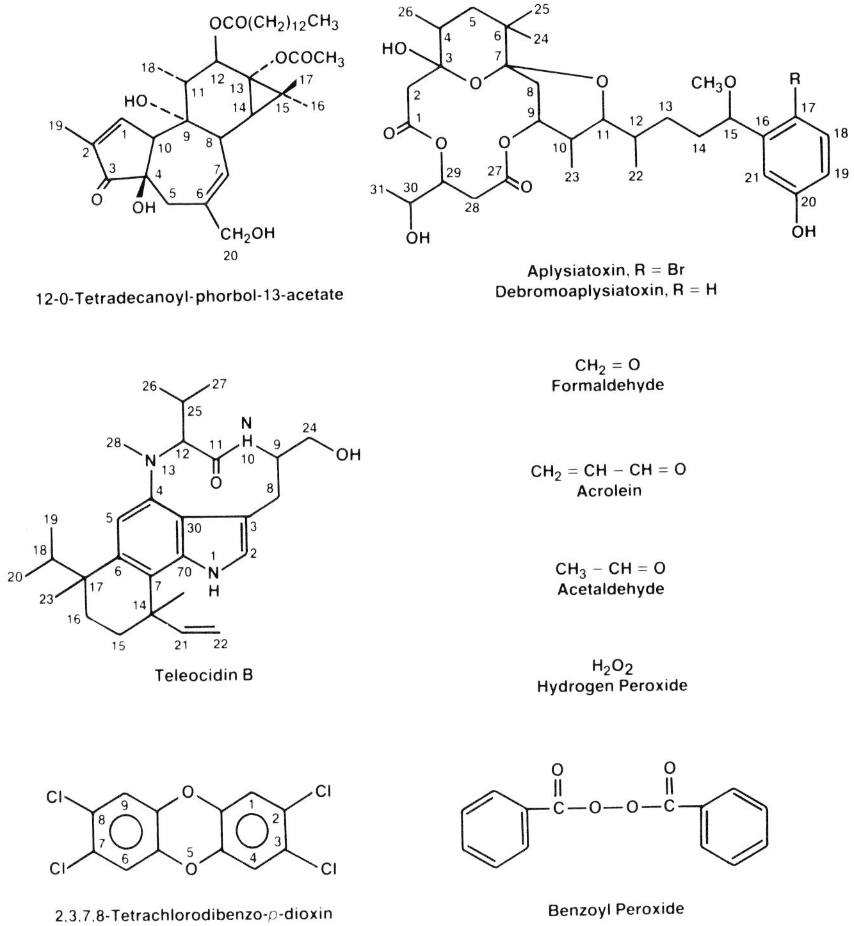

12-0-Tetradecanoyl-phorbol-13-acetate

Aplysiatoxin, R = Br
Debromoaplysiatoxin, R = H

Teleocidin B

$CH_2 = O$
Formaldehyde

$CH_2 = CH - CH = O$
Acrolein

$CH_3 - CH = O$
Acetaldehyde

H_2O_2
Hydrogen Peroxide

2.3.7.8-Tetrachlorodibenzo-*p*-dioxin

Benzoyl Peroxide

FIG. 2. Chemical structures of tumor promoters, aldehydes, peroxides, and dioxins utilized in this study.

MATERIALS AND METHODS

Cells and Media

Normal adult human bronchial tissues were obtained from donors at the time of autopsy. Methods used to establish human bronchial explants and replicative cultures of NHBE have been previously published (12,13). The cells were grown in surface-coated (10 µg/ml fibronectin; 10 µg/ml bovine serum albumin (BSA); 30 µg/ml Vitrogen® collagen) 60 mm plastic culture dishes. LHC-0 was LHC-1 culture medium (13) without epidermal growth factor (EGF).

Clonal Growth Assay

The effects of compounds on cell division were measured using a clonal growth rate assay (13). Five thousand cells were inoculated per 60 mm dish. After 7 to 8 days of incubation in medium containing the test compound or after an initial 6 hr followed by incubation in test compound-free medium for 7 days, the cells were fixed with 10% formalin and stained with 0.25% aqueous crystal violet. The mean number of cells per colony in 18 randomly selected colonies (9 per replicate dish) was determined for each condition tested. To derive the growth rate (population doublings per day), the $\log_2$ of the average number of cells per colony was divided by the number of days of incubation. A computerized image analyzer (Artec 800) was programmed to count the number of cells per colony. Student's t-test was used to evaluate the significance of difference between experimental groups.

Morphological Characteristics

Cell morphology was monitored by phase-contrast microscopy. Twenty thousand cells were seeded per coated 60 mm culture dish. After incubation in LHC-4 medium for 4 days, cells were exposed to the test compound for 6 hr, fixed with 4F/1G (16) for 10 min, and stained with May-Grunwald-Giemsa. The image analyzer was programmed to measure cell area. Two hundred and fifty cells were analyzed for each condition tested.

Cross-Linked Envelope (CLE) Formation

The percentage of cells capable of forming CLE was ascertained by a modification of the method of Sun and Green (22). Cells were inoculated at 50,000 cells/well onto coated 12-well plates (24 mm wells) containing LHC-4. Twenty-four hr later, the number of cells per well was calculated using a grid and the media were replaced with media containing the test compound plus 0.8% agar (LGT agarose, Miles Biochemicals, Elkhorn, IN). After a 6 hr incubation, 2 ml of sodium dodecylsulfate (4%) and dithiothreitol (20 mM) in distilled H_2O was added over the agar. After a further 4 hr incubation at 37°, the number of CLEs per well and percentage of CLE per cell population were then calculated.

Biochemical Assays

DNA and RNA Synthesis

In order to determine the effect of these agents on nucleic acid synthesis, 20,000 cells were inoculated per coated 35 mm culture dish containing serum-free LHC-4 medium supplemented with radioactive deoxythymidine (TdR: 10 nCi [^{14}C]TdR/ml; 52 mCi/mmol) (14). After 2 days of growth, the cultures were rinsed twice with nonradioactive medium, then incubated for 6 hr in isotope-free medium with the agent being tested. For DNA synthesis, the cultures were then incubated for 4 additional hr in medium containing 2 μCi [^{3}H]TdR/ml (75 Ci/mmol), then rinsed twice with phosphate buffered saline (PBS), and finally exposed to 1 ml of 0.2 N NaOH containing 40 μg/ml calf thymus DNA. The cell-NaOH mixture was poured onto a 1 N HCl-soaked glass filter (GF/C; Whatman) that had been rinsed with 100% ethanol, and the radioactivity on the filter was assayed in a scintillation counter. The dpm ratio of ^{3}H/^{14}C was used as a measure of the amount of DNA synthesized, and this value was compared to the ratio obtained for the control cultures. RNA synthesis was measured using the same protocol except [^{3}H]uridine (U) (6 μCi [^{3}H]U/ml, 25.5 Ci/mmol) was substituted for [^{3}H]TdR. [^{3}H]U was added as a 4 hr pulse after incubation of the cells with the agent being tested, and the cells were lysed using a solution of 2% sodium dodecylsulfate, 0.1 mg/ml BSA, and 20 mM HEPES buffered saline, pH 7.6.

For all other biochemical assays, 70-100,000 cells/well were inoculated onto coated 24-well plates (16 mm wells) in 1 ml of LHC-0 or

LHC-4. Twenty-four hr later, media were removed and replaced with 250 µl of fresh media containing the test compounds. ODC, PA, and AHH activities were then assayed as described below.

Ornithine Decarboxylase (ODC) Assay

Media containing test compounds were removed after 6 hr; cells were quickly frozen at –70°. ODC was then quantified by measuring the release of $^{14}CO_2$ from labeled ornithine during a 1 hr incubation (15).

Plasminogen Activator (PA) Assay

PA activity was determined using a modification of a previously described method (11). After 5 hr of incubation with the test compounds, 25 µl of plasminogen (final concentration 0.1 unit/ml) was added and incubation was continued for 1 more hr (a total of 6 hr of incubation with the test compound). Media were removed and centrifuged in an Eppendorf 32000 microfuge for 30 sec to pellet the cells, and 90 µl of medium was incubated with 10 µl of benzyloxy-carbonyl-glycyl-L-prolyl-L-arginyl-[^{14}C]anilide (5 mM, 12.5 mCi/mmol) for 1 hr at 37°. The reaction mixtures were then extracted 3 times each with 2 ml of Econofluor II (New England Nuclear, Boston, MA) and radioactivity assayed. [^{14}C]anilide which has been proteolytically cleaved from the substrate is lipophilic and is extracted into the Econofluor II. The intact substrate is hydrophilic and remains behind when the Econofluor II is removed. A standard curve was made by incubating a range of urokinase concentrations with 0.1 unit/ml plasminogen.

DNA Damage Assays

Cells were exposed to the agents for 1 hr in serum-free medium and subsequently assayed for DNA damage by the alkaline elution technique. Bronchial cells were labeled with [^{14}C]thymidine. L-1210 cells that had received 300 rads were labeled with [^{3}H]thymidine and used as internal standard. The extent of single-strand breaks (SSB) or DPC (DNA:protein crosslinks) per 10^{10} daltons was expressed and calculated as described by Kohn et al. (10).

RESULTS

The agents were initially tested for their mitogenic activity by incubating NHBE cells in culture medium that supports growth at less than an optimal rate (25). Agents were tested over a wide range of concentrations (generally 3-4 log differences). None of the agents were mitogenic.

The IC_{50} was determined by exposing NHBE cells at clonal density, 5000 cells per 60 mm dish, to the agents for either 6 hr followed by incubation in agent-free medium or continuously throughout the 7 day incubation period. In the agents tested in the continuous exposure protocol, aplysiatoxin was the most potent (Table 2). All of these agents (aplysiatoxin, debromoaplysiatoxin, 12-O-tetradecanoyl-phorbol-13-acetate [TPA], and teleocidin B) produced similar morphological changes in the NHBE cells, including increased planar cell surface area, within the first 30 min of exposure to nanomolar concentrations (23,25). PA, CLE, and increased planar area are all useful measures of terminal squamous differentiation. All 3 of the measures were increased following exposure of the NHBE cells to TPA, teleocidin B, and 2,3,7,8-tetrachlorodibenzo-p-dioxin (TCDD) (Tables 3 and 4). In addition, both PA and CLE were increased by aplysiatoxin and debromoaplysiatoxin. The aldehydes and peroxides tested were very potent inducers of CLE formation (Table 4), but only acetaldehyde caused an increase in cell surface area (280%).

To further test the hypothesis that preneoplastic and neoplastic cells are resistant to the induction of terminal squamous differentiation by tumor promoters, we compared the responses of NHBE cells with human lung carcinoma cell lines. As shown in Fig. 3, the carcinomas continue to grow in concentrations of TPA, of up to 100 nM, that inhibit the growth of the NHBE cells by activating their program of terminal differentiation; similar results were obtained with teleocidin B (24). The effects of the aldehydes and peroxides on DNA, i.e., SSB and DPC, are listed in Table 5.

DISCUSSION

Resistance to inducers of terminal differentiation is one of several selective clonal expansion advantages that could lead to selective survival and growth of preneoplastic and neoplastic cells. These inducers of differentiation may be endogenous as well as exogenous compounds. Factors produced by confluent human bronchial epithelial

TABLE 2. Effects of tumor promoters, aldehydes, and cigarette smoke condensate (CSC) on clonal growth rate[a]

Agent	Exposure time	IC_{50}[b]	
Aplysiatoxin	Continuous[c]	30	pM
Debromoaplysiatoxin		100	pM
TPA		300	pM
Teleocidin B		300	pM
TCDD		200	µM
DCDD		250	µM
CSC		10	µg/ml
Benzoyl peroxide	6 hr[d]	56	µM
Formaldehyde		210	µM
Hydrogen peroxide		1.2	mM
Acetaldehyde		10	mM

[a] Population doublings per day (PD/D).
[b] IC_{50}, concentration that causes 50% inhibition of PD/D; concentration for TCDD and DCDD extrapolated from data points from concentrations of 1, 10, and 100 nM (Willey et al., 1984).
[c] Continuous exposure for 7 days to agent.
[d] Six hr exposure to agent followed by 7 days in agent-free media.

cells (14) and factors found in blood-derived serum (14) are examples of endogenous agents that are currently being purified and characterized. NHBE cells are responsive to these inducers as measured by decreased cell growth, increased formation of CLE, and enhanced squamous morphology while carcinoma cell lines continue to grow, in fact, may replicate at a faster rate (14).

Exogenous inducers of terminal differentiation are a diverse group of compounds with varying degrees of selectivity to normal vs. neoplastic cells. Agents with tumor-promoting activity in the mouse skin carcinogenesis model appear to be the most potent inducers of terminal differentiation of NHBE cells currently known. For example, nanomolar quantities of aplysiatoxin, TPA, or teleocidin B are sufficient to rapidly induce plasminogen activator activity and cross-linked envelope formation in the NHBE cells (23,25). Similar observations have been found with cultured human epidermal cells (7,17). However, normal human melanocytes and endometrial stromal cells initiated with carcinogen are stimulated to proliferate by TPA (3,20). Although these 3 tumor promoters all apparently bind to the same membrane receptor, considered to be protein kinase C (see review,

TABLE 3. Effects of tumor promoters on ornithine decarboxylase (ODC) and plasminogen activator (PA) activities in cultured human bronchial epithelial cells

Agent	ODC[a]	PA[a]
Aplysiatoxin (10 nM)	N.D.[c]	310[b]
Debromoaplysiatoxin (10 nM)	N.D.	320[b]
TPA (100 nM)	60[b]	270[b]
Teleocidin B (100 nM)	70[b]	290[b]
Formaldehyde (210 μM)	191[b]	N.D.[c]
Hydrogen peroxide (1.2 mM)	36[b]	N.D.
Benzoyl peroxide (56 μM)	119	N.D.
Formate (30 mM)	22[b]	N.D.
Acetaldehyde (1.2 mM)	61[b]	N.D.
Phorbol (100 nM)	110	130
TCDD (100 nM)	160[b]	150[b]
DCDD (100 nM)	180[b]	180[b]

[a] Percent of control value; typical control ODC value was 1.2 ± 0.5 nmole ^{14}C-ornithine released/hr/mg protein. Control PA value for TPA, teleocidin B, phorbol, DCDD, TCDD, formaldehyde, hydrogen peroxide, formate, benzoyl peroxide, and acetaldehyde was 2.6 ± 1.1 nmol ^{14}C-anilide released/hr/mg protein; control value for aplysiatoxin and debromoaplysiatoxin was 2.3 ± 0.5 nmole ^{14}C-anilide released/hr/mg protein. Six hr exposure to agent.
[b] Significantly different from control value, $p < 0.05$.
[c] Not done.

1), it is important to note that these promoters have strikingly different chemical structures (Fig. 2).

Unlike the results with BDS, enhanced clonal growth rate was not observed in the carcinoma cells exposed to TPA (24). Results consistent with the above hypothesis have been reported by Parkinson and Emmerson (18). They have found that nonpromoting, hyperplastic agents on mouse skin (ethylphenylpropriolate and calcium ionophore A23187), do not have a differential effect on the induction of differentiation in cultured human epidermal cells when compared to squamous cell carcinomas, indicating that these agents enhance differentiation in both normal and neoplastic cells.

Selective clonal expansion advantages may be employed in *in vitro* carcinogenesis studies. Yuspa and coworkers (27) have successfully used relatively high concentrations of calcium ion in serum-containing medium to select resistant mouse epidermal cells. Exposure of mouse epidermal cells to chemical carcinogens increases the number of cells that are resistant to induction of terminal differentiation by culture medium containing a high concentration of calcium ion. These

TABLE 4. Effects of tumor promoters on cell size and formation of cross-linked envelopes (CLE) in cultured human bronchial epithelial cells

Agent	Median cell size[a]	CLE (%)
Solvent control	100	<2[b]
Phorbol (100 mM)	104	0.4 ± 0.3
Formate (30 mM)	80	3 ± 1
Aplysiatoxin (10 nM)	N.D.[b]	17 ± 1[d]
Debromoaplysiatoxin (10 nM)	N.D.	18 ± 3[d]
TPA (100 nM)	150[d]	12 ± 2[d]
Teleocidin B (100 nM)	135[d]	13 ± 1[d]
Formaldehyde (210 µM)	80	12 ± 2[d]
Hydrogen peroxide (1.2 mM)	90	18 ± 4[d]
Benzoyl peroxide (56 µM)	54[d]	15 ± 3[d]
Acetaldehyde (30 mM)	280[d]	7 ± 2[d]
TCDD (100 mM)	121[d]	5 ± 1[d]
DCDD (100 nM)	113[d]	4 ± 1[d]

[a] Percent of control value; control value was $1150 \pm 400 \ \mu^2$ planar surface area. Six hr exposure to test agent.
[b] Control values for different cases range from 0.3 to 2.0%.
[c] N.D., not done.
[d] Significantly different from control, Student's t-test, $p < 0.05$.

resistant cells continue to grow and are operationally considered to be preneoplastic cells. We are also using the concept of selective clonal expansion advantages in carcinogenesis studies of human cells. For example, three selective expansion pressures, i.e., culturing the cells in medium containing BDS, maintaining the cells at high density, i.e., confluence, and suspension of the cells in semisolid media, have allowed the isolation of tumorigenic human bronchial cells following transfection with the H-*ras* oncogene (26). It is of interest that these transformed cells are also resistant to induction of terminal squamous differentiation by TPA.

Because epidemiological and laboratory studies suggest that tobacco smoke has tumor promoting activity, we have initiated studies to identify specific agents in tobacco smoke that induce differentiation in NHBE cells. In the gaseous phase of tobacco smoke, three aldehydes are being investigated (Fig. 2). Acrolein and formaldehyde are each more active than acetaldehyde in causing increases in and formation of CLE in NHBE cells. In the particulate phase of tobacco smoke, the neutral methanol fraction has the most activity in regard to induction

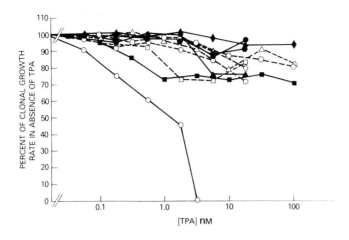

FIG. 3. The effects of TPA on clonal growth rate of normal and neoplastic human lung epithelial cells. For each cell line, cells were inoculated at clonal density in LHC-8 with 1% serum. After 24 hr, the cells were exposed to varying concentrations of TPA in 0.1% DMSO. The medium was changed after 4 days of incubation, and after 7 days, cells were fixed with 10% formalin and stained with 1% crystal violet. Number of cells per colony were counted using an Artec 800 computerized image analyzer. Clonal growth rates were determined as described in the Materials and Methods section. Control clonal growth rates of NHBE cells and each of the cancer cell lines are in parentheses. A-1188 (0.88)●, A-549 (1.05)◆, A-427 (0.35)●, SK Lu-1 (0.41)▲, Calu-1 (0.69)■, NCI H292 (0.70)○, A-1146 (0.45)◊, A-2182 (0.91)○, SW 900 (0.76)△, Calu-6 (0.71)□, NHBE cells (0.95 0, solid line).

TABLE 5. Effects of aldehydes and peroxides on DNA

Agent (mM)	Single Strand Breaks[a]	DNA-Protein Crosslinks[a]
Formaldehyde	1.4	10.8
Formate	< 1.0	< 2.0
Acetaldehyde	< 1.0	< 2.0
Hydrogen peroxide	27.8	< 2.0
Benzoyl peroxide	4.9	5.3

[a] SSB and DPC per 10^{10} daltons; 6 hr exposure to agent.

of differentiation (Willey et al., unpublished results). Results from studies to determine if there is a differential responsiveness between NHBE cells and carinoma cells will be of interest.

In addition to being directly found in tobacco smoke, formaldehyde, acrolein and acetaldehyde are formed by metabolism of both endogenous and exogenous compounds. For example, several carcinogenic N-nitrosamines, including one found in tobacco smoke, N-nitrosodimethylamine, lead to one-to-one stoichiometric generation of alkylcarbonium ion and formaldehyde. Whereas the methylcarbonium ion formed in this reaction is thought to be responsible for the carcinogenicity of N-nitrosamines, a possible contribution of formaldehyde has been largely neglected. In addition to its effects on growth and differentiation, formaldehyde directly damages DNA by causing the formation of DNA-protein cross-links and DNA SSB in human bronchial cells (5). Furthermore, formaldehyde (Table 5) inhibits repair of DNA damage caused by different chemical and physical carcinogens, including ionizing radiation, UV-radiation, BPDE, or N-methyl-N-nitrosourea (5). The removal of O^6-methylguanine and the ligation of γ-ray-induced SSB seem to be preferentially sensitive. A number of mechanisms may be involved in the inhibition of DNA repair by formaldehyde. The high reactivity of the chemical probably causes methylation of chromatin or other proteins including enzymes critical to DNA repair processes. Thus, the potentiating effect of formaldehyde on the cytotoxicity of γ-rays or N-methyl-N-nitrosourea may depend on interaction with enzymes critical for the repair of the respective DNA lesions as demonstrated by the fact that O^6-methylguanine was removed at significantly slower rates in formaldehyde-exposed bronchial fibroblasts and that formaldehyde potentiates the mutagenicity of N-methyl-N-nitrosourea in these normal human cells (5). These and other findings support the hypothesis that aldehydes formed by metabolic pathways of xenobiotic compounds or found in the atmosphere, such as tobacco smoke, may act in concert with other DNA-damaging agents in causing mutations and cancers.

In conclusion, tumor promoters (TPA, teleocidin B, and aplysiatoxin) are potent inducers of terminal squamous differentiation of normal human bronchial epithelial cells *in vitro*. Components of tobacco smoke, including the particulate fraction and aldehydes in the gaseous phase, have some effects similar to the tumor promoters. The specific chemicals in the particulate fraction of tobacco smoke are as yet unknown. Finally, studies are needed to determine the promoting activity of the agents discussed here in human respiratory carcinogenesis.

REFERENCES

1. Blumberg, P. M., Jaken, S., Konig, B., Sharkey, N. A., Leach, K. L., Jeng, A. Y., and Yeh, E. (1984): *Biochem. Pharmacol.*, in press.
2. Doll, R., and Peto, R. (1981): *The Causes of Cancer.* Oxford Press, Oxford.
3. Eisinger, M., and Marko, O. (1982): *Proc. Natl. Acad. Sci. USA*, 79:2018-2022.
4. Grafstrom, R. C., Curren, R., Yang, L., and Harris, C. C. (1984): submitted.
5. Grafstrom, R. C., Fornace, A. J., Jr., Autrup, H., Lechner, J. F., and Harris, C. C. (1983): *Science*, 220:216-218.
6. Grafstrom, R. C., Fornace, A. J., Jr., and Harris, C. C. (1984): *Cancer Res.*, 44:4323-4327.
7. Hawley-Nelson, P., Stanley, J. R., Schmidt, J., Gullino, M., and Yuspa, S. H. (1982): *Expl. Cell Res.*, 137:155-167.
8. International Agency for Research on Cancer (1982): *IARC Monographs on the Evaluation of Carcinogenic Risk of Chemicals to Humans. Some Industrial Dye Stuffs*, Vol 29. IARC, Lyon.
9. International Agency for Research on Cancer (1979): *IARC Monographs on the Evaluation of Carcinogenic Risk of Chemicals to Humans. Some Monomers, Plastics and Synthetic Elastomers and Acrolein*, Vol. 19. IARC, Lyon.
10. Kohn, K. W., Ewig, L. C., Ericson, L. C., and Zwelling, L. A. (19): In: *DNA Repair, A Laboratory Manual of Research Procedures*, edited by E. C. Friedberg, and P. C. Hanawalt, pp. 379-401. Marcel Dekker, New York.
11. Kohn, D. B., Weber, M. J., Carl, P. L., Katzennellenbogen, J. A., and Chakravarty, P. K. (1979): *Anal. Biochem.*, 97:269-276.
12. Lechner, J. F., Haugen, A., Autrup, H., McClendon, I. A., Trump, B. F., and Harris, C. C. (1981): *Cancer Res.*, 41:2294-2304.
13. Lechner, J. F., Haugen, A., McClendon, I. A., and Pettis, E. W. (1982): *In Vitro*, 18:663-642.
14. Lechner, J. F., McClendon, I. A., LaVeck, M. A., Shamsuddin, A. K. M., and Harris, C. C. (1983): *Cancer Res.*, 43:5915-5921.
15. Lichti, W., and Gottesman, M. (1983): *J. Cell Physiol.*, 113:433-439.
16. McDowell, E. M., and Trump, B. F. (1976): *Arch. Pathol. Lab. Med.*, 100:405-414.
17. Parkinson, E. K., and Emmerson, A. (1982): *Carcinogenesis*, 3:525-531.
18. Parkinson, E. K., and Emmerson, A. (1984): *Carcinogenesis*, 5:687-690.
19. Schmid, B. P., Goulding, E., Kitchin, K., and Sanyal, M. K. (1981): *Toxicology*, 22:235-243.
20. Siegfried, J. M., and Kaufman, D. G. (1983): *Int. J. Cancer*, 32:423-429.
21. Slaga, T. J., Fisher, S. M., Weeks, C. E., Klein-Szanto, A. J. P., and Reiners, J. (1981): In: *Mechanisms of Chemical Caricnogenesis*, edited by C. C. Harris, and P. A. Cerutti, pp. 207-227. A. R. Liss, New York.
22. Sun, T.-T., and Green, H. (1976): *Cell*, 9:511-521.
23. Willey, J. C., Moser, C. E., and Harris, C. C. (1984): *Cell Biol. Toxicol.*, in press.
24. Willey, J. C., Moser, C. E., Lechner, J. F., and Harris, C. C. (1984): *Cancer Res.*, in press.
25. Willey, J. C., Saladino, A. J., Ozanne, C., Lechner, J. F., and Harris, C. C. (1984): *Carcinogenesis*, 5:209-215.
26. Yoakum, G. H., Lechner, J. F., Gabrielson, E., Korba, B. E., Malan-Shibley, L., Willey, J. C., Valerio, M., Shamsuddin, A. K. M., Trump, B., and Harris, C. C. (1984): submitted.
27. Yuspa, S. H., Ben, T., Hennings, H., and Lichti, U. (1982): *Cancer Res.*, 42:2344-2349.

Carcinogenesis, Vol. 8, edited by M. J. Mass et al.
Raven Press, New York © 1985.

Heterogeneity in Responses of Human and Rodent Respiratory Epithelial Cells to Tumor Promoters in Culture

Marc J. Mass, *Jill M. Siegfried, *Diane K. Beeman,
and Sharon A. Leavitt

*Carcinogenesis and Metabolism Branch, U.S. Environmental Protection Agency, Research Triangle Park, North Carolina 27711; *Environmental Health Research and Testing, Inc., Research Triangle Park, North Carolina 27709*

The concept that promotion may be an important factor in the etiology of lung cancer with respect to smoking arose when it was suggested that the discontinuance of smoking was associated with a decrease in lung cancer incidence (2). To this phenomenon was drawn the parallel that cessation of application of tumor promoters to carcinogen-initiated mouse skin led to a lower incidence of tumors than did continuous, repeated application of a promoter following carcinogen application (16). This phenomenon has been termed the "reversibility" of tumor promotion. Whether this effect makes a significant contribution to human lung cancer is still not decided, but it is well known that promoters and cocarcinogens are present in cigarette smoke (17,24,28).

A paucity of knowledge exists with regard to the effects of promoters on cells of the pulmonary airways. Because it was previously difficult to deliver substances to respiratory epithelium in an accurate and reproducible manner in experimental systems, studies of promotion in the respiratory tract have lagged far behind those in the skin. Within the past 10 years, difficulties of controlled delivery of precise doses of test agents to respiratory tract epithelium were solved by incorporating agents to be tested into matrices which have defined and measurable characteristics of release of the agent (14). Matrices containing a promoter were fashioned into pellets and inserted into lumens of heterotopic rat tracheal grafts. To date only 12-O-tetradecanoylphorbol-13-acetate (TPA) (22) and asbestos (23) have been tested as promoters in the heterotopic tracheal graft carcinogenesis system; TPA and asbestos exhibit responses concordant with promotion. TPA enhanced tumor yield by greater than 3-fold, and reduced tumor latency under conditions where the initiator, 7,12-dimethyl-benz(a)anthracene, only elicited a 20% incidence of carcinomas. Asbestos also facilitated the appearance of tumors using a dose of initiator that was not inherently carcinogenic.

It has long been recognized that one mechanism of action for tumor promoters might be that they amplify carcinogen-affected populations by the induction of hyperplasia. The presence of a greater number of initiated cells could make more likely the occurrence and observation of a second event which completes the neoplastic phenotype. Another postulated mechanism has its origins in the resistant cell hypothesis of Solt and Farber (3,18). Their method for the induction of hepatocellular carcinomas involves a tumor-initiating exposure to a carcinogen followed by exposures to an agent which is toxic to normal cells. The carcinogen-altered cells proliferate and their numbers are free to expand devoid of competition from normal cells, leading to tumor formation. Yuspa and colleagues (29) have proposed that phorbol esters act as promoters in skin by selectively inducing terminal differentiation in normal cells, thereby killing them. This may lead to relative and eventual absolute enrichment of carcinogen-altered cells that are resistant to the induction of terminal differentiation by a promoter, and consequently, a tumor arises. Thus, two hypotheses have been proposed which may explain the mechanism of action of tumor promoters: 1) non-selective enhancement of cell proliferation in normal and carcinogen-altered cells, and 2) selective inhibiton of proliferation of normal cells allowing unhindered expansion of carcinogen-altered cells.

Clonal assays for the *in vitro* growth of rat tracheal, hamster tracheal, and human bronchial cells are now available which permit assessment of carcinogen-induced cytotoxicity and effects of tumor promoters (6,10,18). In addition, the transformation of rat tracheal epithelial cells in culture is now routinely achieved (13,19,21). We have used these assays for clonal growth to compare the effects of promoters on the commitment to cell proliferation in three species of respiratory epithelium in culture. We have also investigated variation in responses of human bronchial epithelium to phorbol ester tumor promoters and find that responses to 12-O-tetradecanoylphorbol-13-acetate (TPA) are not uniform among individuals.

EFFECT OF TUMOR PROMOTERS ON RAT
TRACHEAL EPITHELIAL CELLS

Normal rat tracheal epithelial (RTE) cells can be grown at low density on a monolayer of Swiss 3T3 cells in Ham's F-12 medium with insulin and hydrocortisone (6), with a colony-forming efficiency (CFE) of about 2-5%. When seeded into culture in the presence of TPA, RTE cells will form colonies at much higher efficiencies; occasionally a maximum of 40% of the RTE cells seeded into culture have been observed to form colonies (11). The average CFE in the presence of TPA is 30%. The concentration response for this effect begins at approximately 1 nM TPA and it saturates at approximately 10 nM TPA (Fig. 1). It appears as if TPA stimulates a specific, limited portion of the epithelial cells isolated. The basal cell population of intact rat tracheal epithelim is approximately 30% of the epithelial cell population (27), and it seems likely that TPA is preferentially stimulating these basal cells to form colonies.

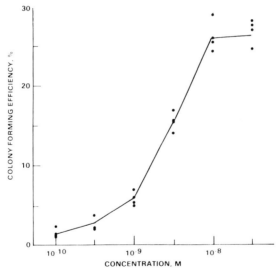

FIG. 1. Relationship between concentration and colony formation of RTE cells seeded in the presence of TPA. Freshly isolated RTE cells (2000/dish) were seeded onto 3T3 cell monolayers in medium containing various TPA concentrations. Modified from ref. 11.

The enhancement of colony formation elicited by TPA is actually inversely related to the ability of untreated control tracheal cells of the same preparation to form colonies of tracheal cells (Fig. 2). In preparations of tracheal cells where the colony forming efficiency is relatively high, treatment with TPA yields an increase in colony formation but the extent of enhancement compared to the initial colony forming efficiency in controls is small In preparations where untreated cells have a low colony forming efficiency, TPA elicits a large apparent increase in the number of colonies. Variations in colony-forming efficiency in untreated cells can result from mechanical trauma during tracheal cell isolation as it is known that physical injury of the epithelium can effectively increase the number of dividing cells (5,9).

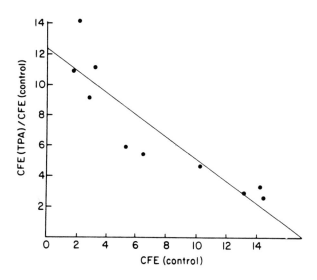

FIG. 2. Colony formation enhancement ratios for TPA-treated versus control RTE cell culture. The extent of enhancement of CFE is the ratio between CFE in TPA-treated and control cultures. Modified from ref. 11.

The marked enhancement of colony formation elicited by TPA was found to be time dependent. Tracheal cells lose their ability to respond to TPA with time in culture. The greatest enhancement of colony formation occurs when TPA is added simultaneously with the seeding of cells into culture. In Fig. 3, TPA was added to a different set of culture dishes every 3 to 4 hr through 48 hr after the initial seeding of cells. After 34 hr in culture TPA has no effect. We have postulated that this initial period of sensitivity to TPA represents a differentiative commitment point during which time the commitment to enter a proliferative mode can be affected by TPA.

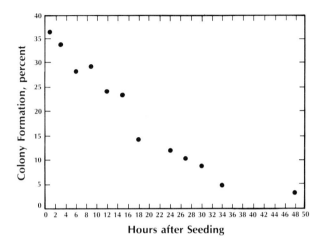

FIG. 3. Effect of delayed TPA addition on colony formation by RTE cells. Cells were seeded onto 3T3 cell monolayers and TPA was added to the culture medium at selected time intervals. Final TPA concentration was 16 nM.

Most cells in the intact tracheal epithelium are thought to be in a non-replicative mode and are thought to be non-participants in the cell cycle, in a G_0 state. TPA appears to be able to cause these normally quiescent cells to enter the cell cycle. During the first 24 hr of culture in the absence of TPA, most cells have not commenced DNA synthesis as evidenced by thymidine labeling (Fig. 4). Refractoriness to TPA is complete at 48 hr when most cells have begun synthesizing DNA. We hypothesized that the commitment event in sensitivity to TPA was related to the onset of DNA synthesis, and that cells that had gone through DNA synthesis in the absence of TPA were refractory to its effect. In order to test this hypothesis, we wanted to determine if it was possible to maintain responsiveness to TPA for greater than 24 to 48 hr by preventing rat tracheal cells from going into DNA synthesis during this time period. Tracheal cells were plated in the presence of the powerful but reversible DNA synthesis inhibitor aphidicolin (1 μg/ml) (26). At the end of 24 or 48 hr the aphidicolin was washed out of the tracheal cell cultures, TPA was added, and the cells were allowed to grow into colonies for 7 days. Inhibition of DNA synthesis by aphidicolin treatment did not preserve responsiveness to TPA (Fig. 5). Thus, it was concluded that traversal of S phase was unrelated to the establishment of refractoriness to TPA. The hypothesis that the TPA responsiveness commitment point lay between the G_1-S border instead of at some point during S phase was also tested. Cells were prevented from entering G_1 from the G_0 state by seeding into culture medium lacking serum for 24 hr. After this time, serum was added to the medium along with TPA. Serum deprivation for 24 hr also did not preserve responsiveness to TPA in these cells (data not shown). We concluded from these experiments that commitment to responsiveness to TPA was probably not cell cycle mediated, and at this time we cannot suggest a mechanism for the time dependence.

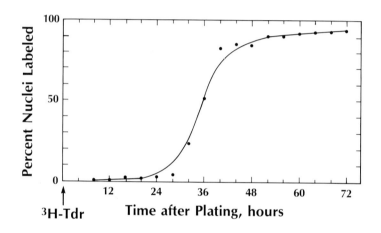

FIG. 4. Continuous [^{3}H]thymidine labeling of RTE cells in culture during the first 72 hr of incubation. Modified from ref. 27.

To determine if responsiveness to TPA, as evidenced by colony formation, was limited to TPA, or if it extended to other phorbol esters, RTE cells were exposed to a series of phorbol esters with various promoting activities in mouse skin (Fig. 6). RTE cells apparently can serve as rather sensitive indicators of the presence of most phorbol ester derivatives. The most potent derivatives are mezerein, TPA, and phorbol didecanoate; the least potent are phorbol diacetate, 4-O-methyl TPA and the parent alcohol phorbol; phorbol dibutyrate and dibenzoate are intermediary in activity. The extent of enhancement of colony formation elicited by each phorbol derivative bears some relationship to

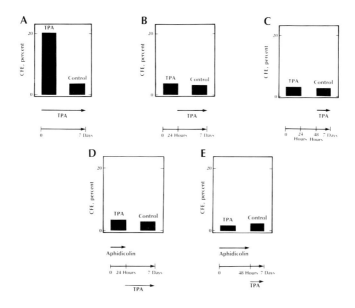

FIG. 5. Effect of aphidicolin on TPA responsiveness in RTE cell cultures. A. TPA (16 nM) was added to RTE cell cultures at the time RTE cells were seeded; B. TPA added 24 hr after RTE cells were seeded; C. TPA added 48 hr after seeding of RTE cells; D. RTE cells seeded into 1 µg/ml aphidicolin. After 24 hr aphidicolin was washed out of cultures and TPA (16 nM) was added; E. Aphidicolin treatment for the first 48 hr of culture, after which it was washed out and TPA (16 nM) was added.

structure-activity relationships for phorbol esters in other systems (1,8). The concentration of phorbol derivative giving half-maximal enhancement of colony formation was calculated (EC_{50}). If it is compared to values derived for phorbol esters in other systems (Table 1) a good correlation is found for some of them including the ability to induce inflammation on the ears of mice, and the inhibition of phorbol dibutyrate binding in membrane fractions of mouse skin. Some correlation is also seen with the EC_{50} in tracheal cells and the ability to act as a promoter in mouse skin but there are some exceptions, notably mezerein.

We have evaluated other non-phorbol esters and inducers of hyperplasia for their ability to elicit increased colony formation in rat tracheal cells. In Table 2 the highest concentration of agent which did not cause cytotoxicity in cultures and the colony forming efficiency in treated and control dishes is shown. Of agents tested, 13 did not

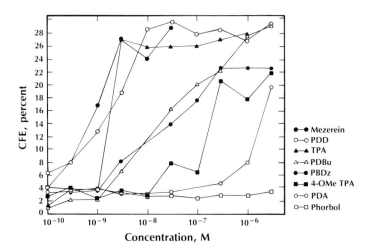

FIG. 6. Structure-activity relationships among phorbol derivatives assessed in RTE cells. Eight phorbol compounds were assayed for their effect on CFE of RTE cells in culture. The phorbol derivatives were included in the culture medium at the time RTE cells were initiated into culture.

TABLE 1. Comparison of potencies of phorbol derivatives

Derivative	EC$_{50}$[a]	ED$_{50}$[b]	Ki[c]	In vivo promoting activity[d]
Mezerein	0.8	30	98	+ +
TPA	2	16	0.74	+ + + +
PDD[e]	3	10	16	+ + +
PDBu	20	67	24	+
PDBz	40	240	82	+
4-O-MeTPA	100	144	–	+ +
PDA	2,000	1,500	3,000	+
Phorbol	> >3,000	>100,000	>8.8 × 10^5	–

[a] Expressed as the concentration in nM needed to induce half maximal enhancement of colony formation of RTE cells; modified from ref. 11.
[b] Dose in pmol that is needed to induce half maximal inflammatory response in mouse ears (8).
[c] Concentration in nM that inhibits specific binding of PDBu in receptor assays using mouse skin homogenates (11).
[d] Relative tumor promoting activity in mouse skin (8).
[e] Abbreviations used: PDD, phorbol didecanoate; PDBu, phorbol dibutyrate; PDBz, phorbol dibenzoate; 4-O-MeTPA, 4-O-methyl TPA; PDA, phorbol diacetate.

enhance colony formation in RTE cells. It is noteworthy that none of these agents are known to compete for binding to the putative TPA receptor. As of yet we have found only one non-phorbol ester tumor promoter that elicits a positive response in the rat tracheal epithelial cell assay for tumor promoters: teleocidin. It appears to be more effective at enhancing colony formation in RTE cells than any of the phorbol derivatives, and it acts at concentrations 10 to 100 fold lower than does TPA (Fig. 7). Teleocidin has been reported to compete as effectively as TPA for phorbol receptors (4,20).

TABLE 2. Non-phorbol ester derivatives inactive when tested for enhancement of colony formation in RTE cells

Compound	Highest concentration (µg/ml)	CFE[a]	Control CFE[a]
Anthralin	0.001	2.2	2.8
Benzoyl peroxide	0.3	3.3	3.3
Butylated hydroxytoluene	10	1.3	0.9
Chloroquinone	3	4.7	4.6
Chrysarobin	1	3.1	2.3
Ethylphenyl propiolate	1	2.5	2.8
Hydroquinone	3	4.4	3.9
Indomethacin	3	3.6	3.1
Ionophore A23187	0.01	6.8	6.9
Limonene	10	2.2	2.3
Mellitin	1	2.7	2.4
Phenobarbital	10	7.1	6.9
Saccharin	10	2.3	2.3

[a] Colony forming efficiency in percent of cells initially seeded.

EFFECT OF TPA ON HAMSTER TRACHEAL EPITHELIAL CELLS IN CULTURE

We have performed limited experiments with tracheal epithelial cells isolated from hamster trachea and inoculated into culture in the presence of TPA. The culture medium used was Ham's F-12 with insulin, hydrocortisone, transferrin, epidermal growth factor, cholera toxin, bovine hypothalamus extract, and culture medium conditioned by 3T3 cells. The serum concentration used was 5%. Hamster tracheal cells differ from rat tracheal cells in that they appear to require a richer culture medium. They also require a thick collagen gel as their substrate. Normal colony forming efficiency was about 2%. The

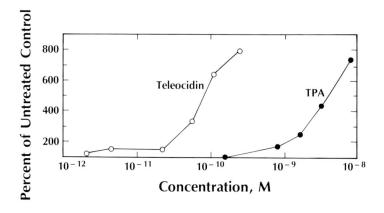

FIG. 7. Comparison of the potencies of teleocidin and TPA on colony formation of RTE cells in primary culture.

addition of TPA to the culture medium at the time of seeding hamster tracheal cells into culture, in contrast to rat tracheal cells, resulted in inhibition of colony formation (Fig. 8).

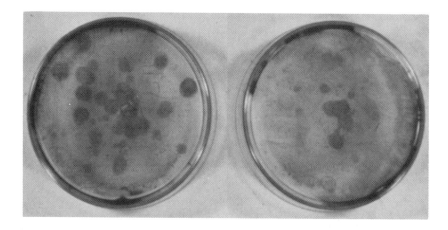

FIG. 8. Effect of 16 nM TPA on the efficiency of colony formation of hamster tracheal epithelial cells. Cells were seeded into dishes in the presence of TPA and grown for 7 days. Left dish is control, right dish treated with TPA.

EFFECT OF PHORBOL ESTERS ON CULTURED
HUMAN BRONCHIAL EPITHELIAL CELLS

Specimens of human bronchial epithelium were derived from either autopsies or from surgical resections of the lung. Pieces of bronchus obtained from tumor patients for studies in explant culture were grossly normal and they did not contain visible tumor growths. The normalcy of the bronchial epithelium was further confirmed by histopathologic examination of paraffin sections of selected portions of the human bronchial specimens. Specimens were transported to our laboratory in chilled Liebovitz L-15 medium. Upon arrival the specimens were cut into 0.25 cm^3 pieces and placed mucosal side down on culture dishes coated with fibronectin and collagen. We initially tried to use epithelial cells dissociated directly from the bronchial fragments but since the specimens were of variable size, depending on the discretion of the surgeon or the pathologist, we could not always isolate enough cells for assays for TPA sensitivity. We consequently enlarged the number of bronchial cells by explant culture of the bronchial fragments. Previous observations in our laboratory with rat tracheal cells and human bronchial cells confirmed that responses to TPA in cells from primary isolations were identical to those in cells from explants. Bronchial cells were allowed to explant for 10-20 days in a serum-free Medium 199 containing 0.66 mM Ca^{++}, epidermal growth factor, hydrocortisone, selenium, insulin, and bovine hypothalamus extract. After this time the tissue fragments were removed from the cultures and the monolayer was allowed to enlarge in a serum-free medium consisting of Ham's F12 with the same constituents as above but also containing cholera toxin. After 3 to 5 days the monolayer was dissociated with trypsin and cells seeded into mitomycin C inactivated 3T3 cells in the same culture medium as above.

Opposite to rat tracheal cells and similar to hamster tracheal cells, we found that TPA was generally inhibitory to colony formation in a concentration-dependent fashion in human bronchial cells plated in the presence of 0.16, 1.6 and 16 nM TPA. Shown in Fig. 9 are responses to TPA in 3 random specimens; the responses to TPA are not uniform.

In order to respresent the variability in inhibitory responses in 19 unique specimens of human bronchus tested, the percent inhibition seen at a TPA concentration of 1.6 nM TPA was plotted as a set of histograms with respect to each respective untreated controls (Fig. 10). The range of variability in inhibitory response spans over a 120-fold range, with no particular clustering patterns. At this time no

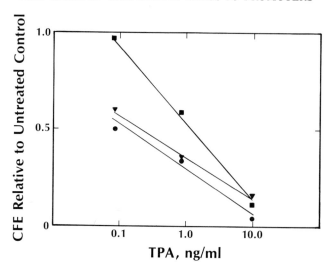

FIG. 9. Responses to TPA in 3 unique specimens of human bronchial cells. Bronchial cells from explants were seeded into culture dishes in the presence of 0.1, 1.0, and 10 ng/ml TPA (0.16 nM, 1.6 nM, 16 nM TPA).

relationship has been observed between inhibition by TPA and whether the specimen was derived from a nontumor or tumor patient, male or female, smoker or non-smoker, and there was no effect of age. However, the pool of specimens is far too small at this time to allow any valid statistical comparisons.

One contribution to the variability in inhibitory response was postulated to be that specimens that did not adapt to culture adequately would be very sensitive to inhibition by TPA, especially if the inhibitory response was a toxic response. However, when the colony-forming efficiency in untreated control cultures was plotted against the extent of inhibition elicited by TPA, no linear relationship was evident (Fig. 11). A linear regression analysis yielded a line with a slope of 0 and a correlation coefficient of 0 indicating that the extent of inhibition by TPA could not be predicted by colony forming efficiency in controls. In the case of RTE cells presented earlier, colony formation in untreated controls very accurately predicted the responses to TPA. We also tested whether the inhibition of colony formation by TPA simply resulted from inhibition of cell attachment, with the result that human bronchial cells attached to their substrate equally well regardless of the presence of TPA in the culture medium (data not shown).

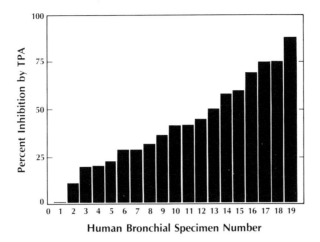

FIG. 10. Response of explanted cells from unique specimens of human bronchus to TPA at 1.6 nM. Specimens were arranged in ascending order of inhibitory response toward TPA; histogram values plotted are the percent inhibition of CFE with respect to the untreated control specimen.

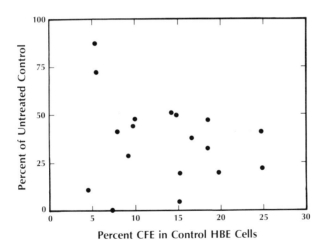

FIG. 11. Cumulative plot of CFE in untreated human bronchial cells versus CFE in human bronchial cells treated with 1.6 nM TPA.

To determine if there were similarities in the manner in which human cells and RTE cells responded to TPA, one specimen was exposed in clonal assays to 7 phorbol derivatives at 10^{-8} M (Table 3).

Mezerein, TPA, and phorbol didecanoate are potent enhancers of colony formation in RTE cells in culture, and at this concentration they enhanced colony formation by 10-fold. Under similar conditions these phorbol esters virtually completely suppressed colony formation in human bronchial cell cultures. Phorbol dibutyrate and dibenzoate were less stimulatory in RTE cells, and were slightly less inhibitory to human bronchial cells at this concentration. 4-O-methyl TPA, the phorbol acetates, and the parent alcohol phorbol - which is generally inactive, very weakly stimulated colony formation in RTE cultures. These derivatives were least inhibitory to colony formation in human bronchial cells. Thus, the structure-activity relationships seen for RTE cells appear to be inverse to that relationship observed for bronchial epithelial cells.

TABLE 3. Comparison of effects of phorbol esters on colony formation of rat tracheal and human bronchial epithelial cells at 10^{-8} M

Derivative	Rat tracheal cells[a]	Human bronchial cells[a]
Mezerein	10	0
TPA	10	0.05
Phorbol didecanoate	10	0
Phorbol dibutyrate	7	0.001
Phorbol dibenzoate	6	0.05
4-O-Methyl TPA	2	0.60
Phorbol di/mono acetate	1.1	0.77
Phorbol	1	0.44

[a] Expressed in % relative to CFE in untreated controls.

Out of 19 specimens tested for the effect of TPA on colony formation, about 95% of these specimens were inhibited from forming colonies by TPA. In one human specimen it was observed that TPA stimulated colony formation approximately 300 percent at 1.6 and 16 nM TPA. This specimen was from a 42-yr old female with a 25 pack year smoking history whose lung was resected for a non-tumorous condition. However, the bronchus was normal. We are continuing to monitor the responses of human bronchial cells to TPA in order to determine the frequencies of these responses. The fact that we found only one specimen of human cells that was enhanced by TPA to form colonies indicates that this is a rare characteristic.

SUMMARY AND CONCLUSIONS

Phorbol ester tumor promoters enhance the ability of primary normal rat tracheal epithelial cells to form colonies in a time-dependent fashion. The potency of phorbol derivatives in inducing this effect is relative to their potency as tumor promoters in mouse epidermis. Agents which do not interact with the putative TPA receptor are not effective. In contrast, both hamster tracheal and human bronchial epithelial cells are inhibited from forming colonies by phorbol esters. The sensitivity of human cells varied among individuals but could not be related to age, smoking history, or presence of a cancerous condition. These results bear some similarity to those of Harris et al. (7) where levels of BP-DNA binding were measured in organ cultures of human bronchus. An interindividual variation of 120-fold was observed in 37 specimens of human bronchus, however, no correlation was apparent between levels of binding and whether the specimens were from patients with cancer. It would be of interest to determine if there is a relationship between carcinogen metabolism or binding and the ability to respond to promoters in specimens from normal and lung cancer patients. It is conceivable that lung cancer arises in individuals that have rare peculiarities in carcinogen metabolism combined with peculiarities in their responses to promoters present in cigarette smoke.

Several conclusions can be drawn from these data. Species vary in response to tumor promoting agents, and the type of response may be a result of the biochemical events which are triggered by interaction with protein kinase C (12) or another cellular receptor. Both responses, that of enhanced growth of epithelial cells observed in the rat, or that of inhibition of growth (induction of terminal differentiation) seen in human (15,25) and hamster epithelial cells are consistent with proposed mechanisms by which tumor promoters may function (3,29). A general enhancement of cell proliferation may lead to fixation or expansion of genetic damage in initiated cells, while induction of terminal differentiation in normal cells could lead to expanded cell proliferation in initiated cells resistant to differentiation controls. This indicates that both responses may be useful in detecting environmental promoting agents. In light of these studies perhaps the hamster trachea may more closely mimic the responses of the human bronchus than does the rat. This is consistent with observations of the difficulty in transforming hamster tracheal epithelium (Dr. Brooke Mossman, personal communication) and human bronchial epithelium compared with rat tissue (13,21). Further studies comparing biological and biochemical responses of these three species to chemical carcinogens may aid in developing *in vitro* transformation models.

ACKNOWLEDGEMENT

We thank Ms. Joye C. Denning for superbly skillful typing of this manuscript.

REFERENCES

1. Delclos, K. B., Nagle, D. S., and Blumberg, P. M. (1980): *Cell*, 19:1025-1032.
2. Doll, R., and Hill, A. B. (1964): *Brit. Med. J.*, 1:1460-1467.
3. Farber, E. (1980): *Biochim. Biophys. Acta*, 605:149-166.
4. Fujiki, H., Suganuma, M., Matsukura, N., Sugimura, T., and Takagama, S. (1982): *Carcinogenesis*, 3:895-898.
5. Gordon, R. E., and Lane, B. P. (1977): *Cell Tissue Kinet.*, 10:171-181.
6. Gray, T. E., Thomassen, D. G., Mass, M. J., and Barrett, J. C. (1983): *In Vitro*, 19:559-570.
7. Harris, C. C., Autrup, H., Conner, R., Barrett, L. A., McDowell, E. M., and Trump, B. F. (1976): *Science*, 194:1067-1069.
8. Kinzel, V., Kreibich, G., Hecker, E., and Süss, R. (1979): *Cancer Res.*, 39:2743-2750.
9. Lane, B. P., and Gordon, R. E. (1974): *Proc. Soc. Exp. Biol. Med.*, 145:1139-1144.
10. Lechner, J. F., Haugen, A., Autrup, H., McClendon, I. A., Trump, B. F., and Harris, C. C. (1981): *Cancer Res.*, 41:2294-2304.
11. Mass, M. J., Nettesheim, P., Gray, T. E., and Barrett, J. C. (1984): *Carcinogenesis*, in press.
12. Niedel, J. E., Kuhn, L. J., and Vanderbark, G. R. (1983): *Proc. Natl. Acad. Sci.*, 80:36-40.
13. Pai, S. B., Steele, V. E., and Nettesheim, P. (1983): *Carcinogenesis*, 4:369-374.
14. Pal, B. C., Topping, D. C., Griesemer, R. A., Nelson, F. R., and Nettesheim, P. (1978): *Cancer Res.*, 38:1376-1383.
15. Parkinson, E. K., and Emmerson, A. (1982): *Carcinogenesis*, 3:525-531.
16. Roe, F. J. C., and Clack, J. (1963): *Brit. J. Cancer*, 17:596-604.
17. Roe, F. J. C., Salaman, M. H., and Cohen, J. (1959): *Brit. J. Cancer*, 13:623-633.
18. Siegfried, J. M., and Nesnow, S. (1984): *Carcinogenesis*, in press.
19. Solt, D., and Farber, E. (1976): *Nature*, 263:701-703.
20. Sugimura, T. (1982): *Gann*, 73:499-507.
21. Thomassen, D. G., Gray, T. E., Mass, M. J., and Barrett, J. C. (1983): *Cancer Res.*, 43:5956-5963.
22. Topping, D. C., and Nettesheim, P. (1980): *Cancer Res.*, 40:4352-4355.
23. Topping, D. C., and Nettesheim, P. (1980): *J. Natl. Cancer Inst.*, 65:625-630.
24. Van Duuren, B. L., Sivak, A., Katz, C., and Melchionne, S. (1971): *J. Natl. Cancer Inst.*, 47:235-240.
25. Willey, J. C., Saladino, A. J., Ozanne, C., Lechner, J. F., and Harris, C. C. (1984): *Carcinogenesis*, 5:209-215.
26. Wist, E., and Prydz, H. (1979): *Nucleic Acids Res.*, 6:1583-1590.

27.   Wu, R., Groelke, J. W., Chang, L. Y., Porter, M. E., Smith, D., and Nettesheim, P. (1983): In: *Growth of Cells in Hormonally Defined Medium*, edited by D. Sirbasku, G. H. Sato, and A. Pardee, pp. 641-656. Cold Spring Harbor Press, New York.

28.   Wynder, E. L., and Hoffmann, D. (1969): *Cancer*, 24:289-301.

29.   Yuspa, S. H., and Morgan, D. L. (1981): *Nature*, 293:72-74.

Carcinogenesis, Vol. 8, edited by M. J. Mass et al.
Raven Press, New York © 1985.

Multistage-Promotion and Carcinogenesis Studies in Rat Tracheal Epithelial Cells in Culture

Vernon E. Steele

Pulmonary Carcinogenesis Laboratory, In Vitro Toxicology Program, Northrop Services, Inc., Research Triangle Park, North Carolina 27709

Human epidemiological evidence has strongly suggested that respiratory tract cancer is a multistage process in which the enhancement process could be due to many mechanisms functioning in concert. Animal studies have allowed us to examine some of these processes in more detail with specific compounds. To further understand the processes of tumor promotion at the cellular and molecular levels, tissue culture models needed to be developed. Two rat tracheal epithelial cell culture systems have been used to provide evidence that tumor promotion or enhancement is a possible mechanism by which respiratory tract tumor incidence is increased by exposure to noncarcinogenic substances (7,12). Specific-pathogen-free Fischer 344 rats were chosen since there is an extremely low background incidence of spontaneous respiratory tract cancer (1). The tracheal epithelium of this rat was chosen because it is histologically similar to human bronchial epithelium and the tumors which arise from this tissue are morphologically similar to human bronchogenic carcinomas. Elsewhere in this volume Dr. Klein-Szanto describes the *in vivo* results of tumor promotion studies using the Fischer 344 rat in the tracheal transplant system. In the studies presented here we have used animals from the same stock in two *in vitro* culture systems.

METHODS

The Tracheal Explant - Cell Culture System

The tracheal explant-cell culture system has been described earlier (4,8). Briefly, Fischer 344 rat tracheas were excised, cut into small explants, placed lumen side up on Gelman TCM filter paper supported by a stainless steel grid in a typical organ culture dish

(Falcon Plastics, Oxnard, CA). The medium used during the organ culture phase was a modified Waymouth's medium originally developed by Dr. Ann Marchok (5). This media contained Waymouth's MB 752/1 media (GIBCO), 2% fetal bovine serum (Microbiological Associates, Bethesda, MD), 0.1 µg/ml insulin (Calbiochem, San Diego, CA), 0.1 µg/ml hydrocortisone (Sigma Chemical Corp., St. Louis, MO), 0.22 mg sodium pyruvate/ml, 0.0178 mg L-alanine/ml, 0.347 mg L-arginine/ml, 0.03 mg L-asparagine:H_2O/ml, 0.021 mg L-serine/ml, 0.25 mg putrescine/ml, 0.5 mg lipoic acid/ml, and 10 mg linoleic acid/ml.

For simplification, single initiators and single promoters were used. The initiator chosen was N-methyl-N'-nitro-N-nitrosoguanidine (MNNG), a direct-acting alkylating agent which has a very short half life under culture conditions. The promoting agent was the phorbol diester, 12-O-tetradecanoylphorbol-13-acetate (TPA). The exposures to MNNG were on Days 3 and 6 for 6 hr each day in serum-free media. The TPA exposures began on Day 9 and were 1 hr in duration every 6 days for 3 weeks again in serum-free medium.

Since previous studies (11) had shown that MNNG concentrations as low as 1 ng/ml produced tumorigenic cell lines in this system; a 10 fold lower concentration, 0.1 ng/ml, was expected to minimize the transformation frequency.

The TPA concentration and exposure duration were chosen since previous studies had shown that shorter exposures to 1 µg/ml of TPA had a maximal effect on cell proliferation (9).

After the last TPA exposure, the explants were removed from organ culture, where little outgrowth of cells occurs and placed on the bottom of tissue culture dishes, where cells rapidly migrate from the explant onto the surface of the dish. At this point the following media changes were made: the insulin was increased to 10 µg/ml, and the fetal bovine serum was increased to 10%. The explants were replanted weekly for 10 weeks to establish primary cultures. Primary cultures were thoroughly examined twice weekly for the appearance of morphologically altered cells. Epithelial cells lines were then established from these cultures as described previously (8).

Cell lines which had reached the fifth passage by a set number of days following carcinogen exposure were inoculated into immunosuppressed isogenic host animals. Each cell line was tested for tumorigenicity by inoculating 10^6 viable cells into each leg of a host animal. The inoculation site was palpated weekly for 4 months for the appearance of tumors.

The Primary Cell Culture System

Epithelial cells were isolated from the tracheas of 10 to 12 week old specific-pathogen-free Fischer 344 rats by the method reported by Wu et al. (15). The lumens of freshly excised tracheas were filled with cold 1% protease (Protease Type VI, Sigma Chemical Co., St. Louis, MO) in Eagle's Minimal Essential Medium (MEM) and incubated overnight at 4°. The cells were collected from the tracheas by washing with MEM containing 10% fetal bovine serum. The cells were plated into collagen coated tissue culture dishes (600 µg/60 mm dish). The seeding density was 10^4 cells/dish. The medium used was a modified Ham's F12 medium as reported by Wu et al. (15). Briefly, a 1:1 mix of Ham's F12 and 3T3-conditioned Dulbecco's Minimal Essential Medium (containing 2% FBS) was used plus the following growth factors: insulin (10 µg/ml), transferrin (5 µg/ml), hydrocortisone (10^{-6} M), bovine hypothalamus extract (0.3%), and gentamicin (50 µg/ml).

The attached epithelial cells were exposed on Day 1 of culture to either 0 or 0.1 µg MNNG/ml of serum free Ham's F12 medium for one hour. Twice weekly from Day 6 to Day 30 the cultures were exposed either to 0 or 0.01 ng TPA/ml in serum-free medium. The final dimethylsulfoxide (DMSO) concentration was 0.2% in all cultures.

At Day 40 the cultures were dissociated and replated into 96 well dishes at various seeding densities from 10^1 to 10^4 cells/well. After 7 days the dishes were fixed and the colonies were counted under a dissecting scope.

Cell numbers and number of epithelial "foci" were also determined at Day 40. Cell numbers were determined by first dissociating the cells with 0.2% trypsin-EDTA (GIBCO) for 10-15 minutes, adding an equal volume of 20% FBS in Hank's balanced salt solution, and pelleting the cells by centrifugation. Direct counts were made of an aliquot of the resuspended cells to determine the total cell number in each dish using a hemacytometer. Epithelial foci were defined as patches of epithelial cells having a cellular density greater than 500 cells/mm^2.

At Day 60 the available cultures were dissociated and replated in 0.3% agarose to assess anchorage independent growth. All cultures were in the second or third passage at this time. The colony forming efficiency in soft agarose was measured by a modification of the MacPherson technique (3). An aliquot of 5×10^4 cells in 1.5 ml of 0.3% agarose was layered on top of a base layer of 0.5% agarose in complete growth medium. The cultures were kept from drying out by adding

0.5 ml of complete medium weekly. After 3 weeks the cultures were scored using a phase microscope. Cultures containing more than 12 colonies were scored as positive. Anchorage independence of cultures was also determined at Day 120.

Determination of DNA Content

Aliquots of cells which were dissociated at Day 40 in the above promotion experiment were fixed in cold ethanol for DNA content analysis as previously described (13). The same procedure was performed at Day 60. The ethanol-fixed cells were centrifuged and an aliquot of fixed diploid tracheal cells was added to one half of the sample. The spiked and unspiked pairs of cultures were handled in parallel so that the diploid peak could be accurately determined. All cultures were stained in Hoechst 33342 (Polysciences, Warrington, PA). Excitation of the bound stain was with the 365 nm line of an argon laser in a flow cytofluorograph. The resultant fluorescent signal was integrated with a 256 channel pulse height analyzer. All samples were run on the same day. In cultures which showed large percentages of 4N signals both the total integrated fluorescence and the pulse time were measured simultaneously. This procedure distinguished between cell doublets and tetraploid cells.

Determination of Keratin Content

Epithelial cells were dissociated from Fischer 344 male rat tracheas as described above. The tracheal cells were plated onto collagen coated dishes containing complete medium containing either 0, 1, 10, or 100 ng of TPA/ml. After six days ^{14}C labeled amino acids were added and the cultures incubated for 24 hr. The cultures were then rinsed three times with phosphate buffered saline (PBS). The final PBS rinse was removed and the cell monolayer frozen over liquid nitrogen. The keratin proteins were removed by extracting the cell lysates twice with a low salt Tris buffer (14) and finally in buffer plus 1% Triton X-100. The pellets were dissolved in sodium dodecylsulfate (SDS) sample buffer and analyzed on a 12% polyacrylamide gel by gel electrophoresis (2,6). The resultant gels were dried and autoradiographed with X-ray film. The keratin proteins were quantitated by placing the exposed and developed X-ray film on a scanning densitometer (Gelman Sciences, Inc., Ann Arbor, MI).

RESULTS AND DISCUSSION

Tracheal Explant - Cell Culture System

Four major events were scored during the course of this study:
1) Time to the appearance of morphologically altered cells
2) Time to the fifth passage of culture
3) Time to expression of tumorigenicity
4) Frequency of tumorigenic cell lines

Table 1 shows the first two of these events. There appears to be no enchancement effect on the overall number of cell lines which were established from exposed primary cultures. Cultures initiated and promoted required on average 77 days less than cultures treated with MNNG alone to first observe morphologically altered cells. These cultures progressed at a faster rate and reached the 5th subculture 114 days before cells treated with MNNG only. Unexpectedly, TPA exposure also induced morphologically altered cells and we were able to establish cell lines from many of these cultures. Control cultures produced no morphologically altered cells and hence no cell lines could be established from them.

TABLE 1. Interval between carcinogen exposure and various stages in the establishment of cell lines from MNNG +/- TPA exposed epithelium

Treatment	No. of cell lines established[a]	Average time from carcinogen exposure (± S.E.)		
		To appearance of morphologically altered cells[b]	To first passage[c]	To fifth passage
0	0	–	–	–
TPA	14	190 ± 21	213 ± 15	287 ± 22
MNNG	10	209 ± 10	242 ± 14	315 ± 12
MNNG + TPA	11	132 ± 11	167 ± 26	201 ± 33

[a] Cell cultures subcultured 5 times were designated as cell lines.
[b] Appearance of small, atypical, rapidly growing cells.
[c] Primary cultures were dissociated for the first time when approximately 10^6 atypical cells were present.

The acceleration in growth was accompanied by an acceleration in tumorigenic potential. Table 2 shows the frequency of tumorigenic cell lines at various times after MNNG exposure. None of the 14 TPA induced cells lines were tumorigenic when tested for up to one year following exposure. In the MNNG alone group only 3 of 10 cell lines were tumorigenic and only after one year. Cell lines in the MNNG + TPA group were established and were tumorigenic as early as 150 days. Nearly all of these cell lines proved to be tumorigenic at much earlier times. After one year when the first few cell lines became tumorigenic in the MNNG alone group over 80% of the cell lines in the MNNG + TPA group were tumorigenic. The tumors which were excised were either squamous cell carcinomas or adenosquamous cell carcinomas. There was no apparent differences in the tumor latency or type of tumor between the promoted and non-promoted groups.

TABLE 2. Tumorigenicity of tracheal epithelial cell lines at various times after MNNG +/− TPA exposure

Time following MNNG exposure (days)	Frequency of tumorigenic cell lines (No. tumorigenic[a]/No. inoculated[b]), (%)					
	TPA		MNNG		MNNG + TPA	
100	0/0	(0)	0/0	(0)	0/0	(0)
150	0/0	(0)	0/0	(0)	1/0	(100)
200	0/0	(0)	0/0	(0)	3/3	(100)
250	0/2	(0)	0/0	(0)	3/4	(75)
310	0/6	(0)	0/2	(0)	6/7	(86)
365	0/14	(0)	3/10	(30)	8/11	(73)

[a] All tumors were malignant carcinomas.
[b] Total number of cell lines which had reached the fifth passage or more by the indicated time point.

The ability of tumor promoters to induce cell lines (10) was further studied by exposing explant cultures to various promoting and non-promoting compounds. Exposures were performed as before. Using several non-promoting compounds and "inactive" TPA analogues, we found that mezerein and acetic acid induced no cell lines, phorbol and 4-O-methyl TPA induced only a very low frequency of cell lines, while TPA induced a high percentage (Table 3). Thus the ability of compounds to induce cell lines in this system appears to correlate well with their *in vivo* promoting ability in mouse skin.

The Primary Cell Culture System

The second culture system which was developed was a tracheal primary cell culture system. The difference between this system and

TABLE 3. Frequency of the establishment of cell lines following exposure of cultured rat tracheal explants to promoters/nonpromoters

Chemical	Concentration (μg/ml)	No. of exposures	No. of cell lines/No. of explants exposed	%
DMSO	0.2%	4	1/15	7
Acetic acid	0.012%	4	0/8	0
Mezerein	1.0	4	0/8	0
4-O-Methyl TPA	1.0	4	1/9	11
Phorbol	1.0	4	2/12	17
TPA	1.0	1	2/8	25
TPA	1.0	4	6/8	75
TPA	0.01	4	5/5	100

the previous one is that only the epithelial cells are exposed to the agents in a monolayer culture condition. This system permits a more direct observation and quantitation of the entire population of exposed cells. A Day 5 colony of epithelial cells growing on a collagen film is shown in Fig. 1. To develop this system the cytotoxicity of TPA was examined using continuous or 1 hr exposures. As shown in Table 4, when TPA exposure was continuous, concentrations higher than 1 μg/ml were 100% toxic. Shorter 1 hr exposures circumvented the toxicity that was seen in chronic exposures. Next, different TPA doses were used to look at the long term growth to find which dose maximized the number of cells which would survive long term culture (Table 5). The experimental protocol is shown in Fig. 2. At Day 20, higher numbers of surviving epithelial colonies per dish were seen in the MNNG exposed cultures but no enhancement by TPA was evident (Table 6). At Day 40, a five fold increase in the number of patches in MNNG treated cultures was again seen, but no enhancement by TPA.

The total cell numbers determined after 40 days is shown in Table 7. While carcinogen treatment significantly enhanced cell numbers compared to control, further treatment of initiated cells with TPA did not increase the Day 40 cell counts.

Upon reseeding these cultures after dissociation, mainly additive effects in colony forming efficiency were observed (Table 8). However, distinct differences in the colony morphology were seen between the control and various exposed cultures in the experiment. The colonies in the control cultures contained large flat cells, while colonies in the TPA and MNNG groups contained smaller more rounded cells. Cells in

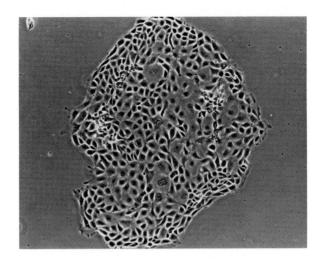

FIG. 1. Morphology of typical rat tracheal epithelial cell colony five days after plating onto a collagen-film-coated tissue culture dish. (Phase contrast, × 100).

TABLE 4.   Differential effect of continuous versus one hour exposures of rat tracheal epithelial cells to TPA[a]

TPA (µg/ml)	% Control CFE[b]	
	Continuous exposure	One hour exposure
0	100	100
0.01	100	ND
0.1	94	94
1.0	119	101
2.0	0	91
5.0	0	114
10.0	0	106

[a] The TPA exposure was begun 24 hr after plating and terminated either after 1 hr or 6 days of exposure. All cultures were fixed and stained six days after the beginning of the exposure.
[b] The control colony forming efficiency ranged from 1 to 3% in these experiments.

TABLE 5. The establishment of cell lines from TPA exposed
rat tracheal epithelial cells in culture

TPA (pg/ml)[a]	No. cell lines established/cultures tested[b]	(%)
0	0/8	(0)
10^{-3}	0/4	(0)
10^{-1}	1/8	(13)
10^{1}	3/9	(33)
10^{3}	3/6	(50)
10^{5}	0/6	(0)

[a] Cell cultures were exposed to various concentrations of TPA in serum-free medium for 1 hr twice weekly from Day 6 to Day 30.

[b] The primary cultures were dissociated on Day 30 and subcultured at least 5 times by Day 90 to form an established cell line.

TRACHEAL PRIMARY EPITHELIAL SYSTEM

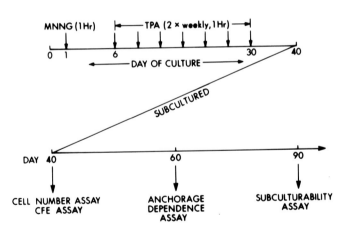

FIG. 2. Experimental protocol for promotion studies using primary cultures of rat tracheal epithelial cells.

TABLE 6.   Effect of MNNG and TPA exposure on colony survival at Days 20 and 40 of culture

Day[a]	Treatment[b]	No. of surviving epithelial colonies/dish (+/− S.D.)	
20	0	0.71	(0.71)
	TPA	1.77	(1.82)
	MNNG	5.48	(2.06)
	MNNG + TPA	4.09	(1.87)
40	0	1.05	(1.11)
	TPA	2.71	(1.45)
	MNNG	5.91	(1.93)
	MNNG + TPA	5.11	(1.64)

[a] The number of days following plating.
[b] 0 treatment was solvent control treatments; MNNG treatment was 0.1 µg/ml on Day 1; TPA treatments were 10 pg/ml twice weekly from Day 6 to Day 30. Means were obtained from 18 to 22 separate cultures. The number of surviving colonies was determined by phase microscopy.

TABLE 7.   Effect of MNNG and TPA exposure on the number of viable cells per culture at Day 40

Treatment[a]	Mean no. of viable cells/culture[b] (+/− S.D.)	
0	0.17	(0.14)
TPA	0.44	(0.32)
MNNG	1.18	(0.52)
MNNG + TPA	1.06	(0.67)

[a] Same as footnote b on Table 6.
[b] Viability was determined by trypan blue exclusion; All treated groups have mean cell numbers significantly higher than the control group ($p < 0.05$, by t-test).

colonies from the MNNG + TPA groups grew in dense colonies and were very heterogeneous.

To assess transformation in all these cultures anchorage independent growth was used (Table 9). Experiment 1 was an experiment in which lower doses were used. There were no notable

TABLE 8. Effect of MNNG and TPA exposure on the colony forming efficiency of rat tracheal epithelial cells at Day 40

Treatment[a]	Colony forming efficiency at various seeding densities[b] (%)		
	625 cells	1250 cells	2500 cells
0	0.02	0.07	0.07
TPA	0.33	0.45	0.32
MNNG	0.11	0.38	0.33
MNNG + TPA	0.70	0.81	0.88

[a] Same as footnote b on Table 6.
[b] At Day 40 the cultures were dissociated and replated at various seeding densities in the 7 mm wells of 96 well dishes. After seven days the colonies were fixed and stained.

differences between the exposure groups in terms of cell numbers or numbers of foci. Also at Day 60 no differences in anchorage independent growth were seen between the treated groups. At Day 120, however, an enhancement of anchorage independence in MNNG+TPA treated cells compared to cultures exposed only to MNNG was obvious. This suggests that at lower promoter doses a longer expression time is required for this phenotype to appear.

In the Experiment 2 where the higher doses were used, it was already evident by Day 60 that anchorage independent growth was enhanced in initiated cells by TPA exposure. At 120 days no further increase was seen.

Induction of Aneuploidy by MNNG and TPA

In a parallel study conducted with Dr. Martin Vanderlaan at Lawrence Livermore Laboratory, the DNA content of these cells in the various exposure groups was examined. Cells with abnormal DNA content were found in many tumors and degree of aneuploidy has been correlated with histopathologic tumor grade.

Samples of the 40 and 60 day-old cultures were fixed and the DNA stained with Hoechst's stain. The fluorescence per cell was then measured with a flow cytometer. The DNA content of freshly isolated cells and Day 40 and 60 control cells had predominately diploid DNA content values (Table 10). TPA exposed cells at Day 40 had DNA contents very similar to controls, but by Day 60 small numbers of aneuploid cells were evident.

TABLE 9.   Effect of MNNG and TPA exposure on anchorage
independent growth of tracheal epithelial cells

Treatment[b]	No. of positive cultures/total cultures tested[a]	
	Day 60	Day 120
Experiment 1		
0	0/9	0/5
TPA	0/10	0/10
MNNG	1/17	1/10
MNNG + TPA	0/16	5/10
Experiment 1		
0	0/7	0/1
TPA	1/15	2/11
MNNG	0/11	1/9
MNNG + TPA	7/13	7/12

[a] Cultures were assayed under a inverted phase microscope and were
scored positive if they had > 12 colonies per dish. Each culture was
independently exposed and maintained.
[b] Treatment of Experiment 1 cultures was as follows: 0, solvent
exposure; TPA, exposed to 10^{-3} pg of TPA/ml; MNNG, exposed to
0.01 µg MNNG/ml; MNNG + TPA, exposed sequentially to MNNG
and TPA. Experiment 2: 0, solvent control; TPA, 10 pg/ml; MNNG,
0.1 µg/ml, MNNG + TPA, sequential exposure.

For cells exposed to MNNG alone the Day 40 DNA content
measurements had a much higher frequency to tetraploid cells and a
significant percentage of aneuploid cells with DNA contents between
2N and 4N were found.   By Day 60 these frequencies were
approximately the same.

Cells derived from cultures exposed to MNNG + TPA had much
higher frequencies of aneuploid cells at Day 40 than cells exposed to
MNNG alone.   However by Day 60 multiple cycling subpopulations
with aneuploid DNA contents were observed.

The appearance of cells with polyploid and aneuploid DNA
contents does not coincide with the development of anchorage
independent or tumorigenic cells, but preceeds their evolution by many
populations doublings (unpublished observations).

These studies suggest that carcinogens may cause chromosomal
instability which appears to be greatly amplified by exposure to TPA.
This process may be an important early step in the process of neoplastic
transformation.

TABLE 10.   Effect of MNNG and TPA treatment on the DNA
content of rat tracheal epithelial cells

Sample		Time in culture (days)	Abnormal peak modes	(Population %)
Control	-1	40	-	
	-2	40	-	
	-3	40	-	
	-4	40	4.4	14
	-5	60	-	
TPA	-1	40	-	
	-2	40	-	
	-3	40	-	
	-4	40	2.8	10
	-5	60	8.0	19
	-6	60	3.4	19
MNNG	-1	40	-	
	-2	40	3.0	20
	-3	40	3.4	34
	-4	40	3.2,6.4	17,5
	-5	60	3.2,6.4,8.0	22,8,8
	-6	60	3.0,6.0	14,7
MNNG + TPA	-1	40	3.2	22
	-2	40	3.2	16
	-3	40	2.4,5.1	21,12
	-4	40	2.7,5.4	17,15
	-5	60	4.2-8.0	50
	-6	60	2.8,3.2	25[a]
			5.6,6,4	21[a]
			8.0	20

[a] Total percent of both peaks.

Promoter Induced Alterations of Gene Expression

A second possible mechanism by which TPA may amplify initiated cells is by altering cellular differentiation (16). The extracted insoluble proteins from the TPA exposed primary cultures were placed on SDS polyacrylamide gels. These insoluble proteins are mainly keratins, and were quantitated by scanning densitometry (Table 11). Eight keratin bands were present in quantifiable proportions. Four keratin bands showed clear dose dependent increases in relative abundance at 0, 1, 10, and 100 ng TPA/ml. These were the 48K, 52K, 56K and 57K dalton keratins. The 100 ng TPA dose induced a greater than 3 fold induction of the 48K dalton keratin, and a greater than 4 fold induction in the

52K dalton keratin. The 57K dalton keratin, not detected in control cultures, was induced in significant proportions by TPA. Keratins greater than 61K daltons were not detected or induced to detectable levels by TPA. The induction of keratin synthesis by TPA in these cells may indicate an change in the normal differentiation processes of these cells. Such changes in normal differentiation could indicate an induction of an atypical proliferative state which could lead to an "immortalization" of the cells. Therefore, initiated cells which would normally be committed to terminal differentiation would enter the proliferative pool and enhance the likelihood of later stages of malignant transformation.

TABLE 11.   Effect of TPA on the synthesis of keratin proteins by rat tracheal epithelial cells

Molecular weight (daltons)	Relative abundance[a] (%) at TPA doses[b] of:			
	0	1	10	100
40K	5	5	25	15
43K (actin)	100	100	100	100
48K	67	133	195	215
51K	20	35	5	5
52K	40	95	148	185
56K	45	85	108	107
57K	0	15	35	50
59K	12	20	20	40
61K	10	15	10	5

[a] Abundance of keratin proteins was standardized with an actin internal standard.
[b] Doses are in ng/ml.

SUMMARY

In summary, two *in vitro* systems with rat tracheal epithelial cells were used to demonstrate that initiated respiratory tract epithelial cells can be promoted or enhanced to transform at a higher frequency by exposure to a noncarcinogenic tumor promoter. The latter two studies suggest possible mechanisms for this enhancement: 1) TPA amplifies the chromosomal instability brought about by initiating doses of carcinogen and 2) TPA alters gene expression and cellular differentiation such that it causes the initiated cell to escape the normal differentiation and senescence process thereby enhancing the proliferative lifespan of initiated cells.

REFERENCES

1. Kuschner, M., and Laskin, S. (1970): In: *Morphology of Experimental Respiratory Carcinogenesis*, edited by P. Nettesheim, M.G. Hanna, and J.W. Deatherage, pp. 203-225. U.S. Atomic Energy Commission Division of Technical Information, Oak Ridge, TN.
2. Nelson, K. G. and Slaga, T. J. (1982): *Cancer Res.*, 42:4176-4181.
3. MacPherson, I. (1973): In: *Tissue Culture*, edited by P. F. Kruse and M. K. Patterson, pp. 276-280. Academic Press, New York.
4. Marchok, A. C., Rhoton, J., Griesemer, R., and Nettesheim, P. (1977): *Cancer Res.*, 37:1811-1821.
5. Marchok, A. C., Rhoton, J., and Nettesheim, P. (1976): *In Vitro*, 12:320.
6. O'Farrrell, P. H. (1975): *J. Biol. Chem.*, 250:4007-4021.
7. Steele, V. E., Beeman, D. K., and Nettesheim, P. (1984): *Cancer Res.*, in press.
8. Steele, V. E., Marchok, A. C., and Nettesheim, P. (1977): *Int. J. Cancer*, 20:234-238.
9. Steele, V. E., Marchok, A. C., and Nettesheim, P. (1978): In: *Mechanisms of Tumor Promotion and Cocarcinogenesis*, edited by T. J. Slaga, R. K. Boutwell, and A. Sivak, pp. 289-300. Raven Press, New York.
10. Steele, V. E., Marchok, A. C., and Nettesheim, P. (1978): *Cancer Res.*, 38:3563-3565.
11. Steele, V. E., Marchok, A. C., and Nettesheim, P. (1979): *Cancer Res.*, 39:3805-3811.
12. Steele, V. E., Marchok, A. C., and Nettesheim, P. (1980): *Int. J. Cancer*, 26:343-348.
13. Vanderlaan, M., Steele, V. E., and Nettesheim, P. (1983): *Carcinogenesis*, 4:721-727.
14. Winter, H., Schweizer, J., and Goerttler, K. (1980): *Carcinogenesis*, 1:391-398.
15. Wu, R., Groelke, J. W., Change, L. Y., Porter, M. E., Smith, D., and Nettesheim, P. (1982): In: *Growth of Cells in Hormonally Defined Media*, edited by D. Sirbasku, G. H. Sato, and A. Pardee, pp. 641-656. Cold Spring Harbor Press, Cold Spring Harbor, NY.
16. Yuspa, S. H., and Morgan, D. L. (1981): *Nature*, 293:72-74.

Carcinogenesis, Vol. 8, edited by M. J. Mass et al.
Raven Press, New York © 1985.

Contrasting Responses of Normal and Transformed Rat Tracheal Epithelial Cells to the Tumor Promoter 12-*O*-Tetradecanoylphorbol-13-Acetate

Paul Nettesheim, Thomas E. Gray, and J. Carl Barrett

Laboratory of Pulmonary Function and Toxicology, National Institute of Environmental Health Sciences, Research Triangle Park, North Carolina 27709

A large body of evidence derived from clinical, epidemiological, and experimental studies suggests that most cancers develop in multiple stages. However, there is still little definitive information concerning the biochemical and molecular characteristics of preneoplastic stages, the number of stages in various experimental or clinical models of carcinogenesis, or the key factors controlling the progression of cells from one preneoplastic stage to another.

In the field of respiratory tract carcinogenesis our knowledge of the stages of neoplastic development is particularly rudimentary. This is somewhat surprising, since researchers studying the major causative agent of human bronchogenic carcinoma, tobacco smoke, have maintained for years that tobacco smoke contains strong tumor promoting agents (26). It has been a tacit assumption that progression through (multiple) stages driven by these promoting agents is an important feature of the pathogenesis of bronchogenic carcinoma. However, little concrete evidence in support of promotion in the development of lung cancer exists. One of the reasons for the slow progress in this field of research is the scarcity of appropriate experimental models suited to define multiple stages and to study the interaction of agents, particularly of initiators and promoters (for discussion and review see ref. 7,10,11).

To facilitate the study of neoplastic development and its modifiers in airway epithelium we have developed a number of experimental models including organ culture and cell culture systems, using the epithelium of rat tracheas (7,10,11). The cell culture models of rat tracheal epithelial (RTE) cells have made it possible to define 3 distinct preneoplastic stages of RTE cell carcinogenesis (for review see ref. 7) which are characterized by changes of *in vitro* growth behavior (Fig. 1).

Normal RTE cells, isolated from adult rats, will undergo 10 to 12 cell divisions in culture, after which proliferation ceases and the cells senesce. In sharp contrast, if the cells have been exposed to a carcinogen (either *in vivo* or in culture), a small number of them will continue to proliferate and form tightly packed, steadily enlarging colonies, termed enhanced growth (EG) variant colonies. These are the primary transformed foci or morphologial transformants of the RTE cell system. In a number of studies we have shown that the cells of these EG variant colonies subsequently undergo progressive changes (see Fig. 1): they become "immortal" transformants, anchorage-independent transformants, and ultimately neoplastic transformants (12,20,21). Neoplastic transformation of RTE cells is divided accordingly into distinct states. It is quite apparent, in viewing the schematic representation given in Fig. 1, that this *in vitro* model provides an excellent opportunity to experimentally approach a variety of problems related to multistage carcinogenesis. The fact that RTE cells can grow at clonal cell density makes it feasible to analyze quantitatively the process of neoplastic transformation at its various stages (4,21). The process of neoplastic development can be studied with RTE cells exposed either *in vivo* or *in vitro* to carcinogens and promoters. The cellular changes induced *in vivo* can be analyzed by the same *in vitro* assays as cells exposed in culture, by isolating cells at various times after exposure and plating them at low density into culture dishes (12,19,20).

Progression of Rat Tracheal Epithelial (RTE) Cells In Vitro and In Vivo

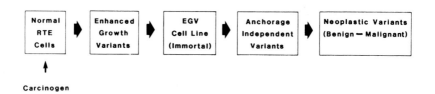

FIG. 1. Sequence of phenotypic changes developing in RTE cell cultures after *in vivo* or *in vitro* exposure to carcinogen. To study modifiers of neoplastic progression cultures are exposed at various stages of transformation to chemicals of interest. EGV = enhanced growth variant.

The first and most obvious question which needed to be answered was whether the epithelium of the conducting airways can be initiated and promoted. The results of several *in vivo* and *in vivo-in vitro* studies showed that the tumor promoter 12-O-tetradecanoylphorbol-13-acetate (TPA) does indeed effectively promote rat tracheal epithelium initiated either with 7,12-dimethylbenz(a)anthracene (DMBA) or N-methyl-N'-nitro-N-nitrosoguanidine (MNNG) (17-19,22).

One of the objectives in our ongoing *in vitro* promotion studies is to determine which stage of neoplastic transformation is susceptible to promoting agents; another goal is to characterize the cellular and biochemical responses elicited by promoters acting on cell populations at different stages of neoplastic transformation. We have previously reported on the effects of TPA treatment during the early post initiation stage, i.e., the first 5 weeks following carcinogen exposure during which the EG-variant colonies form (see Fig. 1). These studies showed that TPA treatment does not increase the number of EG variant colonies (8); but TPA treatment does result in an accelerated appearance of a "late" preneoplastic phenotype, namely the anchorage-independent (ag^+) phenotype (16).

To elucidate the mechanism of this promotion we recently investigated the effects of TPA on RTE cells which have progressed to the second stage of transformation (see Fig. 1) and have become "immortal" (9).

THE EFFECT OF TPA ON NORMAL RTE CELLS AND IMMORTAL RTE CELL VARIANTS

One series of studies was designed to determined the *in vitro* effects of TPA on the proliferative potential of RTE cells. We compared the promoter's effects on normal and immortal, transformed cells using a colony forming assay. This assay measures the proportion of colony forming cells in a cell population and provides an estimate of the relative size of the stem cell pool. The data summarized in Table 1 exemplify the contrasting response patterns of normal and of transformed RTE cells to TPA.

TPA exposure markedly stimulated the colony forming efficiency (CFE) of normal RTE cells. Under the culture conditions used in these studies the colony forming efficiency generally ranged from 2-6%. With TPA present in the culture medium, it was commonly increased by a factor of 5, to a CFE of 25% or more (6). Thus cells which would otherwise not have expressed their ability to proliferate and to form

TABLE 1.   Effect of TPA on the colony forming efficiency of normal
and transformed rat tracheal epithelial cells[a]

TPA concentration ng/ml	Relative survival (%) of RTE cells:	
	Normal	Transformed
0	100	100
0.1	105	80
1.0	150	90
10.0	450	18
100.0	500	0.8

[a] Normal, freshly isolated RTE cells and cells from the transformed RTE cell line EGV-1Cl19 were seeded at low density onto irradiated 3T3 feeder layers and the number of epithelial colonies was counted 8 days later. TPA or solvent were present in the cultures for the duration of the experiment. Data expressed as relative survival, i.e., as % of colony forming cells in solvent control cultures. The colony-forming efficiency of primary RTE cells was 3%; that of the transformed cell line was 25% (9).

colonies were triggered by TPA into replication (see Mass et al., this volume).

The response of transformed RTE cells to TPA exposure was diametrically opposed to that of normal cells. Their colony forming ability was drastically inhibited rather than stimulated. The data in Table 1 show the response of one of the transformed RTE cell lines tested. With 10 ng/ml of TPA the CFE was decreased by more than 80% and at 100 ng/ml by more than 99%. These contrasting effects of TPA on normal and stably transformed RTE cells were highly reproducible. Further studies showed that the majority of immortal RTE cell cultures was sensitive to the inhibition of CFE by TPA (see Table 2). A more detailed account of these studies and of the variables influencing the response to TPA is given elsewhere (9).

Additional experiments were carried out with normal RTE cells to further analyze the effects of TPA (Table 3). To compensate for the increase in CFE due to TPA stimulation, a lower number of cells was plated into the dishes containing TPA. The studies revealed that continuous exposure had little effect on the rate of growth of normal RTE cells. This suggested that the cells might become refractory to the tumor promoter. However this was found not to be the case, because when the cells were subcultured into medium containing TPA, a marked stimulation of the colony forming efficiency was again observed

TABLE 2.   Effect of TPA on the colony forming efficiency (%) of transformed RTE cell lines[a]

Cell line designation		TPA exposure (10 ng/ml)	
		−	+
EGV-1	p9	27.4	0.7
	p28	39.2	0.4
EGV-1Cl19		27.5	0.1
EGV-6	p6	7.2	4.8
EGV-7	p12	15.7	4.3
EGV-8	p7	18.2	0.3
EGV-9	p6	1.8	2.3
	p18	28.1	3.3
EGV-9A1	p5	29.0	0.03
EGV-10	p12	19.9	0.7
EGV-11	p12	16.3	6.7

[a] The EGV cell lines were induced by exposure of primary RTE cell cultures to MNNG or to gamma-irradiation; p = passage number (9).

(see Table 3, two last columns on right). The loss of colony forming ability of normal RTE cells in primary cultures which occurs as the cultures approach the confluent state (4) was not prevented by the presence of TPA. We also studied the formation of cross-linked envelopes (CLE) in the same experiments. Formation of cross-linked envelopes has been used by a number of laboratories as an indicator of terminal differentiation in cultured epithelial cells, and it has been reported that TPA induces CLE formation in a number of cell types including rodent and human skin cells and human bronchial cells (13-15,23-25). We measured spontaneous as well as calcium ionophore-induced CLE formation in control and TPA-treated primary RTE cell cultures and found no evidence of induction of terminal differentiation by TPA. Normal RTE cell cultures had very low CLE formation even when nearly confluent, and TPA exposure caused no significant change (Table 3). Calcium ionophore-induced CLE formation was very high even in sparse RTE cultures but again TPA treatment brought about little change.

In considering the mechanism reponsible for the reduction in colony forming ability of transformed RTE cells exposed to TPA, we examined the possibilities that TPA might either induce terminal differentiation in these cells or, alternatively, toxic cell death. Table 4

TABLE 3.   Effect of TPA on growth rate, cross-linked envelope (CLE) formation, and colony forming cells of normal primary RTE cell cultures[a]

Time of culture in days	TPA exposure	No. of viable cells/dish ($\times 10^6$)	CLE %		CFE % upon replating in presence or absence of TPA	
			Spontaneous	Ionophore induced	– TPA	+ TPA
4	–	0.35	<1.0	72	2.6	7.9
	+	0.42	<1.0	93	4.8	11.5
7	–	0.86	4.0	101	0.1	5.7
	+	1.50	1.4	113	<0.1	7.9
10	–	1.30	0.6	116	<0.1	2.1
	+	1.30	0.1	106	<0.1	2.5

[a] 10^5 freshly isolated, normal RTE cells were plated onto irradiated 3T3 feeder layers into medium without TPA (10^5 cells/dish) or with 10 ng/ml TPA (3×10^4 cells/dish). At indicated time intervals the number of cells per culture and spontaneous and calcium ionophore-induced CLE were determined. At the same time points cells from the primary cultures were replated onto feeders into medium with or without TPA and the CFE was determined (9).

summarizes the results of one of several studies which showed that within 24 hr the number of viable cells dropped rapidly in TPA exposed cultures of transformed RTE cells. This was accompanied by a minor increase in cross-linked envelopes, which was far too small to account for the loss of viable cells. The number of CLE per culture increased from about 2 to 4×10^3 at 2 hr of TPA exposure and from about 3.5 to 4.0×10^3 at 24 hr after TPA exposures. At the same time points the reduction in the number of cells per culture was 6×10^4 and 9×10^4, respectively. These findings lead us to conclude that TPA triggers a rapid cytotoxic response in transformed RTE cells, resulting in loss of viability.

SUMMARY AND CONCLUSION

The data presented here are part of an ongoing effort to examine the response of rat tracheal epithelium to tumor promoting agents and to elucidate the mechanisms of tumor promotion in that epithelial tissue (see Steele, this volume). Previous studies indicated that airway epithelium is responsive to the tumor promoter TPA (6,16) and that TPA can promote the tumor response in rat tracheal epithelium

TABLE 4. Acute effects of TPA on survival and CLE formation of transformed RTE cells[a]

Duration of exposure	TPA exposure	No. of viable cells/dish ($\times 10^5$)	% CLE (spontaneous)
2 hr	−	1.5	1.5
	+	0.9	4.3
24 hr	−	1.8	1.7
	+	0.9	4.3

[a] 2×10^5 transformed cells of the line EGV-1Cl19 were seeded into medium without and with TPA (10 ng/ml). All attached and unattached cells were retrieved at 2 and 24 hr to determine the number viable cells, and the % of cross-linked envelopes (9).

(17-19,22). But what are the mechanisms involved? We have divided this question into two main elements: 1) Which stages of neoplastic development are affected by TPA, i.e., which preneoplastic cell populations are targets for TPA action resulting in the acceleration and enhancement of the process of neoplastic development? 2) What effects does TPA have on various preneoplastic cell populations and how do such effects result in promotion?

The experiments discussed here relate to the second part of the question. They suggested that TPA elicits a marked cytotoxic response in stably transformed RTE cell variants (see Fig. 1). These preneoplastic cell variants are clearly different from untransformed RTE cells which are triggered into cell cycle as indicated by an increase in CFE. This difference between normal and transformed cells is of considerable interest in itself since it points to a fundamental, biochemical alteration in the transformed cells. Evidence exists that transformed RTE cell lines have TPA receptors and that at least some of the reponses elicited by TPA exposure, such as the induction of ornithine decarboxylase activity, are receptor-mediated (5). Whether the cytotoxic response elicited by TPA is receptor-mediated is presently not known.

What role, if any, can the cytotoxic response triggered by TPA in transformed RTE cells play in tumor promotion? At this point it is clearly not possible to extrapolate with any degree of confidence from the cell culture studies to *in vivo* tumor promotion studies. It may nevertheless be useful to formulate testable working hypotheses, based on observations as the ones described here, which can serve as guides for future mechanistic studies. One hypothesis is that the TPA induced death of a sizeable fraction of a preneoplastic cell population may create conditions favorable to the proliferative expansion of the survivors. It would, of course, be important to know whether the cell death is random or selective, that is, whether a particular subpopulation of preneoplastic cells is resistant to the cytotoxic effects of TPA, and, if so, what the basis is for that resistance. At present we have no information on this point except we know that the cell population surviving TPA exposure is somewhat less sensitive to TPA toxicity.

An alternative hypothesis is that TPA causes heritable changes in the initiated or preneoplastic cell population, which predispose these cells to progression towards neoplastic transformation. Evidence has been presented which suggests that such changes might be mediated by free-radical mechanisms, leading to chromosomal damage (1-3). Since the cytotoxic effects of TPA on transformed cells are so prominent in the RTE cell model, it is conceivable that cells surviving the insult have sustained some type of sublethal, heritable damage (either genetic or epigenetic). TPA may not effect neoplastic transformation directly but rather it might cause heritable changes which make the cells prone to undergo secondary alterations resulting in the appearance of the neoplastic phenotype. This could explain the late appearance of neoplastic cells following *in vivo* as well as *in vitro* exposure of RTE cells to TPA (17,22).

A combination of these two hypotheses seems particularly attractive. A heritable change induced by sublethal TPA damage in either a rare cell or a group of cells might clonally expand because of the cell death of surrounding cells and the resulting compensatory hyperplastic response of the altered survivors. Whether such hypothetical mechanisms of tumor promotion have any validity in the promotion of tracheal carcinogenesis remains to be determined by further experimentation.

We believe that the findings presented here suggest two possibly important effects of TPA: 1) TPA may in some cell systems trigger diametrically opposed responses in normal as compared to transformed cells, namely induction of cell replication in the former and induction of cell death in the latter; and 2) the same promoting agent may elicit different responses in cells of different origin, e.g., induction of terminal differentiation in keratinocytes and human bronchial cells (13,14,25) and toxic cell death in rat tracheal cells.

REFERENCES

1. Emerit, J., and Cerutti, P. A. (1981): *Nature*, 293:144-146.
2. Emerit, J., and Cerutti, P. A. (1982): *Proc. Natl. Acad. Sci.* USA, 79:7509-7513.
3. Friedman, J., and Cerutti, P. A. (1983): *Carcinogenesis*, 4:1425-1427.
4. Gray, T. E., Thomassen, D. G., Mass, M. J., and Barrett, J. C. (1983): *In Vitro*, 19:559-570.
5. Jetten, A. M., and Shirley, J. E. (1985): *J. Cell Physiol.*, in press.
6. Mass, M. J., Nettesheim, P., Gray, T. E., and Barrett, J. C. (1984): *Carcinogenesis*, in press.
7. Nettesheim, P., and Barrett, J. C. (1984): In: *CRC Critical Reviews in Toxicology*, Vol. 12, pp. 215-239. CRC Press, Boca Raton, FL.
8. Nettesheim, P., Barrett, J. C., Mass, M. J., Steele, V. E., and Gray, T. E. (1984): In: *Models, Mechanisms and Etiology of Tumor Promotion*, edited by M. Borzonsonyi, N. E. Day, K. Lapis and H. Yamasaki, in press. IARC, Scientific Publ. No. 56, Lyon, France.
9. Nettesheim, P., Gray, T. E., and Barrett, J. C. (1984): *Carcinogenesis*, submitted.
10. Nettesheim, P., and Griesemer, R. A. (1977): In: *Pathogenesis and Therapy of Lung Cancer*, edited by C. C. Harris, pp. 73-188. Marcel Dekker, Inc., New York.
11. Nettesheim, P., and Marchok, A. C. (1983): In: *Advances in Cancer Research*, Vol. 39, edited by G. Klein, and S. Weinhouse, pp. 1-70. Academic Press, New York.
12. Pai, S. B., Steele, V. E., and Nettesheim, P. (1982): *Carcinogenesis*, 3:1201-1206.
13. Parkinson, E. K., and Emmerson, E. (1982): *Carcinogenesis*, 3:525-531.
14. Parkinson, E. K., Gramham, P., and Emmerson, A. (1983): *Carcinogenesis*, 4:857-861
15. Rice, R. H., and Green, H. J. (1978): *J. Cell Biol.*, 76:705-711.
16. Steele, V. E., Beeman, D. K., and Nettesheim, P. (1984): *Cancer Res.*, in press.
17. Steele, V. E., Marchok, A. C., and Nettesheim, P. (1980): *Int. J. Cancer*, 26:343-348.
18. Steele, V. E., and Nettesheim, P. (1983): In: *Mechanisms of Tumor Promotion. Vol. I. Tumor Promotion and Carcinogenesis in Internal Organs*, edited by T. J. Slaga, pp. 91-105. CRC Press, Boca Raton, FL.
19. Terzaghi, M., Klein-Szanto, A. J. P., and Nettesheim, P. (1983): *Cancer Res.*, 43:1461-1466.
20. Terzaghi, M., and Nettesheim, P. (1979): *Cancer Res.*, 39:4003-4010.
21. Thomassen, D. G., Gray, T. E., Mass, M. J., and Barrett, J. C. (1983): *Cancer Res.*, 43:5956-5963.
22. Topping, D. C., and Nettesheim, P. (1980): *Cancer Res.*, 40:4352-4355.
23. Yuspa, S. H., Ben, T. H., and Hennings, H. (1983): Carcinogenesis, 4:1413-1418.
24. Yuspa, S. H., Ben, T. H., Hennings, H., and Lichti, U. (1982): *Cancer Res.*, 42:2344-2349.
25. Willey, J. C., Saladino, A. J., Ozanne, C. H., Lechner, J. F., and Harris, C. C. (1984): *Carcinogenesis*, 5:209-215.
26. Wynder, E. L., and Hoffmann, D., editors (1967): *Tobacco and Tobacco Smoke*. Academic Press, New York.

Carcinogenesis, Vol. 8, edited by M. J. Mass et al.
Raven Press, New York © 1985.

Cocarcinogenic and Tumor Promoting Properties of Asbestos and Other Minerals in Tracheobronchial Epithelium

B. T. Mossman, G. S. Cameron,
and L. P. Yotti

*Department of Pathology, University of Vermont College of Medicine,
Burlington, Vermont 05405*

A number of environmental and occupational particulates are associated with diseases of the respiratory tract in man and experimental animals (reviewed in 38,83). Clearly, the pathogenic potential of each mineral differs. In comparison to other particles and fibers, various types of asbestos are both fibrogenic and carcinogenic (reviewed in 19,43,52). In this regard, occupational exposure to asbestos increases the risk of mesothelioma, a rare tumor of the serosal cells lining the pleural and peritoneal cavities, and bronchogenic carcinoma, a neoplasm arising from the epithelium of the airways. Bronchogenic tumors most commonly are observed in smokers in the general population and are of major concern because of their poor prognosis.

To determine the cellular mechanisms of asbestos-induced toxicity and carcinogenicity in "target" cells of the respiratory tract, we have developed a medley of approaches to assess the interaction of selected minerals with tracheobronchial epithelium *in vitro*. This manuscript provides an overview of our methods and information accumulated thusfar. Results suggest that asbestos resembles a classical tumor promoter, such as 12-O-tetradecanoylphorbol-13-acetate (TPA), in its action on target cells.

MATERIALS AND METHODS

Tracheal Organ Cultures

Tracheal explants are prepared routinely from the tracheas of 6-8 week old female golden Syrian hamsters (41). After sacrifice of animals using Nembutal, the trachea is excised from the larynx to the carina using sterile technique and immersed in Hank's Balanced Salt Solution (HBSS) (GIBCO, Grand Island, NY) containing 100 µg/ml gentamycin and 25 U/ml nystatin. After removal of extraneous tissue by dissection, the tracheal tube is opened along the anatomical discontinuity in the cartilage rings and cut in half. Depending upon the experimental design, the tracheal halves are cultured intact (Fig. 1) or cut into 16 double-ring 4×4 mm^2 explants. The tissues then are grouped in 35 mm petri dishes that are scored to allow adherence of the non-epithelial surface. At this juncture weighed amounts of minerals, alone or coated with polycyclic aromatic hydrocarbons (PAH) (44), are suspended in HBSS at a variety of concentrations (i.e., 0.4-40 mg particle/ml HBSS) and triturated in a syringe before their precipitation on the epithelial surfaces of organ cultures for 1 hr. The tissues then are transferred to dishes containing selected medium (41) with addition of gentamycin (100 µg/ml) and nystatin (25 U/ml) and incubated at 37° in a humidified environment of 5% CO_2--95% air. Medium is added until the epithelial surface is moistened, but not submerged, and is changed twice weekly. Water-soluble carcinogens or carcinogens dissolved in dimethyl sulfoxide (0.1% final concentration in medium) are added to medium directly.

Tracheal Implantation Studies

After a 1-hr exposure to minerals alone and coated with PAH or at intervals after maintenance of carcinogen-exposed tissues *in vitro*, explants are grafted subcutaneously on the backs of syngeneic female weanling hamsters (Fig. 1). To avoid exposure of carcinogens on the epithelial surface of the tracheal implant to the subcutaneous tissue of the recipient, the epithelium of the tracheal segment is sutured along the midline at both ends to the underlying musculature of the host animal. Hamsters are palpated for tumors at 3-week intervals and masses are excised when >5 mm in diameter. To assess premalignant epithelial alterations, implants also are removed and examined at predetermined time intervals after grafting (12,42,44).

Tracheal Epithelial Cell Cultures

An advantage of the organ culture-implantation technique is the preservation of epithelial differentiation and function. Moreover, the normal association of various cell types is preserved. To permit larger numbers of cells for biochemical studies and isolation of cellular

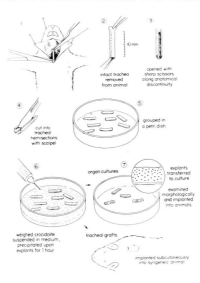

FIG. 1. Procedure for dissection and preparation of hamster tracheal organ cultures and grafts. After exposure to minerals such as crocidolite asbestos, alone or in combination with chemical carcinogens, tissues are either maintained *in vitro* or implanted into syngeneic animals to document the occurrence of tumors. [Reproduced with permission from Wagner, Rom and Merchant (eds.), Health Issues Related to Metal and Nonmetallic Mining, Butterworth Publishers, Boston, p. 125, 1983].

organelles, lines of epithelial cells in monolayer were established from the tracheobronchial epithelium of 2-3 day old hamsters (10). One of these lines, HTE-B, is grown routinely in our laboratory in Ham's F12 medium (GIBCO, Grand Island, NY) with 10% calf serum and can be maintained in serumless medium for periods of less than 24 hr.

Characterization of Minerals

Examination and documentation of the physicochemical properties of selected minerals have been essential in our studies. Accordingly, we have focused on the importance of mineral composition and dimension as important determinants of epithelial cell proliferation, toxicity and carcinogenicity. Thusfar, we have examined comparatively in our bioassays the two most economically important types of asbestos, chrysotile and crocidolite (International Union Against Cancer reference samples; UICC) and a variety of other fibers (glass, attapulgite, erionite, sepiolite) and particles (hematite, carbon, kaolin, glass) (1,7,12,39,42,44,86). To determine whether fibrous geometry is important in biological response, the nonfibrous but chemically identical analogs (antigorite and riebeckite) of chrysotile and crocidolite asbestos, respectively, have been used in a number of experiments (36,86). The mineralogical purity of each preparation has been determined by X-ray diffraction and X-ray energy dispersive spectrometry, whereas morphology and size distributions have been characterized by scanning electron microscopy (SEM).

RESULTS AND DISCUSSION

Minerals as Vehicles for Adsorption of Chemical Carcinogens

In the 1960's, Saffiotti and co-workers reported a high incidence of bronchogenic tumors in hamsters after intratracheal administration of hematite (Fe_2O_3) with the adsorbed PAH, benzo(a)pyrene (BP) (65,66). In contrast, few neoplasms were observed with use of BP alone, and hematite alone was noncarcinogenic. While some have suggested that clearance of BP from the peripheral lung is impeded by hematite (57), autoradiographic studies show BP elutes from the particle surface in the upper airways (24).

Studies at the subcellular level shed some light on the mechanisms of transfer of PAH from particles to cell membranes (27-29). In this regard, Lakowicz and co-workers have measured by fluorimetry the increased transfer of PAH to microsomes and artificial membranes after adsorbance of hydrocarbons to a variety of particulates. Alternatively, dispersions of PAH alone are not taken up readily by membranes. For reasons that are unclear, asbestos fibers are more effective in facilitating transport of hydrocarbons than are particles of silica, carbon and hematite (27-29).

Using autoradiography and liquid scintillation spectrometry, we have examined uptake and retention of BP in tracheal epithelial cells *in vitro* after coating of the hydrocarbon on crocidolite and chrysotile asbestos (14,46). After exposure of cells to BP-coated fibers, approximately 70% of the total BP added enters the cells by 1 hr, and 50% remains intracellular at 8 hr (Fig. 2). In contrast, an initial influx of 20% with retention of only 5% of the initial amount is observed if identical amounts of BP are added to medium. Under the former circumstances, alkylation of DNA by BP, an event critical in transformation, is increased for as long as 5 days.

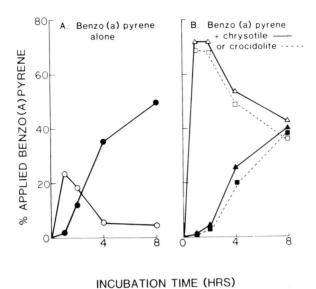

INCUBATION TIME (HRS)

FIG. 2. Quantitation of the uptake and metabolism of benzo(a)pyrene (BP) in hamster tracheal epithelial cells (HTE) after addition of BP alone (A) or equivalent amounts of BP adsorbed to chrysotile and crocidolite asbestos (B). At 1, 2, 4, and 8 hr after exposure of HTE to [^{3}H]BP either solubilized in DMSO (0.1%) in culture medium or coated on asbestos (ca. 2 x 10^{-7}M BP on 3 µg chrysotile or 10 µg crocidolite/ml medium), the cellular content (open symbols) of [^{3}H]BP was measured by scintillation spectrometry. In addition, medium was analyzed to identify the amounts of water-soluble metabolites of BP (closed symbols). [Reproduced with permission from Eastman, Mossman and Bresnick, *Cancer Res.* 43:1251, 1983].

    To address the possible importance of mineral-mediated transfer of PAH in carcinogenesis of the respiratory tract, we adsorbed equivalent amounts of the radiolabeled PAH, 3-methylcholanthrene (3MC), to the surfaces of various particulates including crocidolite asbestos, hematite, kaolin and carbon before their introduction to tracheal organ cultures (44). Negative controls included particles without adsorption of 3MC. After 4 weeks *in vitro*, tissues were implanted into syngeneic hamsters. Whereas no tumors were observed with use of particles alone, tumors, the majority arising from the tracheal epithelium (Fig. 3), appeared with use of all particles and 3MC. A direct relationship was observed between numbers of malignancies

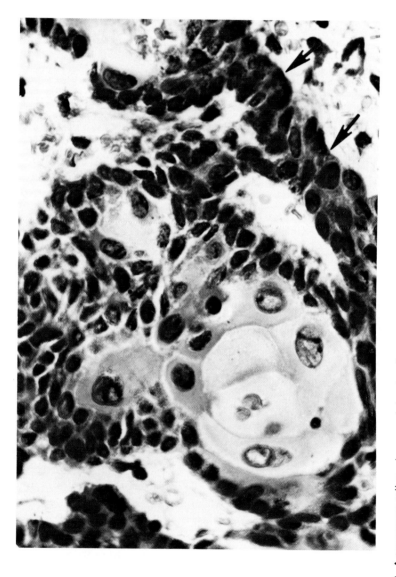

FIG. 3. A squamous cell carcinoma originating from the tracheal epithelium in a hamster tracheal implant exposed *in vitro* to crocidolite asbestos with adsorbed 3-methylcholanthrene (3MC). The tumor cells are protruding into the lumen of the graft. Arrows indicate the basal lamina. Hematoxylin and eosin, × 1,600.

and amounts of 3MC adsorbed to the dusts. Moreover, at highest concentrations of the hydrocarbon, more carcinomas were observed with use of asbestos in comparison to other particles. Future experiments are planned to determine whether other fibrous materials (glass, erionite, etc.) are as (co)carcinogenic as asbestos in this model.

Tumor-Promoting Properties of Asbestos

Classical tumor promoters such as the phorbol esters in mouse skin have various biochemical and morphologic effects on target cells. Over the past few years we have evaluated the ability of asbestos to cause similar proliferative and membrane alterations in tracheobronchial epithelial cells (Table 1). TPA has been used as a 'positive control' in several of these studies (8,30,36). In comparison to TPA, asbestos-induced biologic responses in general are of less magnitude and tend to occur after protracted periods of time (i.e., hours after addition to cultures). Presumably, these observations are related to the fact that asbestos is insoluble--thus, its effects are localized and restricted to cells coming into contact with the fibers. Moreover, uptake of fibers by cells may be integral to cellular response (Fig. 4).

TABLE 1. Biological effects of asbestos on tracheobronchial epithelium resembling those of classical tumor promoters on target cells'

Interaction with plasma membrane
Stimulation of the plasma membrane marker enzyme, Na^+-K^+ ATPase
Release of [^{3}H]arachidonic acid → prostaglandin synthesis
Induction of cell division
Stimulation of polyamine synthesis
Alteration of normal cell differentiation (i.e., squamous metaplasia)
Induction of an inflammatory response
Generation of oxygen free radicals

Interaction of Asbestos with the Plasma Membrane

Empirically it has been known for some time that the initial interaction between an asbestos fiber and a cell occurs at the plasma membrane (5). This interaction is thought to trigger signals which may be important to the subsequent injury or transformation of the target cell.

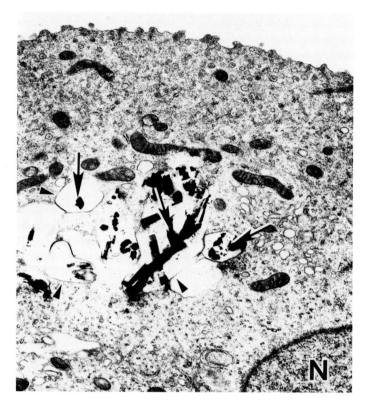

FIG. 4. Transmission electron microscopy (TEM) showing a phagosome containing asbestos in a superficial, nonciliated epithelial cell in organ culture. N = nucleus; arrows = crocidolite asbestos; arrowheads = membranes. Uranyl acetate and lead citrate, × 11,250.

As has been reported with use of TPA in 3T3 cells (73), crocidolite asbestos stimulates the activity of the plasma membrane enzyme, Na^+-K^+ ATPase, in membrane preparations from tracheal epithelial cells (48). Further implicating a role of asbestos in perturbation of membranes are reports showing the binding of positively-charged chrysotile to negatively charged sialic acid residues on red blood cell (RBC) membranes (6,20,23), an event culminating in hemolysis. The consequences of this binding are thought to involve clustering of RBC membrane proteins and alterations in permeability.

Work in this laboratory has indicated that chrysotile interacts with moieties other than sialic acid on the surfaces of tracheobronchial epithelial cells (40,49). After precipitation of chrysotile onto rat tracheal organ cultures, hypersecretion of mucin is observed. To test the hypothesis that chrysotile fibers are interacting with specific carbohydrates on the plasma membrane of mucin-secreting cells, a number of lectins with various specificities were added prior to asbestos. In comparison to other lectins, pretreatment with Conconavalin A (a lectin interacting with α-D-mannose and α-D-glucose) blocked the chrysotile-induced hypersecretion of mucin. These data suggest that interaction of asbestos with specific glycoproteins or glycolipids on the surface of target cells is intrinsic to eventual biological response. Further evidence suggesting the plasma membrane as a target for asbestos fibers is the observation that disialogangliosides and high molecular weight glycoproteins on the cell surface are reduced significantly in Syrian hamster embryo cells exposed to crocidolite, chrysotile, or amosite (58). The authors suggest that asbestos interacts with membrane coenzymes which are responsible for construction and maintenance of cell surface glycolipids and glycoproteins rather than masking or removing these moieties.

Intercellular Communication

The observation that tumor promoters disrupt gap junction-mediated cell to cell communication and the hypothesis that a disruption of cell-cell communication is an important component of the complex of events involved in tumor promotion *in vivo* tumor has been suggested numerous times in the literature (55,63,75,80,84,88). The list of soluble chemicals, i.e. known or suspected tumor promoters, which test positively in assays designed to measure alterations in cell-cell communication, is long and diverse. Included in this list are naturally-occurring chemicals of biological origin [phorbol esters (15)]; environmental pollutants [cigarette tar condensates (21), polybrominated biphenyls (81)]; herbicides and pesticides [DDT, lindane (80)]; chemicals related to nutritional chemistry [polyunsaturated fatty acids (3), bile salts (59)]; medicinal drugs [phenobarbital (80), benzoyl peroxide (74)]; and food additives [saccharin (79)].

To determine whether asbestos blocks intercellular communication as does TPA, we began a series of experiments to determine the effects of chrysotile asbestos upon cell-cell communication (i.e., metabolic cooperation) in V-79 Chinese hamster fibroblasts. Table 2 illustrates the results of an assay utilizing V-79 fibroblasts (6-thioguanine sensitive and 6-thioguanine resistant) co-cultivated in the presence of TPA and varying doses of UICC chrysotile asbestos. As can be seen, metabolic cooperation between the two cell types was effectively blocked by TPA but was unaffected by all concentrations of asbestos.

TABLE 2. The effects of TPA and chrysotile asbestos on cell-cell communication in V79 cells (Chinese hamster lung fibroblasts)[a]

Treatment	CFE[b] of 6TG[r]	% recovery 6TG[r] ± SEM
Control	5.75 ± 0.71	20.9 ± 2.6
TPA (0.1 µg/ml)	27.27 ± 1.10	129.4 ± 5.2
UICC chrysotile (0.05 µg/cm^2)	5.58 ± 1.10	18.4 ± 3.6
UICC chrysotile (0.10 µg/cm^2)	6.50 ± 0.70	22.8 ± 2.4
UICC chrysotile (0.15 µg/cm^2)	5.67 ± 0.63	26.1 ± 2.9
UICC chrysotile (0.20 µg/cm^2)	4.00 ± 0.50	25.0 ± 4.4

[a] V79 Chinese hamster lung fibroblasts were cultured in 60 mm tissue culture dishes in medium D, Eagles Minimal Essential Medium modified to include 1.5 x essential aminio acids, 1.5 x vitamins, and 2 x non-essential amino acids, with 5% fetal calf serum. Two separate cell lines, 6-thioguanine-sensitive (6TG^s) and 6-thioguanine-resistant (6TG^r), were co-cultured in a ratio of 5 x 10^5 to 100. Four hours after cell plating, the medium was removed and fresh medium containing either TPA (0.1 µg/ml) or asbestos (0.5-0.20 µg/cm^2) was added to each plate. 6-Thioguanine (10 µg/ml) was included in all the plates. Treatment groups consisted of 10 plates per group and control groups (6TG^r cells plated alone) consisted of 4 plates. Three days after cell plating the medium was decanted and fresh medium containing 6TG was added to all the plates. Four to 5 days later the colonies were rinsed with 0.85% NaCl, fixed with 95% ethanol and stained with Giemsa. Colonies were scored visually, and evaluated with respect to the colony-forming efficiency (CFE) of 6TG^r cells (mean ± S.E.) plated alone.

[b] CFE determined in presence of 5 x 10^5 6-thioguanine sensitive cells.

To confirm our results in another model of cell-cell communication, we utilized a different biological assay, i.e. the passage of [^{3}H]uridine from cells in contact with one another (61). In this bioassay, V-79 fibroblasts were prelabeled with [^{3}H]uridine (i.e., the donor cells) and co-cultured with V-79 cells containing polystyrene beads (i.e., the recipient cells). Autoradiographs of the mixed cell populations were analyzed to detect communicating cell pairs, i.e., presence of label in cells that had phagocytized polystyrene beads. Whereas 72% of the cell pairs appeared to communicate in untreated cultures (Table 3), TPA reduced the percentage of communicating cells to 35%. However, chrysotile was ineffective in blocking communication between the two cell types. Our results are in agreement with a published report in the literature indicating that mineral dusts (amosite asbestos and silica) do not block metabolic cooperation between V79-4 cells (10).

TABLE 3. The effects of TPA and chrysotile asbestos on ^{3}H-uridine transfer in V79 cells (Chinese hamster lung fibroblasts)[a]

Treatment	Concentration	% cell pairs communicating
Control		72
TPA	0.2 µg/ml	35
UICC chrysotile	0.10 µg/cm^2	71
UICC chrysotile	0.15 µg/cm^2	75
UICC chrysotile	0.20 µg/cm^2	79

[a] Two separate populations of wild type (6TG^5) V79 Chinese hamster lung fibroblasts were established. Recipient cells were grown in 75 cm^2 tissue culture flasks in medium D in the presence of polystyrene monodispersed latex beads (Polysciences, Inc., Warrington, PA). Final bead concentration was 6.2×10^7 beads/ml. Donor cells were grown in 35 mm dishes containing cover slips at a density of 8×10^4 cells per coverslip. The cells were grown overnight and labeled the following morning with tritiated uridine (5 µCi/ml, sp. act. 26 Ci/mM). After a 3-hr period of labeling, the donor cells were washed 4 x with PBS followed by the addition of 1 ml fresh medium D. The recipient cells were then trypsinized and plated on top of the donor cells at a final density of 2.4×10^5 cells per coverslip in the 35 mm dish. Following a 7-hr period of cocultivation, the cells were washed 3 x with PBS, fixed with a 2.5% gluteraldehyde solution for 1 hr, rinsed twice with cold 5% TCA, and allowed to air dry. After drying the coverslips were removed from the dishes, mounted on microscope slides and dipped in NBT-2 (Kodak, Rochester, NY) for autoradiography. The slides were developed 6 days later with D-19 developer (Kodak) and stained with 5% Giemsa. The presence of label in recipient cells with beads was recorded in adjacent pairs of cells and expressed as a percentage of cell pairs communicating.

Several phenomena might explain the lack of effects of asbestos in this assay. For example, asbestos fibers, because they are insoluble in liquids, are unlike other tumor promoting chemicals. Thus, they would contact and affect only a small proportion of cells. Secondly, fibroblasts are not the 'target' cells in bronchogenic carcinoma and therefore may be unresponsive to the tumor-promoting activity of asbestos. Lastly, the phagocytic capacity of V79 cells for asbestos is unclear and phagocytosis of fibers might be essential to disruption of cell-cell communication.

Synthesis of Prostglandins

The process of tumor promotion in mouse skin is characterized by a number of events including stimulation of arachidonic acid metabolism and the subsequent synthesis of prostaglandins. The tumor promoting activity of a number of phorbol compounds seems to correlate with their ability to stimulate this pathway (reviewed in 34). At this juncture, we and others have documented increased release of [³H]arachidonic acid and synthesis of prostaglandins in isolated alveolar macrophages (72), in fibroblast-macrophage co-cultures (18), and in hamster tracheal epithelial cells (8). These studies lend additional support to the idea that asbestos can act as a classical tumor promoter such as TPA.

Proliferative Alterations by Asbestos and Other Minerals

Tumor promoters are hyperplastic agents causing proliferation and amplification of intiated cells. Stimulation of ornithine decarboxylase (ODC), a rate-limiting enzyme in the biosynthesis of polyamines, regulatory molecules in cell division and differentiation, appears to occur concomitantly with proliferative alterations in mouse skin (5). Using incorporation of [³H]thymidine as an indication of DNA synthesis, we have examined by autoradiography proliferative changes in tracheal epithelial cells and explants after addition of asbestos and other minerals (7,30,36,39,86). In addition, ODC activity has been monitored at intervals after exposure of epithelial cells to asbestos or TPA (30,36). Results indicate that various types of fibers (glass, crocidolite, chrysotile) induce both increased DNA synthesis and stimulation of ODC. Alternatively, corresponding nonfibrous analogs (i.e., particles of riebeckite, antigorite, glass) do not cause proliferative alterations.

Induction of Squamous Metaplasia by Asbestiform Fibers

The development of carcinomas is a protracted process preceded by a series of morphological and functional changes in epithelium. In the trachea and bronchus, the normal mucociliary epithelium appears to progress through stages of hyperplasia, squamous metaplasia, dysplasia and carcinoma *in situ*. These changes can be reproduced experimentally in organ cultures of rodent and human tracheas (13,22,31,60). Studies from this laboratory have indicated that crocidolite, amosite and chrysotile asbestos, as well as various types of fiberglass, can induce hyperplastic and metaplastic changes in hamster trachea (45,51,86,87). As indicated above, the fibrous geometry of minerals appears critical in the induction of basal cell hyperplasia and squamous metaplasia--nonfibrous particulates produced no metaplasia in comparison to fibers.

The establishment of hyperplasia and squamous metaplasia in tracheobronchial epithelial cells is not an irreversible process. For example, the administration of analogs of vitamin A (i.e., retinoids) can restore the normal mucociliary epithelium in animals with metaplastic changes induced by a dietary deficiency of vitamin A (37,62,85). Moreover, retinoids can inhibit the occurrence of squamous metaplasia associated with chemical carcinogens (32) and reverse metaplastic changes caused by vitamin A deficiency in tracheal tissues *in vitro* (11).

The observations above are intriguing and suggest a possible prophylatic and/or therapeutic use of retinoids in the prevention of fiber-associated metaplasia. To address this question, we have examined the ability of retinoids to inhibit the development of squamous metaplasia caused by crocidolite and amosite asbestos in hamster tracheal organ cultures (45). Alternatively, the reversal of pre-established metaplasia associated with crocidolite has been documented in this bioassay (9) (Fig. 5). Under both circumstances, the effects of vitamin A are related directly to dosage.

Inflammation and the Importance of Oxygen Free Radicals in Tumor Promotion

The induction of a rapid inflammatory response by phorbol ester tumor promoters in mouse skin appears related directly to their potency (67). In support of this hypothesis, a number of steroidal anti-inflammatory agents inhibit tumor promotion by phorbol compounds. We and others (78) have documented in tracheal grafts massive inflammation after insertion of chrysotile and crocidolite asbestos into the tracheal lumen (Fig. 6). In contrast, nonasbestos minerals (i.e., erionite, hematite, sepiolite) do not induce striking influxes of lymphocytes and polymorphonuclear leukocytes from the host animal (Mossman and Jean, manuscript in preparation).

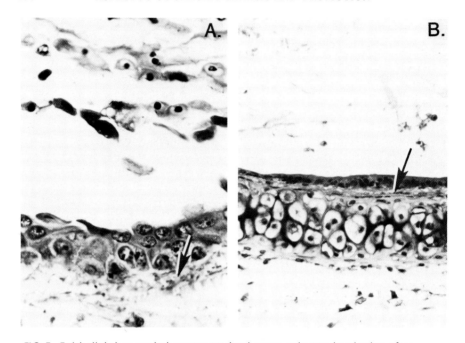

FIG. 5. Epithelial changes in hamster tracheal organ cultures developing after exposure to crocidolite asbestos (A) and crocidolite with subsequent addition of the vitamin A analog, β-retinyl acetate (B). After a 1-hr exposure to crocidolite (4 mg/ml medium), the tissues were maintained for 3 weeks before addition of medium alone (A) or containing β-retinyl acetate (10^{-7}M) (B). At 4 weeks, explants were prepared for histology. Note the squamous epithelium in A and the regenerating columnar epithelium in B. Arrows indicate the basal lamina. Hematoxylin and eosin, A = × 800; B = × 250.

What is the relevance of inflammation to tumor promotion? One school of thought (reviewed in 17) suggests that production of oxygen free radicals, reactive species which can damage DNA and cause membrane perturbations, by inflammatory cell types is intrinsic to tumor promotion. This theory is supported by the observation that antioxidants and scavengers of oxygen free radicals inhibit TPA-mediated cellular alterations and tumor promotion in mouse skin (25,26). Moreover, generators of oxygen free radicals such as benzoyl peroxide act as tumor promoters in the mouse skin bioassay (74).

To determine whether asbestos-induced cell damage is mediated by oxygen free radicals, we have administered scavengers of oxygen free radicals simultaneously with asbestos or fiberglass to tracheal epithelial cells (50,54) and organ cultures (53). Cell damage has been

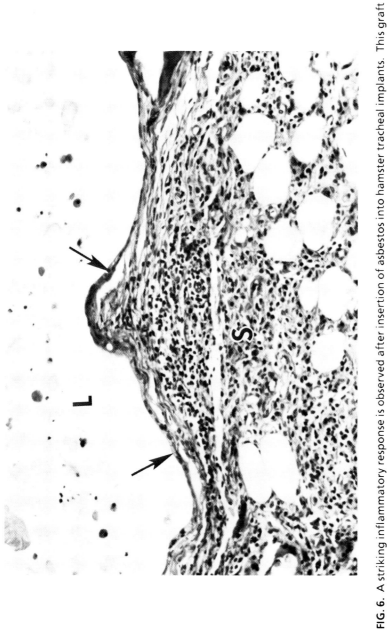

FIG. 6. A striking inflammatory response is observed after insertion of asbestos into hamster tracheal implants. This graft was maintained in a syngeneic hamster for 4 weeks before injection of 100 μg of chrysotile asbestos into the lumen. The trachea was removed and prepared for histology at 40 weeks thereafter. Note the accumulation of inflammatory cells in the submucosa (S) and the lumen (L) of the tissue. The arrows delineate the epithelium. Hematoxylin and eosin, × 1,400.

quantitated over a 24-hr period using a [^{75}Se]methionine incorporation assay in cell cultures (35) and measurement of amounts of the soluble enzyme, lactic dehydrogenase, in the medium of organ cultures (16). After simultaneous introduction with fibers, SOD (the enzyme scavenging superoxide, $O_2^{\pm}$) and scavengers (mannitol, sodium benzoate, dimethylthiourea) of the hydroxyl radical (OH•) inhibit toxicity associated with long fibers (>10 μm) of chrysotile and UICC preparations of chrysotile and crocidolite asbestos, but not toxicity caused by fiberglass or short (≤2 μm) chrysotile. In support of these findings, activity of SOD is increased in tracheal epithelial cells after prolonged addition of UICC asbestos preparations, but not after exposure of cells to fiberglass at comparable concentrations (54,71). Release of $O_2^{\pm}$ into medium also occurs after addition of various fibers to cultures of tracheal epithelial cells and macrophages (16). More generation of $O_2^{\pm}$ is observed with use of long (>10 μm) fibers in epithelial cells whereas production of $O_2^{\pm}$ by the latter cell type appears to be unrelated to fiber type and length.

Results summarized above suggest that short-term (i.e., ≤24 hr) asbestos-induced toxicity is mediated by oxygen free radicals generated presumably after membrane interaction and phagocytosis of fibers. Longer fibers appear to be more toxic to a variety of cells types due to their incomplete phagocytosis leading to prolonged perturbation of the plasma membrane (16).

In recent studies we have explored the effects of SOD and the SOD-mimetic compound Cu(II)(3,5-diisopropyl salicylate)$_2$ (CuDIPS) (33) on inhibition of colony formation by chrysotile asbestos in monolayer cultures of tracheal epithelial cells (Fig. 7). Scavengers were added simultaneously with asbestos at cell plating and colonies of cells were counted to assess cell survival at 7-10 days thereafter. Although complete dose-response studies with other scavengers are warranted, these experiments thus far demonstrate an inability of the scavenging compounds, SOD and CuDIPS, to protect against the long-term effects of asbestos on inhibition of cell growth. To allow additional investigation of the possible importance of oxygen free radicals in asbestos-induced cell proliferation and squamous metaplasia, we are pursuing presently the encapsulation of scavengers in liposomes (82) and coupling to polyethylene glycol (2) to preserve their biologic half-life in medium.

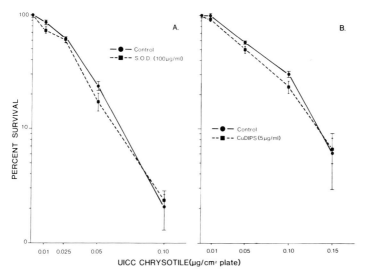

FIG. 7. Toxicity of various concentrations of chrysotile asbestos after addition to HTE cells. Cells were seeded at 2×10^2 in 60 mm dishes and asbestos was added 4 hr after plating. SOD (100 µg/ml) or CuDIPS (5 µg/ml) (i.e., nontoxic concentrations determined previously) was added simultaneously. At 10 days thereafter, plates were fixed in 95% ethanol and stained with Giemsa for determination of numbers of colonies. Data are expressed as Mean ± S.E. in comparison to the percent survival in untreated control cultures. Neither scavenger appears to prevent abestos-associated toxicity.

SUMMARY

Epidemiologic (4,68,69) and experimental (64,70,76) studies document a synergistic effect of asbestos and smoking in the induction of bronchogenic carcinoma. Whereas the increased risk of these cancers in nonsmoking asbestos workers is 4-fold or less in comparison to non-smokers in the general population, individuals who smoke and are exposed to asbestos occupationally have a 80-90 fold increased risk. The observations summarized above provide substantial insight into the interactions between asbestos and chemical carcinogens in cigarette smoke at the cellular level (Fig. 8). On the one hand, asbestos fibers and other particulates appear to act as condensation nuclei for PAH in the occupational setting or environment (56). They then facilitate the transfer of these chemical carcinogens into target cells, i.e., those destined to develop into tumor cells. As a result, the adduct formation of PAH to DNA is encouraged, an event linked intrinsically to initiation of transformation. Alternatively, asbestos appears to enhance and modulate the further development of initiated cells to neoplastic cells by a process resembling tumor promotion in mouse skin. In this regard, the most dramatic example illustrating the importance of asbestos in two-stage carcinogenesis is an experiment by Topping and Nettesheim (77). These investigators inserted the PAH, 7,12-dimethyl-benz(a)anthracene (DMBA) into the lumen of rat trachea which then were implanted on syngeneic animals. Subsequently, chrysotile asbestos was introduced, and grafts were removed for histology when palpable tumors occurred. At non-tumorigenic (i.e., initiating) amounts of DMBA, asbestos promoted the development of malignancies, although two neoplasms were observed with use of asbestos alone. Asbestos was not carcinogenic at these amounts, but a low incidence (5%) of squamous cell carcinoma was observed with use of chrysotile alone at much higher concentrations. These results suggest that asbestos is a weak carcinogen, but more importantly a promoter of carcinogenesis in the respiratory tract. Studies in this laboratory show striking effects of asbestos fibers on cell proliferation and differentiation although these responses appear to occur also after exposure of tracheobronchial cells to nonasbestos fibers including fiberglass.

ACKNOWLEDGEMENTS

This work was supported by grants PHS R01-33501 from the National Cancer Institute and BC-415 from the American Cancer Society. Dr. Cameron is a postdoctoral fellow supported by Environmental Pathology Training grant PHS T32-07122 from the National Institute of Environmental Health Sciences. Dr. Yotti is a postdoctoral fellow supported by Cancer Biology Training grant PHS T32-09286 from the National Cancer Institute. Ms. Rhonda Gilbert, Ms. Lucie Jean, Ms. Joanne Marsh, Ms. Joan Carrassi, and Ms. Judith Kessler provided valuable technical assistance.

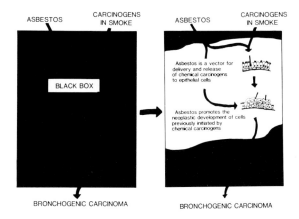

FIG. 8. A hypothetical schema indicating possible interactions between asbestos and chemical carcinogens in the causation of bronchogenic carcinoma. [Supplied by Dr. Craig Woodworth, now at the Department of Microbiology, College of Medicine, Milton-Hershey Medical Center, Hershey, PA].

REFERENCES

1. Adler, K. B., Mossman, B. T., Butler, G., Jean, L., and Craighead, J. E. (1984): *Exp. Lung Res.*, in press.
2. Abuchowski, A., van Es, T., Palczuk, N. C., and Davis, E. F. (1977): *J. Biol. Chem.*, 252:3578-3581.
3. Aylsworth, C. F., Jones, C., Trosko, J. E., Meites, J., and Welsch, C. W. (1984): *J. Natl. Cancer Inst.*, 72:637-646.
4. Berry, G., Newhouse, M. L., and Turok, M. (1972): *Lancet*, 2:476-479.
5. Boutwell, R. K. (1978): In: *Carcinogenesis - A Comprehensive Survey, Vol. 2: Mechanisms of Tumor Promotion and Cocarcinogenesis*, edited by T. J. Slaga, A. Sivak, and R. K. Boutwell, pp. 49-58. Raven Press, New York.
6. Brody, A. R., George, G., and Hill, L. H. (1983): *Lab. Invest.*, 49:468-475.
7. Brown, R. C., Gormley, I. P., Chamberlain, M., and Davies, R., editors (1980): *The In Vitro Effects of Mineral Dusts.* Academic Press, London.
8. Cameron, G. C., and Mossman, B. T. (1984): *Proc. Am. Assoc. Cancer Res.*, 25:143.
9. Cameron, G. S., and Mossman, B. T. (1984): In: *Proceedings of EPA Symposium on Tumor Promotion and Enhancement in the Etiology of Human and Experimental Respiratory Tract Carcinogenesis*, p. 46.
10. Chamberlain, M. (1983): *Environ. Health Perspect.*, 51:5-9.
11. Chopra, D. P. (1983): *Eur. J. Cancer Clin. Oncol.*, 19:847-857.
12. Craighead, J. E., and Mossman, B. T. (1979): *Prog. Exp. Tumor Res.*, 24:48-58.
13. Cocker, T. T., and Sanders, L. L. (1970): *Cancer Res.*, 30:1312-1318.
14. Eastman, A., Mossman, B. T., and Bresnick, E. (1983): *Cancer Res.*, 43:1251-1258.

15. Fitzgerald, D. J., and Murray, A. W. (1980): *Cancer Res.*, 40:2935-2937.
16. Gerhardt, W., Kofoed, B., Westlund, L., and Pavlu, B. (1974): *Scand. J. Clin. Lab. Invest.*, 33:287-306.
17. Goldstein, B., Witz, G., Zimmerman, J., and Gee, C. (1983): In: *Oxygen Radicals and Their Scavenger Systems, Vol. II: Cellular and Medical Aspects*, edited by R. A. Greenwald, and G. Cohen, pp. 321-325. Elsevier Science Publishing, New York.
18. Goldstein, R. H., Miller, K., Glassroth, J., Linscott, R., Snider, G. L., Franzblau, C., and Polgar, P. (1982): *J. Lab. Clin. Med.*, 100:778-785.
19. Harington, J. S. (1976): *Annales d'Anatomie Pathologique*, 21:155-198.
20. Harington, J. S., Miller, K., and Macnab, G. (1971): *Environ. Res.*, 4:95-117.
21. Hartman, T. G., and Rosen, J. E. (1983): *Proc. Natl. Acad. Sci. USA*, 80:5305-5309.
22. Haugen, A., Schafer, P. W., Lechner, J. F., Stoner, G. D., and Trump, B. F. (1982): *Int. J. Cancer*, 30:265-272.
23. Jaurand, M. C., Thomassin, J. H., Baillif, P., Magne, L., Touray, J. C., and Bignon, J. (1980): *Brit. J. Ind. Med.*, 37:169-174.
24. Kennedy, A. R., and Little, J. B. (1974): *Cancer Res.*, 34:1344-1352.
25. Kensler, T. W., Bush, D. M., and Kozumbo, W. J. (1983): *Science*, 221:75-77.
26. Kozumbo, W. J., Seed, J. L., and Kensler, T. W. (1983): *Cancer Res.*, 43:2555-2559.
27. Lakowicz, J. R., and Bevan, D. R. (1979): *Biochemistry*, 18:5170-5176.
28. Lakowicz, J. R., and Bevan, D. R. (1980): *Chem. Biol. Interact.*, 29:129-138.
29. Lakowicz, J. R., McNamara, M., and Steenson, L. (1978): *Science*, 199:305-306.
30. Landesman, J. M., and Mossman, B. T. (1982): *Cancer Res.*, 42:3669-3675.
31. Lane, B. P., and Miller, S. L. (1974): In: *Experimental Lung Cancer: Carcinogenesis and Bioassays*, edited by E. Karbe, and J. F. Park, pp. 507-513. Springer-Verlag, New York.
32. Lasnitzki, I., and Goodman, D. S. (1974): *Cancer Res.*, 34:1564-1571.
33. Leuthauser, S. W. C., Oberley, L. W., Oberley, T. D., Sorenson, J. R. J., and Ramakrishna, K. (1981): *J. Natl. Cancer Inst.*, 66:1077-1081.
34. Levine, L. (1981): *Adv. Cancer Res.*, 35:49-79.
35. Liebold, W., and Bridge, S. (1979): *Immun.-Forsch.*, 155:287-311.
36. Marsh, J. P., and Mossman, B. T. (1984): *Proc. Am. Assoc. Cancer Res.*, 25:143.
37. McDowell, E. M., Keenan, K. P., and Huang, M. (1984): *Virchows Arch. Cell Pathol.*, 45:221-240.
38. Morgan, W. K. C., and Seaton, A. (1975): *Occupational Lung Diseases*. W. B. Saunders Co., Philadelphia.
39. Mossman, B. T., Adler, K. B., and Craighead, J. E. (1978): *Environ. Res.*, 16:110-118.
40. Mossman, B. T., Adler, K. B., Jean, L., and Craighead, J. E. (1982): *Chest*, 81S:23-25S.
41. Mossman, B. T., and Craighead, J. E. (1975): *Proc. Soc. Exp. Biol. Med.*, 149:227-233.
42. Mossman, B. T., and Craighead, J. E. (1979): *Prog. Exp. Tumor Res.*, 24:37-47.
43. Mossman, B. T., and Craighead, J. E. (1981): *Environ. Res.*, 25:269-289.
44. Mossman, B. T., and Craighead, J. E. (1982): In: *Inhaled Particles, V: Ann. Occup. Hyg., Vol. 26.*, pp. 553-567. Pergamon Press, London.
45. Mossman, B. T., Craighead, J. E., and MacPherson, B. V. (1980): *Science*, 207:311-313.

46. Mossman, B. T., Eastman, A., and Bresnick, E. (1983): *Environ. Health Perspect.*, 51:331-335.
47. Mossman, B. T., Ezerman, E. B., Adler, K. B., and Craighead, J. E. (1980): *Cancer Res.*, 40:4403-4409.
48. Mossman, B. T., Halleron, P. A., and Craighead, J. E. (1980): *J. Cell Biol.*, 83:288a.
49. Mossman, B. T., Jean, L., and Landesman, J. M. (1983): *Environ. Health Perspect.*, 51:23-25.
50. Mossman, B. T., and Landesman, J. M. (1983): *Chest*, 83S:50-51S.
51. Mossman, B. T., Ley, B. W., Kessler, J., and Craighead, J. E. (1977): *Lab. Invest.*, 36:131-139.
52. Mossman, B. T., Light, W., and Wei, E. (1983): *Ann. Rev. Pharmacol. Toxicol.*, 23:595-615.
53. Mossman, B. T., and Marsh, J. P. (1984): Submitted for publication.
54. Mossman, B. T., Marsh, J. P., and Shatos, M. A. (1984): Submitted for publication.
55. Murray, A. W., and Fitzgerald, D. J. (1979): *Biochem. Biophys. Res. Comm.*, 91:395-401.
56. Natusch, E. F. S., and Wallace, J. R. (1974): *Science*, 183:202-204.
57. Nettesheim, P. (1972): *Prog. Exp. Tumor Res.*, 16:185-200.
58. Newman, H. A. I., Saat, Y. A., and Hart, R. W. (1980): In: *The In Vitro Effects of Mineral Dusts*, edited by R. C. Brown, M. Chamberlain, R. Davies, and I. P. Gormley, pp. 147-157. Academic Press, London.
59. Noda, K., Umeda, M., and Ono, T. (1981): *Gann.*, 71:614-620.
60. Palekar, L., Kuschner, M., and Laskin, S. (1968): *Cancer Res.*, 28:2098-2104.
61. Pitts, J. D., and Simms, J. W. (1977): *Exp. Cell Res.*, 104:153-163.
62. Port C. D., Baxte, D. W., and Harris, C. C. (1974): In: *Experimental Lung Cancer: Carcinogenesis and Bioassays*, edited by E. Karbe, and J. F. Park, pp. 257-264. Springer-Verlag, New York.
63. Potter, V. R. (1980): *Yale J. Biol. Med.*, 53:367-384.
64. Reeves, A. L., Pylev, L. M., Krivosheeva, L. V., Kulagino, T. F., and Nemenko, B. A. (1974): *Environ. Res.*, 8:178.
65. Saffiotti, U., Cefis, F., and Kolb, L. H. (1968): *Cancer Res.*, 28:104-124.
66. Saffiotti, U., Montesano, R., Sellakumar, A. R., Cefis, F., and Kaufman, D. G. (1972): *Cancer Res.*, 32:1073-1081.
67. Scribner, J. D., and Boutwell, R. K. (1972): *Eur. J. Cancer*, 8:617-621.
68. Selikoff, I. J., Hammond, E. C., and Churg, J. (1968): *J. Am. Med. Assn.*, 204:104-110.
69. Selikoff, I. J., Seidman, H., and Hammond, E. C. (1980): *J. Natl. Cancer Inst.*, 65:507-513.
70. Shabad, L. M., Puro, H. E., and Smith, R. G. (1974): *J. Natl. Cancer Inst.*, 52:1175.
71. Shatos M. A., Marsh, J. P., Woodcock-Mitchell, J., Orfeo, T., Burkhardt, A., and Mossman, B. T. (1984): *Am. Rev. Respir. Dis.*, 129:A151.
72. Sirois, P., Rolla-Pleszczynski, M., and Begin, R. (1980): *Prostagland. Med.*, 5:31-37.
73. Sivak A., Mossman, B. T., and Van Duuren, B. L. (1972): *Biochem. Biophys. Res. Commun.*, 56:605-609.
74. Slaga, T. J., Klein-Szanto, A. J. P., Triplett, L. C., Yotti, L. P., and Trosko, J. E. (1981): *Science*, 213:1023-1025.

75. Slaga, T. J., Sivak, A., and Boutwell, R. K., editors (1978): *Carcinogenesis - A Comprehensive Survey, Vol 2: Mechanisms of Tumor Promotion and Cocarcinogenesis.* Raven Press, New York.

76. Smith, W. E., Miller, L., and Churg, J. (1968): *Proc. Am. Assoc. Cancer Res.,* 9:65.

77. Topping, D. C., and Nettesheim, P. (1980); *J. Natl. Cancer Inst.,* 65:627-630.

78. Topping, D., Nettesheim, P., and Martin, D. (1980); *J. Environ. Path. Toxicol.,* 3:261-275.

79. Trosko, J. E., Dawson, B., Yotti, L. P., and Chang, C. C. (1980): *Nature,* 284:109-110.

80. Trosko, J. E., Yotti, L. P., Warren, S. T., Tsushimoto, G., and Chagn, C. C. (1982): In: *Carcinogenesis - A Comprehensive Survey, Vol. 7: Cocarcinogenesis and Biological Effects of Tumor Promoters,* edited by E. Hecker, N. E. Fusenig, W. Kunz, F. Marks, and H. W. Thielman, pp. 565-585. Raven Press, New York.

81. Tsushimoto, G., Trosko, J. E., Chang, C. C., and Aust, S. D. (1982): *Carcinogenesis,* 3:181-185.

82. Turrens, J. F., Crapo, J. D., and Freeman, B. A. (1984): *J. Clin. Invest.,* 73:87-95.

83. Wagner, W. L., Rom, W. N., and Merchant, J. A., editors (1983): *Health Issues Related to Metal and Nonmetallic Mining.* Butterworth Publishers, Boston.

84. Williams, G. M. (1981) *Food Cosmet. Toxicol.,* 19:577-583.

85. Wolbach, S. B., and Howe, P. R. (1933): *J. Exp. Med.,* 57:511-526.

86. Woodworth, C. D., Mossman, B. T., and Craighead, J. E. (1983): *Cancer Res.,* 43:4906-4912.

87. Woodworth, C. D., Mossman, B. T., and Craighead, J. E. (1983): *Lab. Invest.,* 48:578-584.

88. Yotti, L. P., Chang, C. C., and Trosko, J. E. (1979) *Science,* 206:1089-1091.

Carcinogenesis, Vol. 8, edited by M. J. Mass et al.
Raven Press, New York © 1985.

New Aspects of Tobacco Carcinogenesis

Dietrich Hoffmann, Assieh Melikian, John D. Adams,
Klaus D. Brunnemann, and Nancy J. Haley

*Naylor Dana Institute for Disease Prevention, American Health Foundation,
Valhalla, New York 10595*

Lung cancer is causally associated with cigarette smoking as is well documented in the Surgeon General's Reports on Smoking and Health (26,28). The criteria to establish a causal relationship, in the manner postulated by Robert Koch (30), are in this case: the consistency and strength of the epidemiological data, a dose response effect, the minimal risk for lung cancer of nonsmokers who are not exposed to occupational risk factors, the decrease in cancer incidence upon cessation of smoking and the identification of a variety of agents in the smoke that induce cancer in laboratory animals. Despite the extensive data base for the carcinogenicity of tobacco smoke, some aspects require further elucidation in the laboratory. In this presentation, we will discuss our recent laboratory studies which address some of the unresolved issues and some of the new questions raised. Specifically, they are the following: studies on the cocarcinogenic activity of catechol, the endogenous formation of nicotine-derived carcinogens, and the uptake of tobacco smoke components from polluted respiratory environments by the nonsmokers.

CATECHOLS AS COCARCINOGENS

Early model studies by Van Duuren and Goldschmidt (29) and detailed fractionation experiments by our group have demonstrated that, in mouse skin bioassays, catechols are the major cocarcinogens in tobacco smoke (9). Recently, we have explored the nature of precursors for the pyrosynthesis of catechols during smoking and studied the effect of catechol on benzo(a)pyrene carcinogenesis in mouse skin.

Tobacco Precursors for Catechols in the Smoke

For the precursor study, we extracted tobacco sequentially with hexane and methanol-H_2O and the extracts as well as the extracted residue were pyrolyzed at 650° (4). The analysis of the pyrolysis products demonstrated that the methanol-H_2O extract and the tobacco residue were good precursors for the pyrosynthesis of catechol (Table 1). The methanol-H_2O extract was further fractionated. Subfractions were obtained by high-pressure liquid chromatography (HPLC) and were subsequently pyrolyzed. Fructose, glucose, sucrose and cholorogenic acid, a tobacco polyphenol, were identified as important pyrolytic precursors for catechol.

Analysis of pyrolysis products of the extraction residue showed that cellulose, which comprises 5-12% of the tobacco leaf, is a good pyrolytic precursor for catechol. In order to confirm the findings of the pyrolysis experiments, we added to tobacco either various levels of chlorogenic acid, rutin, or [^{14}C(U)]fructose or [^{14}C(U)]cellulose, isolated from tobacco grown in a $^{14}CO_2$-atmosphere. The cigarettes, so prepared, were smoked and the mainstream smoke was analyzed for catechol. Table 2 presents the estimate of the contribution of a number of individual tobacco constituents to the overall yield of catechol in cigarette smoke. Based on these data, we suggest that pectin, starch, and hemicellulose are also precursors for catechol.

We are now exploring whether derivatization of tobacco polysaccharides can serve as a means of reducing smoke yields of catechols. Although this approach is primarily of academic interest, it has the potential to reduce the levels of the cocarcinogenic catechols in cigarette smoke. This group of compounds is the most important contributor to the carcinogenic potential of tobacco smoke.

The Effect of Catechol on Benzo(a)pyrene (BP)-Metabolism

In order to measure the effect of catechol on the metabolism of BP we treated the skin of mice with acetone solutions containing either 15 µg [^{3}H]BP alone or a mixture of 15 µg [^{3}H]BP with 500 µg of catechol. The mice were sacrificed 30 min, 2, 4, 8 and 24 hr after the treatment. The epidermal layer of the treated skin was separated, homogenized and the organic soluble metabolites were analyzed by HPLC. The aqueous phase was hydrolzyed by β-glucuronidase and aryl sulfatase.

Figure 1 shows that the patterns of disappearance of radioactivity observed in groups treated with [^{3}H]BP alone, and those treated with [^{3}H]BP plus catechol, are similar. This indicates that catechol appears to have no major effect on the removal of [^{3}H]BP from the skin. The middle curve suggests a slight increase in total organic phase radioactivity recovered from the epidermis of mice treated with

TABLE 1. Catechol in pyrolyzates of tobacco and its extracts at 650°

Material pyrolyzed	% of tobacco		μg of catechol in pyrolyzate		% conversion to catechol	
	Bright	1R1	Bright	1R1	Bright	1R1
Whole tobacco	100	100	2230	1590	0.064	0.045
Hexane extract	4	5	5	n.d.[a]	0.003	n.d.
Methanol-H_2O extract	31	31	2090	1900	0.19	0.18
Extracted residue	71	63	2680	1000	0.11	0.046

[a] n.d., not determined

TABLE 2. Estimate of contribution to smoke catechol

Tobacco constituent	% contribution
Chlorogenic acid	13
Fructose + glucose + sucrose	4
Cellulose	7-12
Pectin	n.d.[a]
Starch	n.d.
Hemicellulose	n.d.

[a]n.d., not determined

mixtures of BP and catechol relative to results obtained with BP alone. The lower curves represent the total radioactivity recovered from the aqueous phase. In this case, there appears to be a significant decrease in groups treated with mixtures of [3H]BP and catechol, especially at the 30-min time point, compared to findings upon treatment with [3H]BP alone. This indicates that catechol somehow blocks the detoxification path of BP metabolism. This, in turn, may increase the formation of such metabolites as BP-7,8-diol which can be further converted to diol-epoxides and bind to cellular macromolecules. This concept is reemphasized in Fig. 2 which shows that the total nonpolar metabolites of BP are not greatly influenced by the concurrent treatment of mouse skin with catechol while, at the four time intervals measured, formation of polar metabolites of BP is increased compared to mouse skin treated with BP alone.

Figure 3 details this observation. The left column of each set depicts the nonpolar metabolites with BP-3-OH as a subcolumn. The center column represents the polar metabolites including sulfates and glucuronides of BP, and the right column shows the BP-7,8-diol.

According to these data, especially at the 1/2 and 2-hr time points, the mixture of BP and catechol causes formation of significantly less of the individual polar metabolites and significantly more of the BP-7,8-diol than does BP alone. Currently, we are measuring the BP-DNA adduct formation in mouse skin at several time points in order to verify whether the cocarcinogenicity of catechol can be associated with an increase in the metabolic activation and DNA binding of BP.

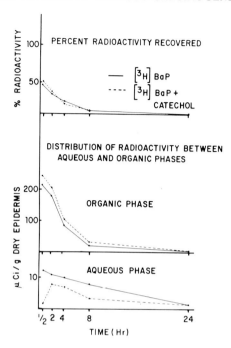

FIG. 1. Recovery of radioactivity from mouse skin with [³H]BP or with [³H]BP plus catechol.

ENDOGENOUS FORMATION OF NICOTINE-DERIVED N-NITROSAMINES

Until a few years ago, our major emphasis in tobacco carcinogenesis had been placed on the identification and quantitation of tumor intiators, tumor promoters, cocarcinogens and organ-specific carcinogens in tobacco products and tobacco smoke, and their mode of action in laboratory animals (18,19). These studies included the documentation of the tobacco-specific N-nitrosamines (TSNA) as a major group of carcinogens in processed tobacco, especially in snuff, and in main- and sidestream smoke of tobacco products (10,16). These nitrosamines are formed primarily from nicotine and, to a limited extent, from the minor tobacco alkaloids (Fig 4; 14). TSNA in tobacco products amount to the highest reported concentrations of nitrosamines in nonoccupational environments. The TSNA can add up to 100 ppm in snuff and to 2.0 µg/cigarette in mainstream smoke (Table 3). Of the

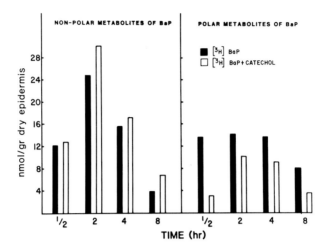

FIG. 2. Polar and nonpolar metabolites in mouse skin treated with [³H]BP or with [³H]BP plus catechol.

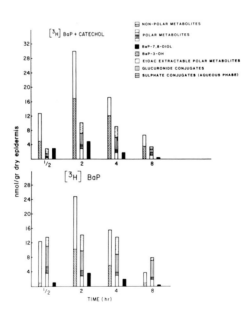

FIG. 3. Metabolites in mouse skin treated with [³H]BP or with [³H]BP plus catechol at different time points.

four TSNA, N'-nitrosonornicotine (NNN) and 4-(methyl-nitrosamino)-1-(3-pyridyl)-1-butanone (NNK) are strong carcinogens in mice, rats and Syrian golden hamsters (10,14,17). In F344 rats, both NNN and NNK induce significant numbers of tumors in the nasal cavity when 9, 3 or 1 mmol/kg is administered intraperitoneally. NNK also causes tumors in the lung and, at the high dose level, in the liver, whereas NNN induces, at the 2 higher dose levels also tumors of the esophagus in addition to tumors of the nasal cavity (Table 4; 17).

FORMATION OF TOBACCO SPECIFIC NITROSAMINES (TSNA)

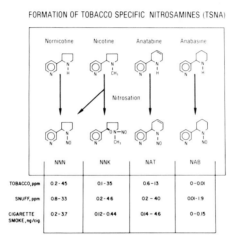

FIG. 4. Formation of tobacco specific nitrosamines (TSNA) from nicotine and minor alkaloids.

A most important observation relates to the fact that these carcinogens can also be formed in the oral cavity during tobacco chewing and snuff dipping (13) and, most likely, from nicotine upon smoke inhalation. It is difficult to document the endogenous formation of NNN and NNK from nicotine upon tobacco smoke inhalation, since it is hardly possible to differentiate between inhaled and endogenously formed nitrosamines and since nicotine, NNN and NNK are metabolized within a few minutes. Furthermore, NNN and NNK form the same metabolites as nicotine (1,10). We are currently developing a method for measuring the concentrations of the TSNA in smokers' blood by utilizing post-labeling techniques. We have already established that snuff and cigarette smoke have measurable potentials for the endogenous formation of nitrosamines (2,15).

TABLE 3. Tobacco-specific N-nitrosamines in chewing tobacco, snuff, and tobacco mainstream smoke

| | Tobacco-specific N-nitrosamines | | |
Tobacco products	NNN	NNK	NAT
Smokeless tobacco (ppm)			
Chewing tobacco - U.S.A.	3.5 - 8.2	0.1 - 3.0	0.5 - 7.0
Chewing tobacco - India	2.4	n.d.[a]	n.d.
Snuff - U.S.A.	0.8 - 89	0.2 - 8.3	0.2 - 4.0[b]
Snuff - Sweden	2.0 - 6.7	0.6 - 1.5	0.9 - 2.4[c]
Snuff - Denmark	4.5 - 8.0	1.4 - 7.0	2.6 - 6.2
Snuff - Bavaria	6.0 - 6.8	1.5 - 1.6	3.9 - 4.4
Mainstream smoke (ng/cig)			
Cigarettes - U.S.A.	120 - 1000	80 - 770	140 - 1000[d]
Cigarettes - Germany	120 - 510	20 - 80	40 - 200
Cigarettes - France	600 - 1000	190 - 220	190 - 200
Little Cigar - U.S.A.	400	160	530
Cigar	3200	1900	1900

[a]n.d., not determined
[b]NAB 0.01 - 1.9 ppm
[c]NAB 0.04 - 0.14 ppm
[d]NAB 120 ng/cigarette

TABLE 4. Numbers and percentages of F344 rats with tumors after treatment with NNN, NNK, or NAT[a]

Treatment group (total dose)	Effective number of rats	% of rats with nasal tumors	% of rats with lung tumors	% of rats with liver tumors	% of rats with esophageal tumors
I. NNN (9.0 mmol/kg)	14 M	86	0	0	29
	15 F	100	7	0	20
II. NNN (3.0 mmol/kg)	15 M	73	33	13	33
	15 F	60	7	0	13
III. NNN (1.0 mmol/kg)	27 M	56	14	0	4
	27 F	44	20	7	4
IV. NNK (9.0 mmol/kg)	15 M	93	93	40	0
	15 F	93	60	33	0
V. NNK (3.0 mmol/kg)	15 M	87	87	27	7
	15 F	80	47	27	0
VI. NNK (1.0 mmol/kg)	27 M	74	85	11	4
	27 F	37	30	15	0
VII. Trioctanoin	26 M	0	0	12	0
	26 F	0	0	4	0

[a]intraperitoneal administration

According to Ohshima and Bartsch (23), proline is endogenously nitrosated to the nonmetabolizing and noncarcinogenic N-nitroso-proline (NPRO) by nitrite furnished as a dietary component. NPRO is excreted exclusively in the urine (23). In order to examine whether endogenous NPRO formation also would occur in smokers, we placed these and a control group of nonsmokers on identical diets (15). On day 3, we collected a 24-hr urine sample and determined the concentration of NPRO. As depicted in Fig. 5, significantly more NPRO was present in urine of cigarette smokers than in that of nonsmokers. The difference in urinary NPRO is further increased upon enriching the diet with proline. The endogenous formation of NPRO is proven by the fact that urinary output of NPRO in the smoker can be diminished to the levels found in urine of nonsmokers when ascorbic acid is added to the diet. The effectiveness of this known inhibitor of N-nitrosation (22) indicates a practical approach for the prevention of endogenous nitrosamine formation including formation of the carcinogenic nicotine-derived nitrosamines. Similar to vitamin C, such inhibition has also been observed for vitamin E. In fact, several studies have strongly indicated that cigarette smokers on vitamin-rich diets have a somewhat reduced risk of cancer compared to those on vitamin-deficient diets (3). The endogenous formation of nitrosamines as a result of snuff-dipping can likely also be inhibited by dietary factors. Recently, we found that 30 snuff-dipping college students had higher concentrations of urinary NPRO than students who are not using tobacco. Students in both groups were on identical diets and had similar physical activities.

The endogenous formation of nicotine-derived carcinogens gains additional significance in considering the apparently syncarcinogenic or cocarcinogenic effects of smoking and asbestos. In model studies, the surface of cellulose acetate, amosite, and β-chrysotile was sprayed with nicotine and subsequently exposed to a stream of either 90 ppm of nitrogen dioxide or to cigarette smoke which contained 280 μg/cigarette of nitrogen oxides. The surface of chrysotile accelerated nitrosamine formation to a significantly greater extent than the surfaces of cellulose acetate and amosite (Fig. 6).

We have found in preliminary studies that instillation of diethanolamine-containing chrysotile into the lungs and subsequent inhalation of an air stream containing 90 ppm of nitrogen dioxide leads to formation of nitrosodiethanolamine. Confirmation of the same reaction by cigarette smoke inhalation experiments would give increased weight to the possibility that endogenous formation of

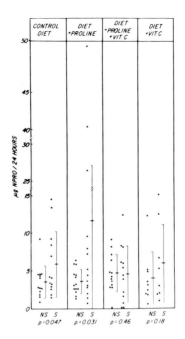

FIG. 5. N-nitrosoproline in 24 hr urine samples of male smokers and nonsmokers.

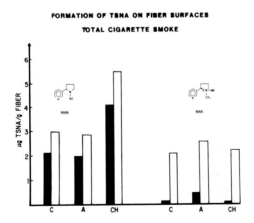

FIG. 6. Formation of TSNA on fibrous surfaces exposed to cigarette smoke.

nicotine-derived nitrosamines plays a role in the increased risk for cancer of the lung of asbestos workers who smoke cigarettes (8,27).

UPTAKE OF TOBACCO SMOKE CONSTITUENTS BY NONSMOKERS IN SMOKE POLLUTED ENVIRONMENTS

Since 1981, a number of epidemiological studies have indicated an increased risk of lung cancer for nonsmoking spouses of cigarette smokers (5,11,12,25). The significance of these findings was questioned in other studies (6,20,21). A major question in the risk assessment concerns the uptake of tobacco smoke by nonsmokers in smoke polluted environments. In order to measure this uptake, we exposed non-smokers under controlled conditions in a small room to various doses of sidestream smoke from cigarettes (Table 5). During this "passive" smoke exposure and after leaving the polluted room, saliva, blood, and urine samples were collected from the volunteers and were analyzed for thiocyanate, nicotine and cotinine. In addition, carboxyhemoglobin (COHb) was determined. The results did not indicate significant increases in thiocyanate and COHb, but did show increases in nicotine and cotinine in all three physiological fluids of the probands. As evident from the data in Table 6, rapid uptake of nicotine is recorded upon exposure to the pollutants and cotinine levels in saliva rise gradually. Upon leaving the smoke polluted room, concentrations of nicotine in saliva decreased quickly, reaching baseline levels after 2-3 hr. Serum cotinine reached values of up to 5 ng/ml which corresponds to only a few percent of the cotinine values measured in the serum of a 1 pack-a-day cigarette smoker (200-300 ng/ml). The urinary excretion of nicotine and possibly that of cotinine indicates a kind of dose response in regard to smoke uptake. These findings suggest that the concentration of nicotine in saliva of nonsmokers can serve as an indicator of recent exposure to sidestream smoke while the urinary levels of nicotine and cotinine can serve as indicators of the long-term exposure of nonsmokers to tobacco smoke.

We are now collecting saliva and urine to determine nicotine and cotinine levels of individuals who are subjected to smoke exposure in various occupational, public and private indoor environments in order to gain information as to their involuntary uptake of tobacco smoke. Comparisons with corresponding data from active cigarette smokers will allow estimates as to the uptake of the carcinogenic particulate matter of tobacco smoke as a result of passive exposure. These data are needed for biochemical validation of epidemiological observations.

TABLE 5. Test laboratory

Size: 16.3 m^3			
Temperature: 22 ± 1°			
Air Exchanges: 6 × per hr			
Pollutants:	Sidestream smoke of 4 concurrently smoked 1R1 reference cigarettes		
Indoor pollution:	Particulate matter	4600	μg/m^3
	Nicotine	280	μg/m^3
	Hydrogen cyanide	56	μg/m^3
	Carbon monoxide	25	ppm
	NO$_x$	0.91	ppm

Other measurements such as that of nitrosoproline in urine and COHb in blood appear less promising as estimates of passive smoke uptake according to our results under controlled laboratory conditions.

Finally, it should be mentioned that there are environmental conditions in which the "passive smoker" may indeed be exposed to relatively high doses of tobacco smoke. Recently, R. A. Greenberg and associates from the Pediatrics Department of the School of Medicine, University of North Carolina in Chapel Hill, in cooperation with our Institute, measured the uptake of nicotine in infants due to maternal smoking (7). The ratio of ng of nicotine or ng of cotinine to mg of creatinine in the urine of infants of nonsmoking mothers reached average values of 7 and 10 respectively, whereas these values in infants of smoking mothers were very significantly higher, namely 85 and 450 (Table 7). The mean nicotine and cotinine levels in the saliva of non-exposed infants were 2.6 and 0.2 mg/ml respectively, whereas the corresponding mean concentrations for the infants of smoking mothers were 30 and 11 ng/ml. This observation indicates that, under certain conditions, the involuntary exposure of tobacco smoke can represent a toxic factor or a risk for respiratory disease in the nonsmoker. In this setting, other measurements for smoke uptake are indicated as well. These would include the cocarcinogenic catechol in saliva and nitrosoproline in the urine. Such data can support epidemiological observations such as those by Preston-Martin, et al. (24) indicating increased risk for childhood brain tumors in children of smoking mothers and observations by Correa et al. (5) pointing to a higher risk

TABLE 6. Nicotine and cotinine levels in saliva, serum and urine of volunteers[a]
(summary of average values)

Time[b] (min)	Saliva (ng/ml)				Serum (ng/ml)	Urine (ng/mg creatinine)					
	Nicotine			Cotinine	Cotinine	Nicotine			Cotinine		
	2[a]	3[a]	4[a]	4[a]	4[a]	2[a]	3[a]	4[a]	2[a]	3[a]	4[a]
Baseline	8	1	3	1.0	0.9	24	20	17	14	14	14
I 40	350	719	830	1.1	0.9						
I 60	430	830	880	2.1	1.2	26	34	84	16	21	28
O 30	76	157	148	1.7	1.8						
O 120	6	17	23	2.5	2.9	40	94	100	21	34	46
O 240	8	2	3	2.0	3.3						
O 300	7	7	7	3.5	3.4	51	58	48	21	38	55

[a]Numbers represent room pollution by smoke of 2, 3, or 4 cigarettes.
[b]I, inside exposure room during pollution; O, outside exposure room after leaving room.
From Greenberg et al., (7).

TABLE 7. Urinary and salivary concentrations of nicotine and cotinine of infants exposed or not exposed to tobacco smoke

Parental Report	Urine		Saliva	
	Nicotine:Creatinine (ng/mg)	Cotinine:Creatinine (ng/mg)	Nicotine (ng/ml)	Cotinine (ng/ml)
Non-Exposed				
Mean	7	19	2.6	0.2
Range	0 - 59	0 - 125	0 - 17.6	0 - 3
	(n = 18)	(n = 18)	(n = 13)	(n = 13)
Exposed				
Mean	85	459	30	11
Range	0 - 370	41 - 1885	0 - 166	(0 - 25)
	(n = 28)	(n = 28)	(n = 29)	(n = 27)
Significance of Difference	p < .0001	p < .0001	p < .0003	p < .0001

Reproduced with permission of the authors and the publishers of the New England Journal of Medicine; taken from Greenberg et al. (1984): New Engl. J. Med., 310:1075-1078.

for lung cancer in smokers whose mothers were cigarette smokers compared to those smokers whose mothers were nonsmokers.

SUMMARY

In tobacco smoke, catechols represent a major group of cocarcinogens. Model studies have indicated that polyphenols and polysaccharides are two major groups of precursors for the catechol formation during smoking. Results from the application of BP together with catechol on mouse skin indicate that the detoxification path of BP metabolism is decreased and the formation of the BP-7,8-diol is increased in comparison to the metabolism pattern observed when BP is applied alone. It remains to be demonstrated that the increased BP-7,8-diol formation leads also to increased formation of BP-DNA adducts in epithelial tissues.

The nicotine-derived N-nitrosamines represent a major group of carcinogens in chewing tobacco, snuff, and tobacco smoke. Their concentrations in processed tobacco and smoke exceed by far those of carcinogenic nitrosamines in other environmental materials. Whereas it has been shown that nicotine gives rise to NNN and NNK during tobacco chewing, the endogenous formation of these potent carcinogens upon smoke inhalation has so far not been demonstrated. However, the formation of N-nitrosoproline in cigarette smokers and snuff dippers proves that smoke and snuff have a measurable potential for the endogenous formation of carcinogenic nitrosamines.

Finally, the data presented here indicate that the individuals subjected to passive smoke exposure under controlled conditions take up measurable amounts of particulate matter. The nicotine level in the saliva of nonsmokers reflect recent passive smoke exposure and levels of nicotine and cotinine in urine reflect the long-term exposure to smoke particulates. The indicators, measured in saliva and serum, make it clear that uptake of particulates due to passive smoke exposure corresponds only to a low percentage (<2%) of the particulates that represent the uptake of a 1 pack-a-day adult smoker.

However, in special settings, such as in the exposure of infants to the smoke pollutants generated by their mothers, uptake of smoke constituents can reach levels which raise concerns as to possible long range toxic effects. A broader base of subjects and a wider range of pollution situations need to be tested in order to substantiate the significance of the dosimetry of uptake executed to date. Such measurements constitute an attempt at more accurate risk assessment for nonsmokers in smoke polluted environments.

ACKNOWLEDGEMENT

Our studies in tobacco carcinogenesis are supported by PHS Grants No. P01-29580 and R01-CA-35607 awarded by the National Cancer Institute.

REFERENCES

1. Adams, J. D., LaVoie, E. J., O'Donnell, M., and Hoffmann, D. (1984): *IARC Sci. Publ.*, in press.
2. Brunnemann, K. D., Scott, J. C., Haley, N. J., and Hoffmann, D. (1984): *IARC Sci. Publ.*, in press.
3. Byers, T., and Graham, S. (1984): *Adv. Cancer Res.*, 41:1-69.
4. Carmella, S. G., Hecht, S.S., Tso, T. C., and Hoffmann, D. (1984): *J. Agric. Food Chem.*, 32:267-273.
5. Correa, P., Pickle, L. W., Fontham, L., Lin, T., and Haenszel, W. (1983): *Lancet*, 2:595-597.
6. Garfinkel, L. (1981): *J. Natl. Cancer Inst.*, 66:1061-1066.
7. Greenberg, R. A., Haley, N. J., Etzel, R. A., and Loda, F. A. (1984): *New Engl. J. Med.*, 310:1075-1078.
8. Hammond, E. C., Selikoff, I. J., and Seidman, H. (1979): *Ann. N.Y. Acad. Sci.* 330:473-490.
9. Hecht, S. S., Carmella, S., Mori, H., and Hoffmann, D. (1981): *J. Natl. Cancer Inst.*, 66:163-169.
10. Hecht, S. S., Castonguay, A., Chung, F.-L., and Hoffmann, D. (1984): *IARC Sci. Publ.*, in press.
11. Hirayama, T. (1981): *Brit. Med. J.*, 1:183-185.
12. Hirayama, T. (1983): *Lancet*, 2:1425-1426.
13. Hoffmann, D., and Adams, J. D. (1981): *Cancer Res.*, 41:4305-4308.
14. Hoffmann, D., Adams, J. D., Brunnemann, K. D., Rivenson, A., and Hecht, S. S. (1982): *IARC Sci. Publ.*, 41:309-318.
15. Hoffmann, D., and Brunnemann, K.D. (1983): *Cancer Res.*, 43:557-574.
16. Hoffmann, D., Brunnemann, K. D., Adams, J. D., and Hecht, S. S. (1984): *IARC Sci. Publ.*, in press.
17. Hoffmann, D., Rivenson, A., Amin, S., and Hecht, S. S. (1984): *J. Cancer Res. Clin. Oncol.*, 108:81-86.
18. Hoffmann, D., Rivenson, A., Hecht, S. S., Hilfrich, J., Kobayashi, N., and Wynder, E. L. (1979): *Prog. Exp. Tumor Res.*, 24:370-390.
19. Hoffmann, D., Wynder, E. L., Rivenson, A., LaVoie, E. J., and Hecht, S. S. (1983): *Prog. Exp. Tumor Res.*, 26:43-67.
20. Kabat, G. C., and Wynder, E. L. (1984): *Cancer*, 53:1214-1221.
21. Koo, L. C., Ho, J. H. C., and Saw, D. (1983): *J. Exp. Clin. Cancer Res.*, 4:365-375.
22. Mirvish, S. S., Wallcave, L., Eagen, M., and Shubik, P. (1972): *Science*, 177:65-68.
23. Ohshima, H., and Bartsch, H. (1981): *Cancer Res.*, 41:3658-3662.

24. Preston-Martin, S., Yu, M. C., Benton, B., and Henderson, B. E. (1982): *Cancer Res.*, 42:5240-5245.

25. Trichopoulos, D., Kalandidi, A., and Sparros, L. (1983): *Lancet*, 2:677-678.

26. U.S. Public Health Service (1964): *Smoking and Health.* Report of the Advisory Committee to the Surgeon General of the Public Health Service. DHEW Publ. (PHS) 1103, 387 pp.

27. U.S. Public Health Service (1979): *Smoking and Health.* A Report of the Surgeon General of the Public Health Service. DHEW Publ. (PHS) 78-50066, 1136 pp.

28. U.S. Public Health Service (1982): *The Health Consequences of Smoking - Cancer.* A Report of the Surgeon General. DHHS Publ. (PHS) 82-50179, 322 pp.

29. Van Duuren, B. L., and Goldschmidt, B. M. (1976): *J. Natl. Cancer Inst.*, 56:1237-1242.

30. Wynder, E. L., and Day, E. (1961): *J. Am. Med. Assoc.*, 175:997-999.

Carcinogenesis, Vol. 8, edited by M. J. Mass et al.
Raven Press, New York © 1985.

Studies on the Tumor Initiating, Tumor Promoting, and Tumor Co-Initiating Properties of Respiratory Carcinogens

Stephen Nesnow, *Larry L. Triplett, and *,[1]Thomas J. Slaga

*Carcinogenesis and Metabolism Branch, Genetic Toxicology Division, Health Effects Research Laboratory, U.S. Environmental Protection Agency, Research Triangle Park, North Carolina 27711; *Biology Division, Oak Ridge National Laboratory, Oak Ridge, Tennessee 37831*

We have been interested for several years in studying the tumorigenic and carcinogenic properties of respiratory carcinogens, with major emphasis on complex environmental mixtures (10-13). With mouse skin as the bioassay model, the multifaceted behavior of these chemicals and mixtures can be elucidated using the protocols of tumor initiation, tumor promotion, tumor co-initiation, and complete carcinogenesis. Reviews of mouse skin carcinogenesis have stressed the multistage nature of this process (15,16), the qualitative and quantitative relationships between tumor initiation and complete carcinogenesis, chemical, strain and tissue specificity towards the tumor initiating and tumor promoting properties of chemicals, and biochemical and biological properties related to tumor promotion and progression (15,16). In chemical-based reviews of mouse skin tumorigenesis, it is clear that although a multitude of functionally different chemicals have been examined, the major portion of the data base is comprised of studies relating to polycyclic aromatic hydrocarbons (PAH) and their derivatives (10,14). Studies with complex mixtures also provide a major data base in the mouse skin system, as this tissue is unusually responsive to the tumorigenic and carcinogenic effects of combustion products (11,13,14).

In an earlier review of mouse skin tumorigenesis, we suggested that further evaluation should be undertaken to expand the data base on the tumor-initiating effects of respiratory carcinogens, using several well-known animal and human respiratory carcinogens to probe the

[1]Present Address: The University of Texas System Cancer Center, Research Division, Smithville, Texas 78957

sensitivity of mouse skin as an assay to detect these chemicals (10). The first part of this report describes the results of these experiments.

In addition to studies with individual respiratory carcinogens, we have been evaluating the tumorigenic and carcinogenic effects of complex environmental mixtures. One of the goals of this research program is to compare the potency of human respiratory carcinogens based on epidemiological data with the bioassay potency data obtained from mouse skin tumor initiation and mouse skin complete carcinogenesis experiments as well as the bioassay potency data obtained from short-term genetic toxicology bioassays. Three human respiratory carcinogens were used: emissions from coke ovens, emissions from roofing tar pots, and cigarette smoke. When the potency obtained from mouse skin tumor initiation experiments of these materials was compared with the potency based on human respiratory cancer, a surprisingly close correlation was observed. Over a potency range of 1 to 1,000, the relative incidence of human lung tumors correlated well with the incidence of mouse skin papillomas and carcinomas (1,8). Due to these unique findings, additional experiments were undertaken to evaluate the tumor-promoting and tumor-co-initiating properties of these human respiratory carcinogens. The remainder of this report will describe the results of these studies.

MATERIALS AND METHODS

Sample Generation and Collection

The details of the sample preparation have been reported elsewhere (11,13). The diesel sample was obtained from a 1973 preproduction Nissan-Datsun 220C and represents a dichloromethane extract of diesel particulates collected on a Pallflex fiber glass filter. The coke oven sample is a dichloromethane extract of coke oven material collected from a separator located between the gas collector and the primary coolers at a coke oven battery at Republic Steel, Gadsden, AL. In previous reports, this sample has been referred to as the coke oven main sample (12,13). The roofing tar sample is a dichloromethane extract of roofing tar emissions produced by heating coal tar based pitch at 182-193° in a conventional tar pot and collecting the emissions in a Teflon sock in a bag-house. The cigarette smoke condensate sample was produced from Kentucky R1 cigarettes utilizing a smoking machine and was collected in an acetone-Dry Ice bath.

Mouse Skin Tumorigenesis

Seven- to nine-week-old SENCAR mice (16) bred at the Oak Ridge National Laboratory were used (80 mice of each sex per treatment group). Animals were housed in plastic cages (10 per cage) under yellow light with hardwood chip bedding, fed Purina chow and water ad libitum, and maintained at 22-23° with 10 changes of air per hour. Only mice in the resting hair growth cycle were used. Unless otherwise noted, all treatments were performed using 200 µl of spectral-grade acetone.

Under the tumor initiation protocol, mice were treated with a single topical administration of the test agent, unless otherwise noted. One week after treatment, mice were treated topically, twice weekly with 2 µg of 12-O-tetradecanoylphorbol-13-acetate (TPA). Under the tumor promotion protocol, mice were treated with benzo(a)pyrene (B(a)P) (50.5 µg/mouse) and after one week were treated weekly with the test agents, except for the 4,000-µg/mouse dose that was administered as two weekly doses of 2,000 µg/mouse. Under the tumor co-initiation protocol, mice were treated with both B(a)P (50.5 µg/mouse) and test agent and were subsequently treated twice weekly with TPA (2 µg/mouse).

Skin tumor formation was recorded weekly. Papillomas >2 mm in diameter and carcinomas were included in the cumulative total if they persisted one week or longer. The tumors were verified by standard histological methods.

Survival was >90% in the tumor co-initiation experiments and in the tumor promotion experiments up to week 31.

RESULTS

Tumor Initiation Studies

Using the mouse skin tumor initiation protocol, the potential tumor-initiating activities of four suspect human respiratory carcinogens were evaluated: the metal salts beryllium sulfate, nickel sulfate, and potassium dichromate and 4,4'-methylene bis(2-chloroaniline) (MOCA). In order to maximize the effects of the metal salts, they were administered to the mice by intraperitoneal (i.p.) injection in saline. The mice were subsequently dermally treated twice weekly with TPA for 26 weeks. Except for potassium dichromate, there was no overt toxicity due to treatment with the metal salts. The highest dose chosen for each was approximately 1/5 of the LD_{50}. Potassium dichromate was completely lethal to these mice at 5,000 μg/mouse. Over a dose range of 0.01-10.0 μg/mouse (beryllium sulfate, Table 1); 0.1-400 μg/mouse (nickel sulfate, Table 2); or 50-1,000 μg/mouse (potassium dichromate, Table 3), none of these chemicals induced significant numbers of mouse skin papillomas. MOCA was administered by dermal application to the dorsal area of mice; these mice were subsequently treated twice weekly with TPA. Over a dose range of 100-200,000 μg/mouse, MOCA did not induce significant numbers of mouse skin papillomas (Table 4).

Tumor Promotion Studies

In order to compare the tumor-promoting activity of the complex mixtures, coke oven and roofing tar, an experiment was performed in which these materials were applied to SENCAR mice previously initiated with 50.5 μg of B(a)P. Over a dose range of 100-5,000 μg/mouse, coke oven and roofing tar were applied weekly to groups of 40 male and 40 female B(a)P-initiated mice. The mice were scored weekly for the appearance of papillomas and squamous cell carcinomas. The data for combined sexes from the 27th week of the experiment are presented in Fig. 1. On a mass basis, the coke oven sample was approximately four times as active as a tumor promoter as the roofing tar sample. Comparison of these results with those obtained from mice initiated with 50.5 μg of B(a)P and promoted with B(a)P (12.6-252 μg/wk/mouse) indicates that on a mass basis, B(a)P is 15.9 times as active as coke oven and 80 times as active as roofing tar.

A comparison was performed between mice treated once with B(a)P and subsequently treated weekly with coke oven or roofing tar and mice treated weekly only with coke oven or roofing tar. Data are presented in Fig. 2 for the coke oven studies when scoring was performed for squamous cell carcinoma formation at week 37. Over a dose range of 1,000-4,000 μg/wk/mouse, mice treated with coke oven alone were more susceptible to carcinoma formation than mice treated once with 50.5 μg of B(a)P and subsequently treated weekly with coke oven. Similar increases were seen in the same animals when they were scored at weeks 30 or 31 for papillomas per mouse (Fig. 3) or for the number of mice bearing papillomas (Fig. 4). However, using the same experimental procedures with roofing tar, the inverse effect was seen. Mice treated once with B(a)P and subsequently treated weekly with 1,000-4,000 μg/wk/mouse of roofing tar bore more papillomas (Fig. 5)

TABLE 1. Mouse skin tumor initiation by beryllium sulfate

Dose, µg[a]	Number of mice surviving		Mice bearing papillomas, percent	
	M	F	M	F
0	40	36	10	11
0.01	39	38	8	18
0.10	39	37	8	22
1.0	37	39	0	18
5.0	38	38	5	18
10.0	36	39	8	21
B(a)P, 50.5	38	39	68	74

[a] Intraperitoneal administration. Mice dermally promoted with TPA.

TABLE 2. Mouse skin tumor initiation by nickel sulfate

Dose, µg[a]	Number of mice surviving		Mice bearing papillomas, percent	
	M	F	M	F
0	40	36	10	11
0.1	39	39	13	15
1.0	40	40	5	8
50	39	40	10	3
100	40	39	5	3
400	40	39	5	8
B(a)P, 50.5	39	39	97	95

[a] Intraperitoneal administration. Mice dermally promoted with TPA.

TABLE 3. Mouse skin tumor initiation by potassium dichromate

Dose, µg[a]	Number of mice surviving		Mice bearing papillomas, percent	
	M	F	M	F
0	40	36	10	11
50	38	40	18	8
100	40	40	5	8
500	38	41	5	7
1,000	37	31	11	10
B(a)P, 50.5	39	39	97	95

[a] Intraperitoneal administration. Mice dermally promoted with TPA.

TABLE 4. Mouse skin tumor initiation by MOCA

Dose, µg[a]	Number of mice surviving		Mice bearing papillomas, percent	
	M	F	M	F
0	40	36	10	11
100	35	38	6	3
1,000	39	39	23	15
10,000	38	39	5	5
100,000	38	40	16	15
200,000	37	37	14	5
B(a)P, 25.2	39	39	90	94

[a] Dermal administration. Mice dermally promoted with TPA.

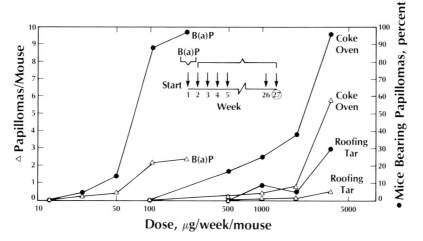

FIG. 1. Comparison of the tumorigenic activities of complex mixtures to B(a)P on B(a)P-initiated SENCAR mouse skin. Benzo(a)pyrene-initiated mice (50.5 µg/mouse) were subsequently treated weekly (except for the 4,000-µg/wk/mouse dose, which was administered as twice weekly doses of 2,000 µg/mouse) with either B(a)P, coke oven, or roofing tar. The circled week number represents the week of scoring.

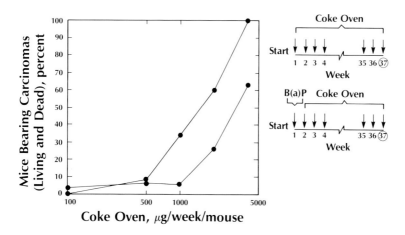

FIG. 2. Formation of squamous cell carcinomas in mice treated weekly with coke oven for 37 wk or treated once with B(a)P (50.5 µg/mouse) and subsequently treated weekly for 36 wk with coke oven. The 4,000-µg/wk/mouse dose was administered as twice weekly doses of 2,000 µg/mouse. Mice were scored on week 37. In B(a)P-initiated mice, the same results were obtained at weeks 37 and 38.

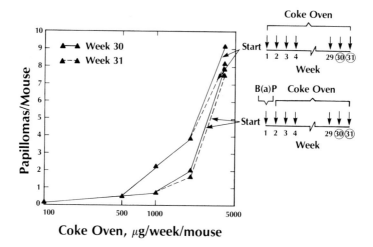

FIG. 3. Skin papilloma multiplicity in mice treated weekly with coke oven for 30 or 31 wk or treated once with B(a)P (50.5 µg/mouse) and subsequently treated weekly with coke oven for 30 or 31 wk. The 4,000-µg/wk/mouse dose was administered as twice weekly doses of 2,000 µg/mouse.

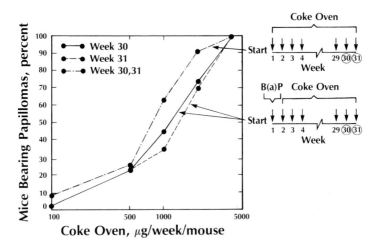

FIG. 4. Skin papilloma incidence in mice treated weekly with coke oven for 30 or 31 wk or treated once with B(a)P (50.5 µg/mouse) and subsequently treated weekly with coke oven for 30 or 31 wk. The 4,000-µg/wk/mouse dose was administered as twice weekly doses of 2,000 µg/mouse.

and had a higher papilloma incidence (Fig. 6) than mice treated weekly only with roofing tar when scored at week 30 or 31 of the experiment.

Tumor Co-Initiation Studies

Tumor co-initiation studies were performed in groups of 40 male and 40 female SENCAR mice by co-administering the test agent with 50.5 µg/mouse of B(a)P, a component of each of the complex mixtures studied. After one week, these mice were treated twice weekly with TPA for up to 30 wk. Papilloma formation was recorded weekly, and the results presented in the following figures are the combination of the results from both the male and female mice.

Experiments were first performed with a PAH known to be found in each of these complex mixtures: pyrene. Using the tumor co-inititiation protocol, pyrene was found to exert a synergistic effect with B(a)P (Fig. 7,8). Pryene is inactive as a tumor initiator at the doses examined; however, when co-administered with B(a)P at 200 or 400 µg/mouse, it produced significant increases in papillomas per mouse (Fig. 7) and smaller increases in papilloma incidence (Fig. 8) compared to mice treated with B(a)P alone. The lower dose of pyrene produced a 50% increase, while the higher dose produced a 100% increase based on tumor multiplicity.

Cigarette smoke condensate was evaluated as a tumor co-initiator and was also found to induce a synergistic effect with B(a)P (Fig. 9 to 11). These effects could only be observed during the early weeks of the studies. Cigarette smoke condensate co-administered with B(a)P at doses of 500-10,000 µg/mouse produced increased papilloma responses compared to B(a)P-treated mice (Fig. 9). Unlike pyrene, however, cigarette smoke condensate did produce a slight tumorigenic response at 1,000 and 2,000 µg/mouse. An examination of the temporal synergistic effects of cigarette smoke condensate with B(a)P at 1,000 and 2,000 µg/mouse with both appropriate controls can be seen in Fig. 10 and 11.

Roofing tar was examined for its ability to induce a synergistic effect with B(a)P as a tumor co-initiator in SENCAR mouse skin. The effects of roofing tar in combination with B(a)P are shown in Fig. 12 to 15. In terms of papilloma incidence, roofing tar exhibited a dose-related effect from 1,000-10,000 µg/mouse in SENCAR mice co-initiated with 50.5 µg B(a)P/mouse (Fig. 12). Unlike pyrene and like cigarette smoke condensate, roofing tar did produce a tumorigenic effect when administered alone to mice as a tumor initiator. At 2,000 µg

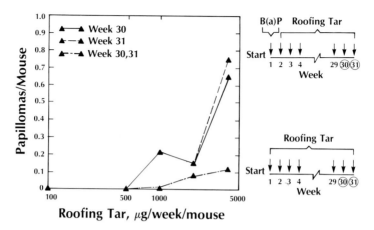

FIG. 5. Skin papilloma multiplicity in mice treated weekly with roofing tar for 30 or 31 wk or treated once with B(a)P (50.5 µg/mouse) and subsequently treated weekly with roofing tar for 30 or 31 wk. The 4,000-µg/wk/mouse dose was administered as twice weekly doses of 2,000 µg/mouse.

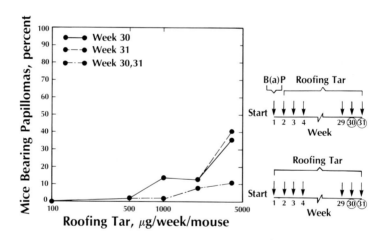

FIG. 6. Skin papilloma incidence in mice treated weekly with roofing tar for 30 or 31 wk or treated once with B(a)P (50.5 µg/mouse) and subsequently treated weekly with roofing tar for 30 or 31 wk. The 4,000-µg/wk/mouse dose was administered as twice weekly doses of 2,000 µg/mouse.

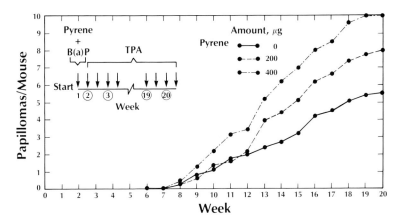

FIG. 7. Synergistic effects of pyrene and B(a)P in SENCAR mice co-initiated with these PAH and promoted with TPA. Data reported as papillomas per mouse. Pyrene has no effect as a tumor initiator at these doses.

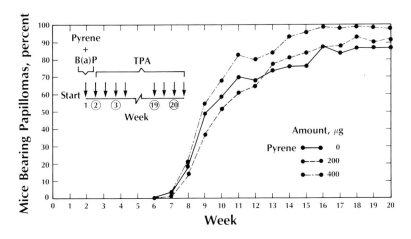

FIG. 8. Synergistic effects of pyrene and B(a)P in SENCAR mice co-initiated with these PAH and promoted with TPA. Data reported as percent of mice bearing papillomas. Pyrene has no effect as a tumor initiator at these doses.

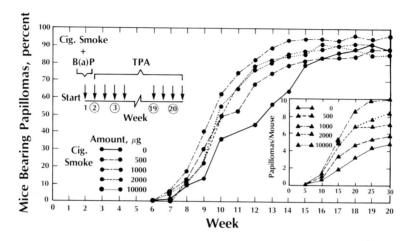

FIG. 9. Mouse skin tumor co-initiation studies with cigarette smoke condensate and B(a)P. Mice were co-initiated with these two agents and subsequently promoted with TPA.

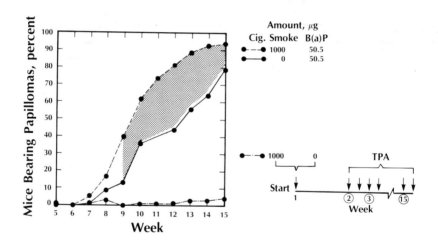

FIG. 10. Temporal synergistic effects of cigarette smoke condensate and B(a)P in the tumor co-initiation protocol. Mice were treated once with cigarette smoke condensate (1,000 µg/mouse) or B(a)P (50.5 µg/mouse) or were treated once with a combination of cigarette smoke condensate and B(a)P. All mice were promoted with TPA.

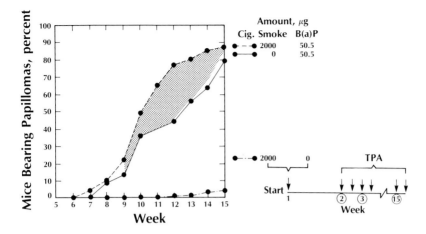

FIG. 11. Temporal synergistic effects of cigarette smoke condensate and B(a)P in the tumor co-initiation protocol. Mice were treated once with cigarette smoke condensate (2,000 μg/mouse) or B(a)P (50.5 μg/mouse) or were treated once with a combination of cigarette smoke condensate and B(a)P. All mice were promoted with TPA.

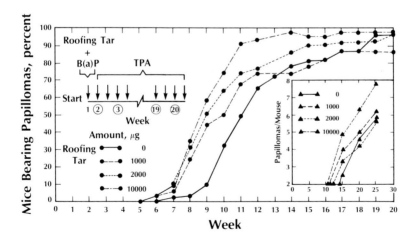

FIG. 12. Mouse skin tumor co-initiation studies with roofing tar and B(a)P. Mice were co-initiated with these two agents and subsequently promoted with TPA.

roofing tar/mouse with B(a)P, a synergistic effect was observed at weeks 8-10 of the experiment (Fig. 13); at later time points, this effect was reduced. Similar effects were measured at the 10,000-μg/mouse dose level for both papilloma incidence (Fig. 14) and multiplicity (Fig. 15).

Diesel was examined for possible synergistic effects with B(a)P on SENCAR mouse skin as a tumor co-initiator (Fig. 16,17). When co-administered with 50.5 μg B(a)P/mouse, diesel at 2,000-10,000 μg/mouse had no demonstrable effect (Fig. 16). However, when considering that both B(a)P and diesel (10,000 μg/mouse) can induce significant tumor-initiating effects by themselves, as indicated in Fig. 17, the fact that their combined effects are not additive indicate that diesel and B(a)P are antagonistic as tumor co-initiators in SENCAR mice.

DISCUSSION

The ability of mouse skin to identify carcinogens that act on respiratory tract tissue is of importance, as this system is commonly used to investigate the activity of complex environmental mixtures isolated from airborne emissions. Extrapolations of the results from mouse skin experimentation to the human respiratory situation are strengthened by the findings that human and animal respiratory carcinogens are also active on mouse skin. It has recently been shown that the relative potency of three complex mixture human respiratory carcinogens obtained from mouse skin tumor initiation studies is approximately equal to their relative potency as human carcinogens (1,8). The studies presented herein were performed to explore the sensitivity of the mouse skin system to known human and animal respiratory carcinogens as single agents. The three metal salts examined were negative at the doses utilized using the i.p. route of administration. MOCA was also not active as a mouse skin tumor initiator when topically administered. A summary of the known human and animal respiratory carcinogens and their activity in mouse skin is presented in Table 5. Of the 11 chemicals or mixtures evaluated in the mouse skin system, 7 were positive. Of the four inactive agents, three were metal salts. These findings suggest that mouse skin can be used to evaluate complex mixtures for carcinogenic activity, especially if they contain PAH. However, mouse skin should not be used to evaluate metal salts or mixtures that contain sufficient quantities of metal salts.

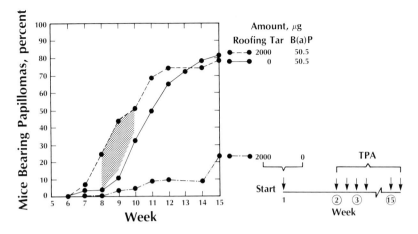

FIG. 13. Temporal synergistic effects of roofing tar and B(a)P in the tumor co-initiation protocol. Mice were treated once with roofing tar (2,000 µg/mouse) or B(a)P (50.5 µg/mouse) or were treated once with a combination of roofing tar and B(a)P. All mice were promoted with TPA.

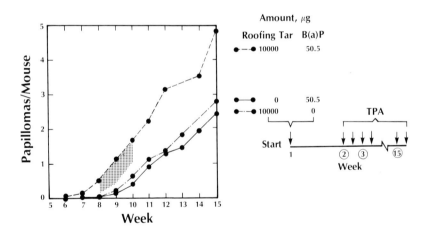

FIG. 14. Temporal synergistic effects of roofing tar and B(a)P in the tumor co-initiation protocol. Mice were treated once with roofing tar (10,000 µg/mouse) or B(a)P (50.5 µg/mouse) or were treated once with a combination of roofing tar and B(a)P. All mice were promoted with TPA. Data are reported as papillomas per mouse.

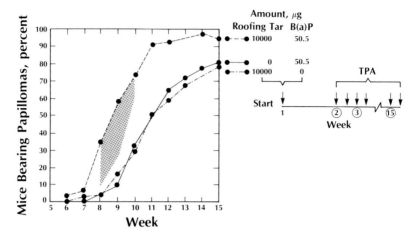

FIG. 15. Temporal synergistic effects of roofing tar and B(a)P in the tumor co-initiation protocol. Mice were treated once with roofing tar (10,000 µg/mouse) or B(a)P (50.5 µg/mouse) or were treated once with a combination of roofing tar and B(a)P. All mice were promoted with TPA. Data are reported as percent of the mice bearing papillomas.

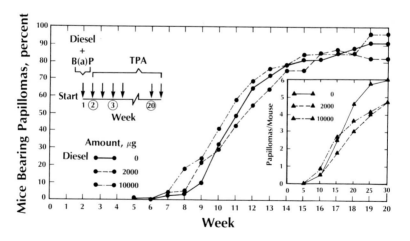

FIG. 16. Mouse skin tumor co-initiation studies with diesel and B(a)P. Mice were co-initiated with these two agents and subsequently promoted with TPA.

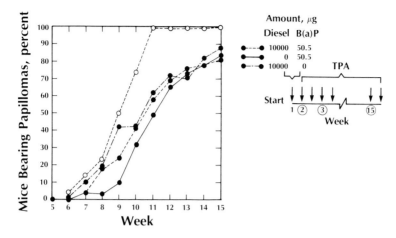

FIG. 17. Temporal potential antagonistic effects of diesel and B(a)P in the tumor co-initiation protocol. Mice were treated once with diesel (10,000 µg/mouse) or B(a)P (50.5 µg/mouse) or were treated once with a combination of diesel and B(a)P. All mice were promoted with TPA. Data are reported as percent of the mice bearing papillomas. The line connecting the open circles represents the expected additive effects of both diesel and B(a)P.

A tumor promoter is defined as an agent that is capable of enhancing the tumorigenic effects of other chemicals and that has for the most part no tumorigenic activity by itself. In general, tumor promoters also have the characteristics of being epigenetic in mechanism and inducing reversible changes, at least in the early stages of their action (15,17). Since we have previously determined that coke oven and roofing tar are complete carcinogens on SENCAR mouse skin, they can be considered to possess both tumor-initiating and tumor-promoting activities (12,13). However, the experimental verification of these conclusions is difficult to establish using the standard tumor initiation/tumor promotion protocol, since they are tumorigenic agents. One of the hallmarks of mouse skin tumor promotion is the early formation of large numbers of papillomas that begin to partially regress after 30 weeks of TPA treatment. Large numbers of papillomas per mouse were observed in coke oven-promoted, B(a)P-initiated mice (Fig. 3), providing direct experimental evidence for the tumor-promoting activity of coke oven. Similar effects were not observed with roofing tar. As a result, the results obtained from the experiments using the tumor promotion protocol can be thought of as sequential syncarcinogenesis, as described by Williams (17).

TABLE 5. Response of respiratory carcinogens in the mouse skin tumorigenesis bioassay system

Chemical	Occupational respiratory carcinogen[a]	Animal respiratory carcinogen[a]	Mouse skin tumorigen[b]
Arsenic	+		
Asbestos	+	+	
Beryllium	+	+	– ?[c]
Carbamates		+	+
Chloromethyl ethers	+	+	+
Chromium	+		– ?[c]
Cigarette smoke	+	+	+[d]
Coke oven	+		+[d]
Isopropyl oil	+		
MOCA	+	+	– ?[c]
Mustard gas	+	+	
Nickel	+	+	– ?[c]
Nitrosamines		+	
PAH	+	+	+
Roofing tar	+		+[d]
Quinolines		+	+
Vinyl chloride	+	+	

[a] Data from (1,3).

[b] Data from (9,14). Includes both tumor initiation and complete carcinogenesis studies.

[c] Based on data presented in this article and limited to the doses employed and the routes of administration utilized.

[d] Data from (13).

The anticarcinogenic effect in mice treated once with B(a)P and then treated weekly with coke oven compared to mice treated weekly only with coke oven, and the syncarcinogenic effect observed with roofing tar, may be explained in terms of DNA adducts. It is reasonable to assume that there are a finite number of sites on the DNA in which PAH-activated species can interact. It is also assumed that the first treatment the mice receive saturates or nearly saturates these potential sites on the DNA. Therefore, the resultant effects of these treatments in terms of tumors is reflected in the efficiency or potency of the adducts in producing tumors. In the case of coke oven, it would seem that adducts produced by coke oven are more productive towards tumor formation than adducts produced by B(a)P. Therefore, mice first treated with B(a)P and then treated with coke oven will exhibit fewer tumors than mice treated only with coke oven. The same argument can be made for roofing tar, in which adducts produced by roofing tar are less efficient or potent in producing tumors than B(a)P. Therefore, mice first treated with B(a)P and then treated with roofing tar will exhibit more tumors than mice treated only with roofing tar. The content of B(a)P in each of these mixtures (1380 ppm, coke oven; 889 ppm, roofing tar) does not contribute to the tumorigenic activities observed in these experiments (1).

The synergistic effects observed with cigarette smoke condensate and roofing tar are in concert with the determination of chemicals in these samples that are known to exert these activities. 1-Methylindole, 9-ethylcarbazole, and catechol have previously been identified as enhancers of mouse skin tumorigenesis and are present in cigarette smoke condensate (6,7). Pyrene is present in both cigarette smoke condensate and roofing tar (J. Lewtas, personal communication) and produces synergistic effects with B(a)P (Fig. 7,8). In addition to pyrene, roofing tar contains carbazole and methylcarbazoles, both potential cocarcinogens (J. Lewtas, personal communication).

The anticarcinogenic effects observed with combined treatment of mice with diesel and B(a)P can be explained by alterations in the metabolism/detoxification of B(a)P that is induced by diesel. Haugen and Peak (5) have reported that fractions from coal-derived oil suppressed the rat liver S9 metabolism, covalent DNA binding, and bacterial mutagenic activity of B(a)P.

It is clear from this work and the work of others that B(a)P content cannot account for all of or even a major portion of the tumorigenic activity of coke oven, roofing tar, or diesel. Chemical class fractionation of these mixtures and subsequent bioassay of the fractions in *Salmonella typhimurium* for mutagenic activity has shown that fractions containing the mutagenic activity are not the fractions that contain the greatest mass. More importantly, for each complex mixture, the fraction that contained B(a)P had <22% of the total mutagenic activity of the unfractionated mixture (2). From tumor initiation studies, B(a)P can account for up to approximately 30% of the tumorigenic activity of coke oven, roofing tar, or diesel (Fig. 18). Grimmer et al. (4) have reported that B(a)P accounts for only 2.4% of the total carcinogenicity of automobile exhaust condensate. Therefore, other carcinogens, cocarcinogens, and syncarcinogens must play a major role in the carcinogenic activity of these complex environmental mixtures.

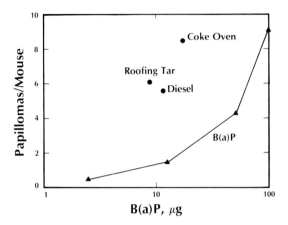

FIG. 18. Mouse skin tumor initiation: relationship between B(a)P content and tumorigenic effects. SENCAR mice were initiated with 10 mg of each complex mixture and promoted with TPA. For the B(a)P data, mice were initiated with various doses of B(a)P and promoted with TPA.

REFERENCES

1. Albert, R., Lewtas, J., Nesnow, S., Thorslund, T., and Anderson, E. (1983): *Risk Anal.*, 3:101-117.
2. Austin, A. C., Claxton, L. D., and Lewtas, J. (1984): *Environ. Mutagen.*, in press.
3. Frank, A. L. (1978): In: *Pathogenesis and Therapy of Lung Cancer*, edited by C. C. Harris, pp. 25-51. Marcel Dekker, New York.
4. Grimmer, G., Brune, H., Deutsch-Wenzel, R., Dettbarn, G., and Misfeld, J. (1984): *J. Natl. Cancer Inst.*, 72:733-739.
5. Haugen, D. A., and Peak, M. J. (1983): *Mutat. Res.*, 116:257-269.
6. Hoffmann, D., Melikian, A., Adams, J. D., Brunnemann, K. D., and Haley, N. J. (1985): In: *Carcinogenesis - A Comprehensive Survey, Cancer of the Respiratory Tract: Predisposing Factors*, edited by M. J. Mass, D. G. Kaufman, J. A. Siegfried, V. E. Steele, and S. Nesnow. Raven Press, New York, in press.
7. Hoffmann, D., and Wynder, E. L. (1971): *Cancer*, 27:848-864.
8. Lewtas, J., Nesnow, S., and Albert, R. (1983): *Risk Anal.*, 3:133-137.
9. Nesnow, S., Argus, M., Bergman, H., Chu, K., Frith, C., Helmes, T., McGaughey, R., Ray, V., Slaga, T. J., Tennant, R., and Weisburger, E. (1985): *Mutat. Res.*, in press.
10. Nesnow, S., Triplett, L. L., and Slaga, T. J. (1981): In: *Short-Term Bioassays in the Analysis of Complex Environmental Mixtures II*, edited by M. D. Waters,

S. S. Sandhu, J. Lewtas Huisingh, L. Claxton, and S. Nesnow, pp. 277-297. Plenum Press, New York.

11. Nesnow, S., Triplett, L. L., and Slaga, T.J. (1982): *J. Natl. Cancer Inst.*, 68:829-834.

12. Nesnow, S., Triplett, L. L., and Slaga, T. J. (1983): In: *Short-Term Bioassays in the Analysis of Complex Environmental Mixtures III*, edited by M. D. Waters, S. S. Sandhu, J. Lewtas, L. Claxton, N. Chernoff, and S. Nesnow, pp. 367-390. Plenum Press, New York.

13. Nesnow, S., Triplett, L. L., and Slaga, T. J. (1983): *Environ. Health Perspect.*, 47:255-268.

14. Pereira, M. (1982): *J. Am. Coll. Toxicol.*, 1:47-82.

15. Slaga, T. J., and Klein-Szanto, J. P. (1983): *Cancer Invest.*, 1:425-436.

16. Slaga, T. J., and Nesnow, S. (1985): In: *Handbook of Carcinogen Testing*, edited by H. A. Milman, Noyes Publications, New York, in press.

17. Williams, G. M. (1985): In: *Carcinogenesis - A Comprehensive Survey, Cancer of the Respiratory Tract: Predisposing Factors*, edited by M. J. Mass, D. G. Kaufman, J. M. Siegfried, V. E. Steele, and S. Nesnow. Raven Press, New York, in press.

Carcinogenesis, Vol. 8, edited by M. J. Mass et al.
Raven Press, New York © 1985.

Promotion-Like Enhancement of Transformed Phenotypes in Human Endometrial Stromal Cells

Jill M. Siegfried, *Karen G. Nelson, and *David G. Kaufman

*Carcinogenesis and Metabolism Section, Environmental Health Research and Testing, Inc.,
Research Triangle Park, North Carolina 27709; *Department of Pathology, University of North
Carolina, Chapel Hill, North Carolina 27514*

The multi-stage nature of carcinogenesis has been well-documented in animal models (5,29,32) and in human tumor development (2,25,30,31). Progressive stages of alteration leading to transformation have also been documented in cultured cells following carcinogen administration (3,18).

In two-stage models of carcinogenesis, expression of transformation following a sub-threshold exposure to a carcinogen has been brought about by administration of promoting agents such as phorbol esters (1,5,36), bile acids (26) and artifical sweeteners (7,16). *In vitro*, homones (13) and phorbol esters (19,23,37) have been used to enhance expression of transformation. The ability of 12-O-tetradecanoylphorbol-13-acetate (TPA) to enhance progression through premalignant stages has also been demonstrated by O'Brien et al. (28) in Syrian hamster embryo cells, by Steele et al. (35) in rat tracheal epithelial cells and by Wigley (39) in murine submandibular gland epithelial cells.

In order to investigate the role that tumor promotion may play in human cancer, we have attempted to determine whether promotion can be demonstrated in cultured human cells. Human endometrial stromal cells were chosen for these studies. Our laboratory has previously demonstrated (9,17) that a series of phenotypic alterations resembling those found in human endometrial sarcomas can be elicited in stromal cells repeatedly exposed to N-methyl-N'-nitro-N-nitrosoguanidine (MNNG). The alterations documented were increased saturation density, altered morphology, increased γ-glutamyltranspeptidase (GGT) expression, and altered growth requirements. These phenotypes were acquired in a stepwise manner which was primarily dependent on cumulative carcinogen exposure (9).

We selected two compounds from these studies, the prototype tumor promoter, TPA, and diethylstilbestrol (DES), an agent associated with vaginal adenocarcinoma in women exposed *in utero* (12,14,15). The mechanism by which DES acts is unclear. It was not mutagenic in the Ames test (11) and did not produce mutations in Syrian hamster embryo cells (4,21), although transformation could be demonstrated. Recently DES has been shown to act as a promoter in the C3H10T$\frac{1}{2}$ cell system (20). Both TPA and DES may cause chromosomal damage through superoxide production, especially through oxygen activated during arachidonic acid oxidation (8,22). Such a mechanism could serve to magnify genetic alterations brought about by an initiating agent. The results reported here demonstrate that both TPA and DES enhance expression of premalignant phenotypes in human endometrial stromal cells. The endpoints measured included: GGT expression, clonal growth in selective media, and morphology. In addition, attempts were made to explore the mechanism by which enhancement was brought about. These studies have been described previously (33,34).

MATERIALS AND METHODS

Two Stage Protocol

Human endometrial stomal cell cultures were established from hysterectomy specimens (10,38). Tissue culture reagents were obtained from Grand Island Biological Co. (Grand Island,.NY), except for fetal bovine serum, which was obtained from Sterile Systems, Inc. (Logan, UT). After establishment as primary cultures in CMRL-1066 medium with 10 mM glutamine, 5 µg/ml insulin, 25 mM HEPES, 100 U/ml penicillin, 100 µg/ml streptomycin, and 10% fetal bovine serum for 3 weeks, stromal cells were plated at clonal density (15 cells/cm^2) in DMEM medium supplemented with 4 mM glutamine, the above concentrations of insulin, HEPES, penicillin, and streptomycin, and 20% fetal bovine serum. Stromal cells were allowed to grow one week into small colonies of 10-15 cells and were then exposed to MNNG. Fresh solutions of MNNG (Sigma Chemical Co., St. Louis, MO) were prepared in reagent grade acetone (Aldrich Chemical Co., Milwaukee, WI) immediately before use.

Cultures were washed with Hanks' balanced salt solution (Grand Island Biological Co.) and fresh solution was added to each plate.

Cultures received carcinogen or acetone alone (0.1% final concentration); cultures were incubated at 37° for 30 min, after which carcinogen solution was replaced by DMEM medium containing serum. After MNNG treatment, cultures were allowed to grow to confluence with weekly medium changes for 8-10 weeks. Medium was supplemented with 0.1 μM DES (Sigma Chemical Co.), 0.01 μg/ml TPA (PL Biochemicals, Milwaukee, WI), or ethanol vehicle beginning one week after MNNG. DES stock solutions were prepared in 70% ethanol and stored at 4°. TPA stock solutions were prepared in absolute ethanol and stored at -70°. After confluence was reached, cultures were analyzed for phenotypic changes. DES or TPA was not present during these assays.

For some studies, frozen cultures which had previously been repeatedly treated with MNNG (1.0 μg/ml) or acetone at a cell density of 5000 cells/cm^2 were reconstituted and continuously cultured in TPA, DES or ethanol for up to 6 months.

Analysis of Growth Characteristics

GGT activity was demonstrated histochemically (10). Slides were prepared by seeding cells onto 2-well Lab Tek slides (Miles Laboratories, Naperville, IL) and allowing them to propagate for 1 week. After staining, 10 random fields were viewed at 200× on each slide. The number of positive cells was determined visually.

Colony forming ability was evaluated by plating a single cell suspension of 500 cells/dish onto 60 mm tissue culture dishes. Cells were allowed to grow for 14 days, after which dishes were fixed in methanol:acetic acid (9:1) and stained with 10% Giemsa in phosphate buffered saline (Fisher Scientific, Pittsburgh, PA). Colonies larger than 10 cells were counted since, in this assay, stromal cells have a doubling time of 4 days. Three different media were used in these assays: DMEM (which supports the clonal growth of normal cells), CMRL-1066 (which does not support the clonal growth of normal cells), and DMEM, containing reduced calcium (which also does not support the growth of normal cells). Use of these different media conditions has been described previously (10,17). Reduced calcium medium was prepared by using a DMEM formulation which did not contain CaCl$_2$, and substituted Na pantothentate for Ca pantothentate. This was supplemented with serum which had been treated with Chelex (BioRad Laboratories, Richmond, CA) to remove calcium. This treatment did not impair the ability of serum to support growth at normal calcium concentration. This medium with Chelex-treated fetal bovine serum was found to contain no more than 1 µg/ml calcium. Normal DMEM and CMRL-1066 were also supplemented with 20% fetal bovine serum. Colonies were counted under a dissecting microscope (40×). Colony-forming ability was calculated as the number of colonies formed divided by the number of cells plated, multiplied by 100. The average value for groups of three plates were determined in each case.

Homonal Effects of DES on Endometrial Cultures

DNA synthesis was measured by monitoring [³H]thymidine incorporation at 24, 48 and 96 hr after addition of DES. Triplicate dishes containing 10^5 stromal cells were plated 3 days before DES addition in DMEM with normal calcium. A two-hour pulse with [³H]thymidine was used; incorporation was linear over this time. [Methyl-³H]thymidine (5 µCi/dish) was added in saline and cells were incubated at 37°. Cultures were then put on ice, washed 4 times with cold saline, and macromolecules were precipitated onto dishes with 5 ml of 5% trichloroacetic acid. The dishes were washed 4 times with 95% ethanol. After the dishes were air dried, the DNA was dissolved by incubating with 3 N NaOH at 37° for 24 hr. The absorbance of each sample was measured at 280 nm, and the data were expressed as cpm/absorbance unit.

Lactate dehydrogenase (LDH) isoenzymes were anlayzed by agarose gel electrophoresis. To obtain extracts containing LDH, confluent cultures were disrupted with 0.25 M sucrose-0.15 M NaCl solution and triturated with a 25 gauge needle. Cytosol was separated by centrifugation at 15,000 rpm for 20 min. Cytosol (1 µl) was placed in sample wells of 1% agarose gels. Isoenzymes were separated at 250 V for 1 hr in a buffer consisting of 50 mM Tris, 12 mM citrate, and 25 mM barbital. Isoenzymes were detected with a prepared stain (Sigma Chemical Co.).

RESULTS

GGT Expression

Enhanced GGT expression was demonstrated histochemically in cultures exposed chronically to TPA (Table 1) or DES (Table 2). Chronic medium supplementation with TPA for 3 months brought about increased GGT expression in cultures which otherwise showed no differences from controls. In cells initiated with 1 exposure to MNNG (1 μg/ml), TPA treatment caused a 3.5-fold increase (p < 0.05) in the number of GGT-positive cells. After 6 exposures to MNNG, TPA treatment caused a 10.4-fold increase (p < 0.05) in this parameter.

TABLE 1. GGT expression in stromal cell cultures after chronic TPA treatment[a]

Cumulative number of MNNG exposures (1 μg/ml)[b]	TPA 0.01 μg/ml[c]	Percent positive cells
0	−	2.0 ± 1.0
	+	3.1 ± 1.0
1	−	2.8 ± 1.0
	+	11.0 ± 3.0[d]
6	−	3.4 ± 1.0
	+	32.4 ± 3.4[d]

[a] Stromal cells were exposed to 0.01 μg/ml TPA for 3 months following return to culture from liquid N_2 storage. Cultures were then tested for GGT activity as described in MATERIALS AND METHODS. Data are expressed as mean percent positive cells ± S.E.M.
[b] Dissolved in acetone.
[c] Dissolved in ethanol.
[d] p < 0.05, one way analysis of variance. Modified from Siegfried and Kaufman (33).

Changes in GGT expression were observed after chronic DES treatment, as shown in Table 2. MNNG or DES treatment alone did not bring about a significant change in the percentage of GGT-positive cells as compared to untreated controls, but the combined treatment of MNNG followed by DES did bring about a significent increase. The mean increase was 4.0-fold (p < 0.001) over that seen with MNNG alone and 5.0-fold over that seen with DES alone. In general the extent of histological reaction was also greater in cultures which received combined MNNG and DES or TPA treatment compared to any of the other conditions.

Growth in Restrictive Media

DES or TPA treatment for 8 weeks also increased the number of cells which were capable of clonal growth in 2 restrictive media (Table 3). Human endometrial stromal cells normally have strong

TABLE 2. GGT expression in stromal cell cultures after
chronic DES treatment[a]

MNNG (2 μg/ml)[b]	DES 0.1 μM[c]	Percent positive cells
−	−	7.8 ± 2.7
−	+	14.4 ± 5.4
+	−	18.0 ± 2.5
+	+	71.6 ± 17.5[d]

[a] Stromal cells were exposed to MNNG at colony-forming density and grown to confluence with or without DES and then tested for GGT activity as described in MATERIALS AND METHODS. Data are expressed as mean percent positive cells ± S.E.M.
[b] Dissolved in acetone.
[c] Dissolved in ethanol.
[d] $p < 0.001$, one way analysis of variance. Modified from Siegfried et al. (34).

dependence on calcium for cell division, and in CMRL medium, undergo predecidual differentiation similar to that seen at the end of the menstrual cycle. Stromal sarcomas, on the other hand, are able to divide in reduced calcium and can also form colonies in CMRL medium. After repeated carcinogen treatment, cells capable of forming colonies under these two conditions can also be demonstrated (9,17).

Both DES and TPA enchanced the ability of cells pretreated with MNNG to form colonies in the 2 media. In CMRL media, control cultures contained an occasional positive colony, and exposure to DES for 8 weeks did not alter this incidence. TPA, however, did cause an increase in the number of uninitiated cells able to form colonies in CMRL. This was not as great as the increase seen with combined MNNG and TPA, although it was statistically significant. Carcinogen treatment alone also increased the incidence of positive cells in these 2 assays, but this was not significant at any concentration. Exposure to MNNG followed by DES or TPA brought about a much higher incidence of positive cells compared to controls especially at MNNG concentrations of 3.5 and 5.0 μg/ml. DES treatment alone did not alter the number of positive cells compared to controls.

Morphologic Alterations

Chronic treatment with DES or TPA brought about alterations in morphology in cultures initiated with MNNG, but not in control

TABLE 3. Effect of DES and TPA on colony formation in restrictive media[a]

			Mean number colonies per 500 cell plated	
MNNG µg/ml[b]	DES 0.1 µM[c]	TPA 0.1 µg/ml[c]	CMRL	DMEM 1 µg/ml Ca^{+2}
0	−	−	0.40 ± 0.35	0 ± 0
0	−	+	4.77 ± 2.69[d]	0 ± 0
0	+	−	0.37 ± 0.32	0 ± 0
2.0	−	−	1.80 ± 0.20	0 ± 0
2.0	−	+	4.30 ± 0.45[f]	0.1 ± 0.1
2.0	+	−	5.33 ± 0.53[e]	0 ± 0
3.5	−	−	1.16 ± 0.39	0 ± 0
3.5	−	+	9.01 ± 1.00[f]	0.35 ± 0.30
3.5	+	−	18.10 ± 2.77[f]	3.62 ± 1.85[f]
5.0	−	−	1.08 ± 0.20	0.13 ± 0.01
5.0	−	+	18.3 ± 0.25[f]	2.60 ± 0.50[e]
5.0	+	−	7.59 ± 3.00[f]	7.11 ± 0.24[f]

[a] Stromal cells were exposed to MNNG at colony-forming density and grown to confluence in the presence or absence of DES or TPA. Cultures were then tested for ability to form colonies as described in MATERIALS AND METHODS.
[b] Dissolved in acetone.
[c] Dissolved in ethanol.
[d] $p < 0.05$; one way analysis of variance. Modified from Siegfried and Kaufman (33) and Siegfried et al. (34).
[e] $p < 0.01$.
[f] $p < 0.001$.

cultures. Cellular crowding, decreased cell size, and nuclear abnormalities were observed between 4-8 weeks after beginning exposure to DES in carcinogen-treated cultures (Fig. 1). Control cultures showed little morphologic change with DES (Fig. 1A,B), while in cells pretreated with MNNG, pronounced differences in morphology were observed. The extent of change was dependent upon total carcinogen exposure. In cultures which had been exposed once to MNNG (1 µg/ml), DES brought about modest crowding (Fig. 1C,D). In cultures exposed six times to MNNG (1 µg/ml), DES treatment brought about pronounced crowding and bizarre nuclear shapes (Fig. 1E,F). Ethanol vehicle induced no morphologic alterations. Similar changes occurred with TPA treatment over a span of 8-12 weeks.

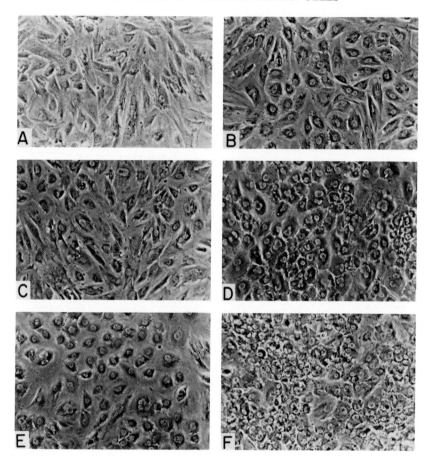

FIG. 1. Morphology of human stromal cell cultures after chronic treatment with DES or ethanol (8 weeks). A. Acetone-treated control cells which received ethanol treatment; B. Acetone-treated control cells which received 0.1 μM DES; C. MNNG-treated cells (1 μg/ml, one exposure) which received ethanol treatment; D. Culture identical to that in C which received 0.1 μM DES; E. MNNG-treated cells (1 μg/ml, six exposures) which received ethanol treatment; F. Culture identical to that in E which received 0.1 μm DES.

Evidence for Selection of Altered Cells by TPA

Moolgavkar and Knudson (24) have suggested that tumor promotion may be viewed as expansion of the "initiated" stem cell population, which may lead to an increased probability of tumor expression. Likewise Yuspa and Morgan (41) have documented the ability of TPA to induce terminal differentiation in epidermal epithelial cells from normal, but not carcinogen-treated mouse skin. O'Brien et al. (28) have also reported that TPA prevented Syrian hamster embryo cells exposed to benzo(a)pyrene in culture, but not control cells, from undergoing senescence.

Based on this evidence, we postulated that TPA may bring about promotion of carcinogenesis in human endometrial stromal cells by selectively allowing altered cells to proliferate, while impeding the proliferative capacity of normal cells. We tested this hypothesis by determining the fraction of cells capable of clonal growth in initiated and noninitiated cultures following chronic TPA exposure (0.01 µg/ml). These measurements were performed at monthly intervals; the most pronounced effect was observed at 6 months (Table 4). These studies utilized DMEM medium with standard concentrations of calcium and fetal bovine serum; under these conditions, the growth of both normal and carcinogen-treated cultures is supported. The percentage of uninitiated control cells which were capable of forming colonies was profoundly decreased by TPA treatment; over a 10-fold decrease was observed. In contrast, the proportion of the initiated cell population treated with TPA which was capable of forming colonies in comparison to matched cultures not treated with promoter steadily rose with increasing cumulative exposure to MNNG. This is best illustrated by comparing the ratio of colony-forming efficiency of vehicle-treated to TPA-treated cultures for each MNNG exposure group (Table 4). Differences among the 4 groups were not due to a change in the number of cells which attached to the tissue culture plates; this percentage was consistent within each treatment group (data not shown). Rather, the differences appear to reflect a change in the number of individual cells which survive and form a colony after plating.

Estrogenic Effects of DES

We did not observe that DES caused similar terminal differentiation of noninitiated stromal cells. Colony-forming efficiency in nonrestrictive medium was unchanged by chronic DES exposure

TABLE 4.   Effect of chronic TPA treatment on colony-forming ability in permissive medium[a]

Cumulative number of MNNG exposures (1 µg/ml)[b]	TPA 0.01 µg/ml[c]	Colony-forming efficiency[d]	Ratio[e]
0	−	12.5 ± 0.01	0.07
	+	0.9 ± 0.20	
1	−	18.3 ± 1.00	0.70
	+	12.8 ± 0.01	
6	−	7.1 ± 0.70	1.14
	+	8.1 ± 0.60	
10	−	17.1 ± 0.40	1.65
	+	28.3 ± 2.30	

[a] Stromal cells were treated repeatedly with MNNG and stored in liquid N_2. Following return to culture, cells were maintained in chronic TPA for 6 months. Colony-forming ability was measured in DMEM with normal calcium, in which stromal cells usually demonstrate a colony-forming efficiency of 10-15%.
[b] Dissolved in acetone.
[c] Dissolved in ethanol.
[d] Data are expressed as colony-forming efficiency ± S.E.M.
[e] Ratio of colony-forming efficiency of TPA cultures to that of vehicle control at each number of MNNG exposures. Modified from Siegfried and Kaufman (33).

(data not shown).   We therefore investigated whether hormonal responses might play a role in promotion of transformed phenotypes by DES. No growth-stimulating effect of acute DES exposure could be observed in several different assays. DES had no effect on thymidine incorporation into DNA (Table 5) over a 96-hr period. Likewise, acute DES treatment over a concentration range of 0.001-10.0 µM produced only a slight decrease in colony-forming efficiency of stromal cells (34). Measurements of growth rates also showed no change with DES administration (data not shown). DES treatment did cause changes in LDH isoenzyme patterns, which are known to vary during the menstrual cycle.   In endometrial tissue from proliferative phase specimens, we have found a higher proportion of LDH1 and LDH2, the heart forms of LDH, than of the muscle forms, LDH4 and LDH5. A shift toward the muscle forms was observed in primary endometrial tissue from a secretory phase specimen (27).

Over time in culture, the LDH pattern resembled that of secretory phase, but DES administration shifted the LDH pattern to that of

TABLE 5. [^{3}H]-Thymidine incorporation into DNA

Treatment	Hours after DES addition[a]		
	24	48	96
Ethanol	2025 ± 825	8000 ± 800	2430 ± 245
DES, 0.1 μM	3005 ± 405	10250 ± 2150	1280 ± 510

[a] Data are expressed as cpm/absorbance unit at 280 nm ± S.E.M.
Modified from Siegfried et al. (34).

proliferative phase (Fig. 2), as reflected by a decrease in LDH4 and LDH5. This was true of acetone-treated cells as well as MNNG-treated cultures, and was found in cultures in which DES enhanced preneoplastic changes. In cultures derived from 4 different individuals, a similar effect was observed, but to varying extents. There was not a correlation, however, between ability of DES to induce a shift in LDH isoenzyme pattern and ability to enhance preneoplastic phenotypes.

DISCUSSION

TPA and DES have been shown to facilitate the expression of several phenotypic changes associated with transformation in human endometrial stromal cells exposed first to a direct-acting carcinogen. Both TPA and DES were capable of decreasing the threshold MNNG concentration required for expression of morphologic atypia, GGT expression, and colony-forming ability in restrictive media. The time course and extent of changes were similar with both agents, and with both agents the extent of alteration observed was dependent on the concentration of the "initiating" agent, MNNG. Chronic administration of either promoting agent alone produced only slight changes in these parameters. TPA did cause an increase in the number of control cells capable of forming colonies in CMRL medium but the effect was smaller than that of combined MNNG and TPA, and may reflect an effect of TPA on the differentiation pathway of stromal cells.

Although we have not been successful in confirming the malignancy of highly altered cultures in nude mice, we have found that cultured human uterine sarcomas share several of their characteristics (9,17). For example, ability to form colonies in CMRL and low calcium media were both expressed by uterine sarcomas *in vitro*. These results suggest that promotion of transformation can be demonstrated in

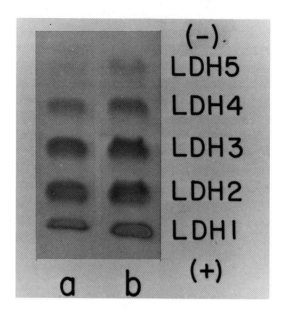

FIG. 2. Agarose gel electophoretic separation of LDH isoenzymes. A. DES treatment, 0.1 µM; B. Ethanol vehicle.

human cells, which would imply that a two-stage model of tumorigenesis may be operative in the development of human tumors.

A fundamental mechanistic question concerning tumor promotion is whether promoters enhance carcinogenesis by directly causing further genetic or epigenetic alterations in "initiated" cells or whether they act indirectly by providing conditions which allow the expansion of the "initiated" population in preference to unaltered cells, thus increasing the probability of tumor development. Our experiments with TPA indicate that a selective mechanism may act, at least in part, to produce enhancement of phenotypic changes by phorbol esters. The growth potential of cells which have not been "initiated" with carcinogen, as measured by colony-forming efficiency, was decreased 10-fold upon prolonged exposure to TPA. Such an effect was maximal after 6 months, but was also observed in some cultures after only 3 months of continuous TPA exposure. The growth potential of cells from carcinogen-treated cultures, on the other hand, was stimulated by prolonged TPA, generally in proportion to the cumulative amount of carcinogen used. In studies reported elsewhere (33), we have also reported a difference in sensitivity between "initiated" and normal stromal cell cultures to morphologic changes induced by acute TPA exposure. MNNG-treated cultures showed a heightened response and a lower threshold compared to controls, and did not become refractory as control cells did (33). This indicates an altered response to promoters in cells exposed to carcinogen but which otherwise are indistinguishable from controls.

Evidence for a selective mechanism was not found with DES. Growth of stromal cells in non-restrictive medium was not affected in culture by either acute or long-term exposure to DES, in MNNG-treated or control cultures. Shifts in LDH isoenzyme pattern after DES exposure were found, indicating that this hormone-like response was present in culture, but the response was similar in control and MNNG-treated cultures.

REFERENCES

1. Armuth, V., and Berenblum, T. (1972): *Cancer Res.*, 32:2259-2262.
2. Auerbach, O., Stout, A. P., Hammond, E. C., and Garfinkel, L. (1961): *New Engl. J. Med.*, 265:253-267.
3. Barrett, J. C. (1979): *Prog. Exp. Tumor Res.*, 24:17-27.
4. Barrett, J. C., Wong, A., and McLachlan, J. A. (1981): *Science*, 212:1402-1404.
5. Boutwell, R. K. (1964): *Prog. Exp. Tumor Res.*, 4:207-250.
6. Cerutti, P. A., and Emerit, I. (1981): *Nature*, 293:144-146.
7. Cohen, S. M., Arai, M., Jacobs, J. B., and Friedell, G. H. (1979): *Cancer Res.*, 39:1207-1217.
8. Degen, G. H., Eling, J .E., and McLachlan, J. A. (1982): *Cancer Res.*, 42:919-923.
9. Dorman, B. H., Siegfried, J. M., and Kaufman, D. G. (1983): *Cancer Res.*, 43:3348-3357.
10. Dorman, B. H., Varma, V. A., Siegfried, J. M., Melin, S. A., Adamec, T. A., Norton, C. R., and Kaufman, D. G. (1982): *In Vitro*, 18:919-928.
11. Forsberg, J. G. (1979): *Arch. Toxicol.*, Suppl. 2:263-274.
12. Greenwald, P., Barlow, J. J., Nasca, P. C., and Burnett, W. S. (1971): *Engl. J. Med.*, 285:390-392.
13. Guernsey, D. L. (1980): *Nature* (Lond.), 288:591-592.
14. Herbst, A. L., Paskanzer, D. C., Robboy, S. J., Friedlander, L., and Scully, R. E. (1975): *New Engl. J. Med.*, 292:334-339.
15. Herbst, A. L., Ulfelder, H., and Paskanzer, D. C. (1971): *New Engl. J. Med.*, 284:878-881.
16. Hicks, R. M., Wakefield, J. St. J., and Chowaniec, J. (1975): *Chem.-Biol. Interact.*, 11:225-283.

17. Kaufman, D. G., Siegfired, J. M., Dorman, B. H., Nelson, K. G., and Walton, L. A. (1983): In: *Human Carcinogenesis*, edited by C. C. Harris, and H. Autrup, pp. 469-508. Academic Press, New York.
18. Knowles, M. A., and Franks, L. M. (1977): *Cancer Res.*, 37:3917-3924.
19. Lasne, C., Gentil, A., and Chouroulinkov, I. (1974): *Nature* (Lond.), 247:490-491.
20. Lillehaug, J. R., and Djurhuers, R. (1982): *Carcionogenesis*, 3:797-799.
21. McLachlan, J. A., Wong, A., Degen, G. H., and Barrett, J. C. (1982); *Cancer Res.*, 42:3040-3045.
22. Metzler, M., and McLachlan, J. A. (1978): *Biochem. Biophys. Res. Commun.*, 85:874-884.
23. Mondal, S., Brankow, D., and Heidelberger, C. (1976): *Cancer Res.*, 36:2254-2260.
24. Moolgavkar, S. H., and Knudson, A. G. (1981): *J. Natl. Cancer Inst.*, 66:1037-1052.
25. Muto, J., Bussey, H. J. R., and Morson, B. C. (1975): *Cancer* (Phila.), 36:2251-2270.
26. Narisawa, T., Hagadia, N. E., Weisburger, J. H., and Wynder, E. L. (1974): *J. Natl. Cancer Inst.*, 53:1093-1097.
27. Nelson, K. G., Siegfried, J. M., Siegel, G. P., Martin, J. L., and Kaufman, D. G. (1984): *Carcinogenesis*, in press.
28. O'Brien, T. G., Saladik, D., and Diamond, L. (1982): *Cancer Res.*, 42:1233-1238.
29. Peraino, C., Fry, R. J. M., Saffeldt, E., and Kisieleski, W. E. (1973): *Cancer Res.*, 33:2201-2209.
30. Richart, R. M. (1963): *Am. J. Obst. Gynec.*, 86:703-712.
31. Saccomanno, G., Archer, V. E., Auerbach, O., Saunders, R. P., and Brennan, L. (1974): *Cancer*, 33:256-270.
32. Schreiber, H., Saccomanno, G., Martin, D. H., and Brennan, L. (1974): *Cancer Res.*, 34:689-698.
33. Siegfried, J. M., and Kaufman, D. G. (1983): *Int. J. Cancer*, 32:423-429.
34. Siegfried, J. M., Nelson, K. G., Martin, J. L., and Kaufman, D. G. (1984): *Carcinogenesis*, in press.
35. Steele, V. E., Marchok, A. C., and Nettesheim, P. (1980): *Int. J. Cancer*, 26:343-348.
36. Terzaghi, M., Klein-Szanto, A., and Nettesheim, P. (1983): *Cancer Res.*, 43:1461-1466.
37. Traul, K. A., Hink, R. J., Kachevsky, V., and Wolff, J. S. (1981): *J. Natl. Cancer Inst.*, 66:171-175.
38. Varma, V. A., Melin, S. A., Ademec, T. A., Dorman, B. H., Siegfried, J. M., Walton, L. A., Carney, C. N., Norton, C. R., and Kaufaman, D. G. (1982); *In Vitro*, 18:911-918.
39. Wigley, C. B. (1983): *Carcinogenesis*, 4:101-106.
40. Yuspa, S. H., and Morgan, D. L. (1981): *Nature* (Lond.), 293:72-74.

Carcinogenesis, Vol. 8, edited by M. J. Mass et al.
Raven Press, New York © 1985.

Reactive Oxygen Dependent Activation of Polycyclic Hydrocarbons by Phorbol Ester-Stimulated Human Polymorphonuclear Leukocytes

M. A. Trush, J. L. Seed, and T. W. Kensler

*Johns Hopkins School of Hygiene and Public Health,
Baltimore, Maryland 21205*

The actions of most mutagens or carcinogens can be attributed to biotransformation from relatively inert chemicals to highly reactive metabolites capable of interacting with biological molecules (6,21). It is generally acknowledged that ultimate carcinogenic metabolites are electrophilic reactants and that the initiation of chemical carcinogenesis is closely linked with the formation of specific carcinogen-DNA adducts. Polycyclic aromatic hydrocarbons (PAHs) represent an important and diverse class of environmental carcinogens. Benzo(a)pyrene (BP) is one of the best studied PAHs and has been particularly useful in dissecting the relationship between metabolic activation and chemical carcinogenesis. Activation of BP involves a specific sequence of reactions resulting in the generation of a bay region diol epoxide that is mutagenic, elicits the transformation of cells in culture, and is carcinogenic *in vivo* (6). This diol epoxide can be formed from the penultimate metabolite, BP-7,8-dihydrodiol, through the catalytic actions of microsomal cytochrome P-450, or by an oxidant generated during lipid peroxidation or the peroxidase component of prostaglandin synthesis (9,10). This metabolism of BP-7,8-dihydrodiol results not only in the carcinogenic BP-7,8-dihydrodiol-9,10-epoxide, but in the formation of a 9,10-dioxetane intermediate which decomposes with the emission of photons, as indicated by chemiluminescence (CL) (25). The interaction of BP-7,8-dihydrodiol with singlet oxygen ($^1O_2$) generated by chemical systems also results in CL with an emission spectrum identical to that observed with rat liver microsomes (25). Fig. 1 illustrates these reactions. Because this CL reaction exhibits site specificity, it has been proposed that the generation of CL is an indirect indication of the metabolic activation of a PAH at the 9,10 position (11).

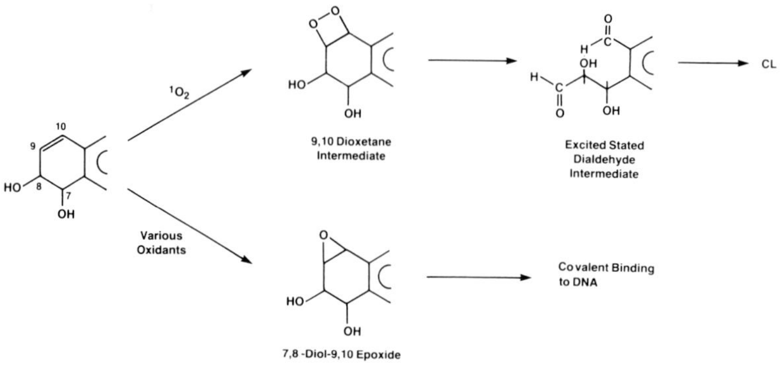

FIG. 1. Proposed reaction pathways for the generation of chemiluminescent and genotoxic metabolites from polycyclic aromatic hydrocarbons.

Increased generation of free radicals such as the superoxide anion (O_2^-) and hydroxyl radical ($\cdot OH$) are characteristic of activated inflammatory cells, including polymorphonuclear leukocytes (PMNs) (1,31). Through the catalytic actions of myeloperoxidase (MPO) the reactivity of O_2^- and H_2O_2 are amplified by the generation of an O_2 metabolite or complex with singlet oxygen-like reactivity (1). Inasmuch as PMNs generate a spectrum of oxidants, it is possible that the elaboration of oxyradicals by PMNs could also mediate the metabolic activation of pulmonary carcinogens (24). Such an activation mechanism could provide an explanation as to how neoplasms often develop at sites of ongoing inflammation (8). The purpose of this study is to demonstrate that PMNs can elicit CL from PAHs, that this reactive oxygen-dependent reaction is site specific and that the PAHs are metabolically activated to genotoxic derivatives as a result of this interaction.

MATERIALS AND METHODS

Cell Isolation

Blood obtained from normal health volunteers was centrifuged at $150 \times g$ for 10 min, afterwhich, the plasma and buffy coat were discarded. The remaining leukocytes and erythrocytes were mixed with an equal volume of 6% dextran and incubated in inverted syringes for 45 min at 37° (30). The upper leukocyte-rich fractions were ejected through a 16 gauge needle (90° bend), pooled and spun at $150 \times g$ for

5 min at 4°. Contaminating erythrocytes were lysed by adding cold
0.155 M NH_4Cl, 0.01 M $KHCO_3$ and 0.1 mM EDTA buffer (pH 7.4).
PMNs were washed, resuspended in phosphate-buffered saline with
0.1% glucose and counted on a hemacytometer. This procedure yielded
a preparation of PMNs that were >95% pure.

Measurement of Chemiluminescence (CL) Responses

CL responses were monitored using an ambient temperature
liquid scintillation spectrometer (Model 3003, Packard Instrument Co.)
operated in the out-of-coincidence mode (20). The counter was set as
follows: gain, 100%; window A to ∞ with discriminators set at 0 to 1000
and input selector 1 + 2. Experiments were begun by incubating
7×10^6 PMNs in 3 ml of PBS plus 0.1% glucose for 10 min at 37° in dark
adapted polyethylene vials. After the background CL of each vial was
determined, the PAH (3 µM) or vehicle (dimethyl sulfoxide [DMSO];
0.1%) was added, any response noted and the reactions initiated by
addition of 12-O-tetradecanoylphorbol-13-acetate (TPA) (15). The final
concentration of TPA was 162 nM. CL was monitored for 0.2 min at 75-
sec intervals and vials were maintained at 37° between counting. All
additions to the vials as well as the CL counting procedure were
performed in a darkened room. Results are expressed as counts/unit
time minus background. Data are presented as peak (maximum)
responses and temporal response curves.

Covalent Binding to DNA

[^{3}H]BP-7,8-dihydrodiol (3 µM, 367 mCi/mmole) was incubated
with 1×10^7 PMNs and 1.5 mg calf thymus DNA at 37° for 60 min in a
total volume of 3 ml. After 60 min, the PMNs were removed by
centrifugation at 150 × g and the supernatant extracted by shaking
with an equal volume of phenolic reagent (phenol/hydroquino-
line/isoamyl alcohol; 100:8:11) for 20 min (10). The phases were
separated by centrifugation at 10,000 × g for 20 min and the phenolic
layer was removed and discarded. The aqueous layer was reextracted
with 3 ml chloroform reagent (chloroform/isoamyl alcohol; 24:1) until
background radioactivity was achieved (generally 5 washes). The
aqueous layer was then washed with 3 ml of water saturated ether to
remove residual solvents. The DNA-containing aqueous layer was
precipitated with cold ethanol overnight at –20°. The DNA precipitates
were removed, dried under N_2, redissolved in 0.1 M potassium

phosphate buffer, and DNA-bound radioactivity determined. The concentration of DNA was determined by the diphenylamine reaction (5). Data are expressed as pmol of [^{3}H]BP-7,8-dihydrodiol bound per mg of DNA.

Mutagenesis Assay

The mutagenesis assay was conducted as described by Ames et al. (2). *Salmonella typhimurium* strain TA100 was cultured overnight in 5 ml of nutrient broth, then centrifuged at 1000 × g, and the bacterial pellet was resuspended in an equal volume of Dulbecco's PBS. This washing step was repeated three times in order to remove any chemotactic proteins from the bacteria. The *Salmonella* (300 µl) were then incubated with 2 × 10^6 PMNs, the indicated PAH at 10 µM concentration, with or without 162 nM TPA, in a total volume of 3 ml. After 1 hr of incubation at 37°, 1 ml of the incubation medium was transferred to soft agar containing 0.05 mM histidine and biotin, and then poured on a minimal agar plate. Revertant colonies were determined after 72 hr of incubation at 37°.

Materials

The PAHs used in this study were provided through the National Cancer Institute Chemical Respository (IIT Research Institute, Chicago, IL). 7,8-dihydro-BP was a generous gift from Dr. Donald Jerina, NIH, Bethesda, MD. [^{3}H]BP-7,8-dihydrodiol (367 mCi/mmole) was purchased from Midwest Research Institute, Kansas City, MO. Superoxide dismutase, zymosan, TPA, and calf thymus DNA were obtained from Sigma Chemical Co., St. Louis, MO, and sodium azide from Nutritional Biochemists, Cleveland, OH. Dextran (100-2000,000 M.W.) was purchased from Polysciences Inc., Warrington, PA. The biomimetic superoxide dismutase Cu(II)(3,5-diisopropylsalicyclic acid)$_2$ (CuDIPS) was synthesized as previously described (16). The Dulbecco's PBS (pH 7.4) consisted of the following (in g/L): NaCl (8.0); Na$_2$HPO$_4$ (2.16); KCl (0.2); KH$_2$PO$_4$ (0.2); CaCl$_2$ · 2H$_2$0 (0.1); MgSO$_4$ · 6H$_2$O (0.1) and glucose (1.0).

RESULTS

The oxidation of BP-7,8-dihydrodiol by ^{1}O$_2$ results in a 9,10-dioxetane intermediate which decomposes with the emission of photons as indicated by CL (Fig. 1). Since PMNs generate an oxidant with chemical reactivity similar to $^1O_2$ (1), we examined whether the interaction of BP-7,8-dihydrodiol with phorbol ester stimulated PMNs resulted in enhanced CL. The results of this experiment are illustrated in Fig. 2. Significant CL was observed from BP-7,8-dihydrodiol within 0.2 min following the addition of TPA, which peaked by 2.5 min and then slowly dissipated. Enhanced CL (2-fold greater than the TPA response) was observed at 0.3 μM, and there was a linear relationship between the concentration of BP-7-8-dihydrodiol and the generation of CL. The peak CL response from BP-7,8-dihydrodiol was 7 times greater than that of BP which is in agreement with their respective responses with $^1O_2$-generating systems (26).

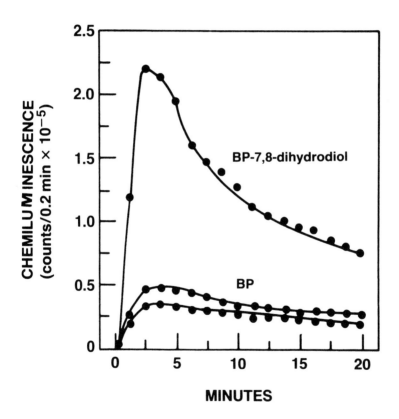

FIG. 2. Chemiluminescence responses of 3 μM BP-7,8-dihydrodiol and BP in the presence of TPA-stimulated PMNs.

When superoxide dismutase (50 µg/ml), the biomimetic superoxide dismutase CuDIPS (0.5 µM), or azide (1.0 mM) was included in the admixture the CL response from BP-7,8-dihydrodiol was inhibited 97, 90 and 98%, respectively. The effect of azide indicates that the oxidant involved in the formation of the dioxetane intermediate was primarily myeloperoxidase-derived in accord with observations implicating the involvement of this enzyme in the PMN-mediated CL from luminol and imipramine (7,29). In addition to the above agents, butylated hydroxyanisole (0.1 mM), indomethacin (0.15 mM) and ellagic acid (2.5 µM) all inhibited the CL response greater than 90%. All of these compounds inhibited the CL response to TPA in the absence of any PAH, indicating that they either prevented the generation of, or scavenged the oxidant responsible for the formation of the dioxetane intermediate, rather than interacting with this intermediate directly.

The various CL responses of the PAHs illustrated in Fig. 3 demonstrated that there was a site specificity to this reaction (Table 1). In addition to *trans* BP-7,8-dihydrodiol, *cis* BP-7,8-dihydrodiol and 7,8-dihydro-BP were chemiluminescent substrates whereas companion derivatives lacking a double bond at the 9,10 position, namely 9,10-dihydro-BP and BP-7,8-dihydrodiol-9,10-dihydro, were not. BP and its 7,8-quinone derivative yielded only slight CL responses. These results indicate that the PMNs generate a reactive species, dependent on O_2^- and the activity of myeloperoxidase, which oxidizes PAHs at the 9,10 double bond yielding a dioxetane intermediate.

Those compounds which we observed to be chemiluminescent in the presence of stimulated PMNs have all been shown to be mutagenic when activated by a purified cytochrome P-448 system (34). Likewise, those derivatives which were not chemiluminescent, were not mutagenic. This relationship suggests that in addition to the 9,10-dioxetane intermediate that other reactive intermediates, such as the 9,10-epoxide of BP, may be formed from PAHs as a result of their interaction with PMNs. Concordantly, coincubation with either resting or TPA-stimulated PMNs produced significant covalent binding of [3H]BP-7,8-dihydrodiol to calf thymus DNA (Table 2). Approximately 8-fold more binding was observed in the presence of activated PMNs. CuDIPS (1.0 µM) inhibited this binding by 60% while azide (1.0 mM) inhibited binding by 83% indicating that this activation to an alkylating metabolite was also reactive oxygen-dependent. The biological effects of the formation of this PAH-DNA adduct are reflected in the ability of BP-7,8-dihydrodiol to elicit mutagenesis in *Salmonella typhimurium* TA100 (Table 2), and to induce sister chromatid

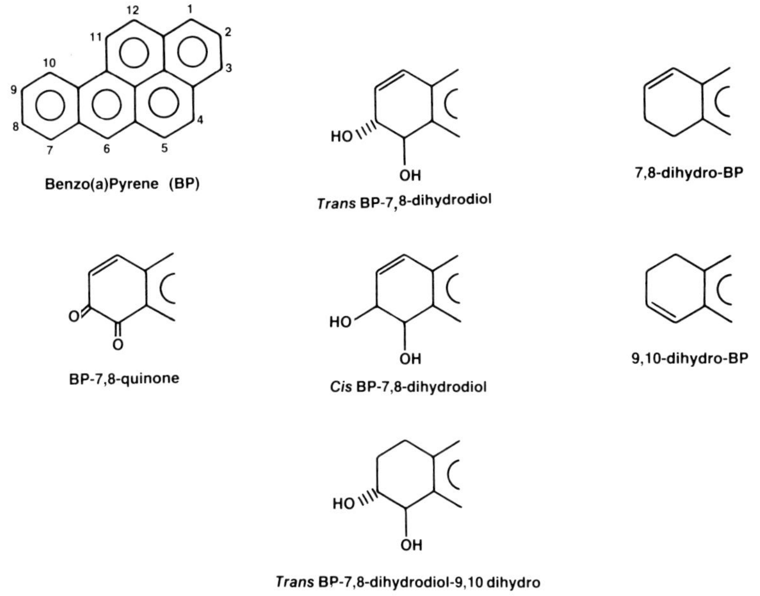

FIG. 3. Structures of various polycyclic aromatic hydrocarbons.

TABLE 1. Chemiluminescent response of various polycyclic aromatic hydrocarbons in the presence of TPA-stimulated PMNs

Compound[a]	Peak CL (Counts/0.2 min) $\times 10^{-4}$
None	3.2[b]
BP	4.3
BP-7,8-quinone	4.4
trans BP-7,8-dihydrodiol	27.6
cis BP-7,8-dihydrodiol	17.7
trans BP-7,8-dihydrodiol-9,10-dihydro	3.6
7,8-dihydro BP	49.2
9,10-dihydro BP	2.7

[a]Each compound was tested at 3 μM.
[b]Means of triplicate determinations.

exchanges (SCE) in V-79 cells (unpublished observation). In the presence of TPA-stimulated PMNs *cis* BP-7,8-dihydrodiol and 7,8-dihydro-BP were also mutagenic to the *Salmonella* whereas under these conditions, BP, BP-7,8-quinone, 9,10-dihydro-BP, and *trans* BP-7,8-dihydrodiol-9,10-dihydro were not. Resting PMNs or phorbol ester-stimulated PMNs were not mutagenic to *Salmonella* TA100. Since BP-7,8-dihydrodiol is not directly genotoxic, it can be concluded that PMNs mediate the metabolic activation of this class of caricnogens. On the basis of the structure-activity considerations this activation occurred at the 9,10 position.

TABLE 2. Genotoxic effects of BP-7,8-dihydrodiol in the presence of PMNs

Additions to PMNs	Covalent binding[a] pmol/mg DNA	Mutagenesis[a] histidine revertants
None	---	79
TPA	---	70
BP-7,8-dihydrodiol	0.79	95
TPA, BP-7,8-dihydrodiol	6.06	249

[a]Means of triplicate determinations.

DISCUSSION

It is becoming increasingly apparent that the simultaneous or sequential exposure of tissues to an agent can enhance or promote the toxicological response induced by another agent. A classic example of such an interaction is the promotion by phorbol esters of epidermal carcinogenesis following application of an initiating agent (25). The induction of cancer by chemicals is represented by stages of cellular evolution from normal through preneoplastic and premalignant to a highly malignant state that have been operationally defined as initiation, promotion, and progression (14). Experimental and epidemiological evidence has been provided which suggests that a multistage process is also pertinent to the development of lung cancer (22). The increased risk to lung cancer of asbestos workers who smoke probably best exemplifies this process (27). Asbestos exposure elicits the recruitment and accumulation of inflammatory cells, including PMNs, into the lung (4). Interestingly, a number of human malignancies have been shown to be associated with sites of ongoing inflammation and infection (8,24).

Reactive oxygen has been implicated in the multiple stages of carcinogenesis (17,18), and interest is expanding on the role of reactive oxygen-dependent reactions mediated by PMNs in carcinogenesis. DNA damage has been implicated in the actions of tumor promoters (3), and PMNs have recently been shown to elicit reactive oxygen-dependent genetic lesions in bacterial and mammalian cells (32,33). Thus, under conditions where there is an accumulation of metabolically stimulated PMNs, they could facilitate the promotion of initiated cells (Fig. 4). For example, rats with chronic murine pneumonia have been shown to have a much higher incidence of lung tumors relative to pathogen-free animals (24 versus 7) following initiation with nitrosamine (22).

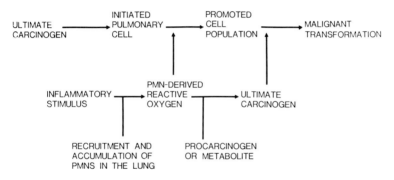

FIG. 4. Proposed mechanisms by which an inflammatory stimulus and subsequent PMN activation could contribute to the etiology of lung cancer.

Another interaction of relevance to pulmonary carcinogenesis is the reactive oxygen-dependent metabolic activation of carcinogens such as PAHs to genotoxic derivatives. While the metabolic activation of carcinogens to electrophilic DNA-binding reactants has usually been associated with the initiation of carcinogenesis, recent observations suggest that such a reaction may also be important in the progression of benign tumors to malignancy (13). PMNs have been shown to oxidize chemicals (19,28,29), and in this study we have demonstrated that metabolically stimulated PMNs can activate carcinogenic PAHs to genotoxic metabolites via a reactive oxygen-dependent reaction. Depending upon the temporal relationship between exposure to carcinogen and the appearance of PMNs, such an interaction could be relevant to the initiation or the progression of the promoted cell population to malignancy (Fig. 4). Neutrophils are rarely found in the alveolar structure of normal nonsmokers, but are found in high proportions in individuals with interstitial and familial fibrosis and with asbestosis. Thus, those individuals who because of occupation and/or lifestyle are exposed to pulmonary carcinogens and who have superimposed on this an inflammatory problem could be at greater risk. Interestingly, asbestos not only elicits the accumulation of PMNs in the lung but also stimulates their redox metabolism (12,23).

ACKNOWLEDGEMENTS

We gratefully acknowledge the financial support of the American Cancer Society, Maryland division and grant SIG-3, and the National Institutes of Health ES00454. We also thank Patricia Egner and Marletta Regner for their excellent assistance.

REFERENCES

1. Allen, R. C. (1980): In: *The Reticuloendothelial System, Vol. 2*, edited by A. J. Sbarra and R. Strauss, pp. 309-338. Plenum Press, New York.
2. Ames, B. N., McCann, J., and Yamaski, E. (1975): *Mutat. Res.*, 31:347-364.
3. Birnboim, H. W. (1982): *Science*, 215:1247-1249.
4. Bozelka, B. E., Sestini, P., Hammad, Y., Lenzini, L., Gaumer, H. R., and Salvaggio, J. E. (1983): *Chest*, 83s:9s-10s.
5. Burton, K. A. (1956): *Biochem. J.*, 62:315-323.
6. Conney, A. H. (1982): *Cancer Res.*, 42:4875-4917.
7. DeChatelet, L. R., Long, G. W., Shirley, P. S., Bass, D. A., Thomas, M. J., Henderson, R. W., and Cohen, M. S. (1982): *J. Immunol.*, 129:1589-1594.
8. Demopoulos, H. B., Peitronigro, D. D., and Seligman, M. L. (1983): *J. Am. Coll. Toxicol.*, 2:173-184.
9. Dix, T. A., and Marnett, L. J. (1983): *Science*, 221:77-79.
10. Gelboin, H. V. (1969): *Cancer Res.*, 29:1272-1276.
11. Hamman, J. P., Seliger, H. H., and Posner, G. H. (1981): *Proc. Natl. Acad. Sci. USA*, 78:940-942.
12. Hatch, G. E., Gardner, D. E., and Menzel, D. L. (1980): *Environ. Res.*, 23:121-136.
13. Hennings, H., Shores, R., Wenk, M. L., Spangler, E. F., Tarone, R., and Yuspa, S. H. (1983): *Nature*, 304:67-69.
14. Hicks, R. M. (1983): *Carcinogenesis*, 4:1209-1214.
15. Kensler, T. W., and Trush, M. A. (1981): *Cancer Res.*, 41:216-222.
16. Kensler, T. W., and Trush, M. A. (1983): *Biochem. Pharmacol.*, 32:3485-3487.
17. Kensler, T. W., and Trush, M. A. (1984): *Environ. Mutagenesis*, 6:593-616.
18. Kensler, T. W. and Trush, M. A. (1984): In: *Superoxide Dismutase, Vol. III: Pathological States*, edited by L. W. Oberley, in press. CRC Press, Boca Raton, FL.
19. Klebanoff, S. J. (1977): *J. Exp. Med.*, 145:983-998.

20. Marnett, L. J. (1981): *Life Sci.*, 29:531-546.
21. Miller, J. A. (1970): *Cancer Res.*, 30:559-576.
22. Nettesheim, P., Topping, D. C., and Jamasbi, R. (1981): *Ann. Rev. Pharmacol. Toxicol.*, 21:133-163.
23. Rola-Pleszcyzynski, M., Rivest, D., and Berardi, M. (1984): *Environ. Res.*, 33:1-6.
24. Roman-Franco, A. A. (1982): *J. Theor. Biol.*, 97:543-555.
25. Slaga, T. J. (1983): *Environ. Health Perspect.*, 50:3-14.
26. Seliger, H. H., Thompson, A., Hamman, J. P. and Posner, G. H. (1982): *Photochem. Photobiol.*, 36:359-362.
27. Selikoff, I. J., Hammond, E. C., and Churg, J. (1968): *J. Am. Med. Assoc.*, 204:106-112.
28. Trush, M. A. (1984): *Toxicol. Lett.* 20:297-302.
29. Trush, M. A., Reasor, M. J., Wilson, M. E., and VanDyke, K. (1984): *Biochem. Pharmacol.*, 33:1401-1410.
30. Trush, M. A., Wilson, M. E., and VanDyke, K. (1978): In: *Methods in Enzymology, Vol. 57*, edited by M. DeLuca, pp. 462-494. Academic Press, New York.
31. Weiss, S. J., and LoBuglio, A. F. (1982): *Lab. Invest.*, 47:5-18.
32. Weitberg, A. B., Weitzman, S. A., Destrempes, M., Latt, S. A., and Stossel, T. P. (1983): *New Engl. J. Med.*, 308:26-30.
33. Weitzman, S. A., and Stossel, T. P. (1982): *J. Immunol.*, 128:2770-2772.
34. Wood, A. W., Levin, W., Lu, A. Y. H., Ryan, D., West, S. B., Yagi, H., Mah, H. D., Jerina, D. M., and Conney, A. H. (1977): *Mol. Pharmacol.*, 13:1116-1125.

Carcinogenesis, Vol. 8, edited by M. J. Mass et al.
Raven Press, New York © 1985.

Effects of Ethanol, Phenol, Formaldehyde, and Selected Metabolites on Metabolic Cooperation Between Chinese Hamster V79 Lung Fibroblasts

A. Russell Malcolm, *Lesley J. Mills, and †James E. Trosko

*Biological Effects Division, Environmental Research Laboratory, U.S. Environmental Protection Agency, Narragansett, Rhode Island 02882; *Department of Microbiology, University of Rhode Island, Kingston, Rhode Island 02881; †Department of Pediatrics and Human Development, College of Human Medicine, Michigan State University, East Lansing, Michigan 48824*

Since the discovery of two-stage (initiation/promotion) carcinogenesis (98), multistage carcinogenesis has been demonstrated in liver (86), colon (92), bladder (15,48), pancreas (67), mammary gland (6,18,51), stomach (40), and several organs comprising the respiratory tract (5,10,107,123-125,148). Moreover, recent investigations (41,109) confirm and extend Boutwell's observations (11) that tumor promotion on mouse skin is itself a multistage process.

The respiratory tract is continuously exposed to complex mixtures of chemicals which include carcinogens, cocarcinogens and tumor promoters (77,116,117). 12-O-tetradecanoylphorbol-13-acetate (TPA) (72,103,116,124,125), some retinoids (119), and asbestos (125) are promoters of respiratory tract carcinogenesis in animal models. Some tobacco leaf extracts (9,137,152), whole tobacco smoke condensate (42), and selected fractions of whole tobacco smoke condensate are reported (21,94,150,152) to promote tumor development on mouse skin. More importantly, epidemiologic studies implicate smoking (49,50,135), ethanol consumption in combination with other factors (59,62,73,149), and occupational exposure to asbestos (101,102,140) in cocarcinogenic or tumor-promoting effects in the respiratory and upper alimentary tracts of humans. These findings have stimulated increased interest in the role of cocarcinogens and promoters in cancer etiology and in the development of short-term tests for their detection.

Tumor promoters induce a broad spectrum of cellular effects and several such effects are being investigated for their utility in screening tests. Included are chromosomal alterations in eukaryotic cells (55,84), promoter-induced transformation of intiated cells *in vitro* (23,74,106), effects on cell metabolism (43,61), viral induction (155), induction of oxygen radicals (126), and many others (68). It was recently discovered (76,154) that phorbol ester tumor promoters inhibit metabolic cooperation (exchange of low (1000 daltons or less) molecular weight signals *via* permeable gap junctions between cells) *in vitro*. This discovery suggests a potential role for metabolic cooperation (MC) in tumor promotion, and a possible short-term assay for tumor promoters. Mechanistically, if initiated cells are deficient in critical regulatory messages, suppression of MC could prevent receipt of such signals from competent neighboring cells and perhaps facilitate the clonal expansion of initated cell populations (127,132,154).

While it is unclear if inhibition of MC is necessary for tumor promotion, correlation studies from several laboratories show that many structurally diverse promoters inhibit MC. Included are anthralin (132,138), benzoyl peroxide (60,111), butylated hydroxytoluene (70,71,132,147,148), dinitrofluorobenzene (9,142), selected fatty acids (2,127,130,132), bile acids (91,132), synthetic gonadal steroids (153), surfactants (99,104,132), artificial sweeteners such as saccharin and cyclamate (22,48,71), environmentally-important chemicals such as DDT (87,134,145), polybrominated biphenyls (54,128), polychlorinated biphenyls (89,133), di-(2-ethylhexyl) phthalate (70,71,141), and trisodium nitrilotriacetate (47,70,71). In this paper, we briefly describe the MC assay and summarize test results for some chemicals implicated in respiratory tract carcinogenesis.

MATERIALS AND METHODS

Metabolic Cooperation Assay

The principle underlying the MC assay and an experimental protocol have been published (127,131,154). Briefly, mycoplasma-free, mutant (HGPRT⁻) and wild-type (HGPRT⁺) Chinese hamster V79 lung fibroblasts were used in all experiments. Cells were grown in antibiotic-free Eagle's Minimum Essential Medium modified for the MC assay as originally described (154). Cell cultures were grown at 37° in humidified incubators containing 5% CO_2 in air. Experimentally, mutant and wild-type cells were co-cultivated in the presence of the test chemical and 6-thioguanine (6TG), a mutant cell selective agent. One hundred mutant (HGPRT⁻, 6TG-resistant) and 400,000 wild-type (HGPRT⁺, 6TG-sensitive) cells in 4 to 5 ml of medium were inoculated into each of several 60 × 15 mm disposable plastic tissue culture dishes (15 dishes per dose). After incubating 4 hr for cell attachment, the test chemical and 6TG were added and incubation continued another two to four days. The medium was then replaced with fresh medium containing only 6TG. Incubation was continued another three to four days for colony development. Each test chemical was generally evaluated at five different concentrations selected from initial cytotoxicity tests, and permitting at least 70% relative survival. Survival was estimated by the number of mutant cells per dish developing into macroscopic colonies. Dishes were fixed with ethanol, stained with crystal violet, and colonies counted either electronically or by hand.

HGPRT⁻ mutants are deficient in the enzyme hypoxan-thineguanine phosphoribosyltransferase (HGPRTase), a purine salvage enzyme catalyzing the conversion of purine bases into their corresponding ribonucleotides that become incorporated into new DNA (19). HGPRTase also catalyzes the conversion of certain purine analogs, such as 6TG, into nucleotides which are lethal upon incorporation into DNA. Because plasma membranes are generally impermeable to phosphorylated compounds, nucleotides tend to become incorporated into the DNA of those cells within which they arise (52,63). Consequently, 6TG is lethal to HGPRT⁺ but not HGPRT⁻ cells, providing the two cell types do not establish physical contact. If contact occurs, gap junctions form and the toxic 6TG metabolite is transferred from HGPRT⁺ to HGPRT⁻ cells, killing both cells. This interaction between co-cultivated HGPRT⁺ and HGPRT⁻ cells provides a convenient way to identify substances which affect MC. The MC assay may thus be considered as a reconstructed selection experiment in which mutation cell survival relative to control is determined by the effects of test chemicals on MC. Because V79 hamster cells have a limited capacity to metabolize xenobiotic compounds (14), and no exogenous metabolizing system is currently used with the assay, observed responses are assumed to result from the direct action of unmetabolized test chemcials.

Cytotoxicity Assay

Prior to assessing the effects of chemicals on MC, doses permitting at least 70% survival in treated cell populations were estimated from preliminary cytotoxicity tests. For chemicals in Table 1, except formaldehyde and formic acid, tests were conducted with only mutant cells, as originally specified (131,154). Toxicity tests employing only mutant cells, however, do not duplicate the experimental conditions (HGPRT⁻ cells co-cultivated with many HGPRT⁺ cells) under which effects on MC are measured; therefore, such tests only estimate cytoxicity under the conditions of higher cell density present in MC assays. The absence of HGPRT⁺ cells effectively increases toxicant concentration per cell, with possible increases in cytotoxicity. To estimate the cytotoxicity of formaldehyde and formic acid, a modified toxicity test employing co-cultivated HGPRT⁻ and HGPRT⁺ cells was used. In these tests, the HGPRT⁻ cells were also deficient for MC (6). In the presence of HGPRT⁺ cells, the survival of (HGPRT⁻, MC⁻) mutants should be primarily a function of test agent cytotoxicity. If true, this type of toxicity test should render a more realistic estimate of the cytotoxicity present in MC tests, providing the (HGPRT⁻, MC⁻) mutants respond to the test chemical in approximately the same way as the (HGPRT⁻, MC⁺) mutants used in actual experiments.

RESULTS AND DISCUSSION

Chemicals had either no effect on MC, inhibited MC, or enhanced it (Table 1). Chemicals had no effect on MC if mutant recovery was not statistically different (131) from that in the solvent control. MC was inhibited if mutant recovery was statistically greater in any test situation relative to the solvent control. Enhancement of MC occurred when mutant recovery in any test situation was statistically less than that in the solvent control.

Positive Controls

TPA, a potent promoter of mouse skin tumors (7,46,112,136,138), induced almost complete mutant recovery at 1 ng/ml (71). Phorbol dibutyrate (PDBu), a weaker promoter of mouse skin tumors (110), also induced almost complete mutant recovery, but at 10 ng/ml (70). These results are similar to those reported by others (154), and further suggest that the phorbol esters inhibit MC approximately in proportion to their promoting activity. Besides promoting tumor development in mouse skin, TPA promotes adenocarcinomas in hamster lung following single or multiple intubation of benzo(a)pyrene (103), enhances carcinogenesis in cultured respiratory epithelium (115), and has a promoting-like effect on tracheal carcinogenesis in rats (124).

TABLE 1. Effect of test chemicals on metabolic cooperation (mutant survival) at maximally effective concentration[a]

Compound metabolite	Concentration (μg/ml)	Cytotoxicity (average % RS)	Metabolic cooperation assay		
			(Average % MR)	MR (EX)/MR (CT)	Effect
TPA	0.001	84	84	7.7	I (strong)
PDBu	0.01	98	81	7.2	I (strong)
ETOH	20000.0	75	41	3.9	I (weak)
DMSO	20000.0	87	52	4.1	I (weak)
Formaldehyde	1.25	85	22	2.2	I
Formic acid	200.0	72	9	0.9	N
Phenol	250.0	75	17	1.1	N
Catechol	2.5	77	45	2.3	I
Quinol	1.5	71	29	2.3	I
Hydroxyquinol	2.0	74	29	2.0	I
1,4-Benzoquinone	2.5	87	27	2.7	I
2-Methoxyhphenol	70.0	88	2	0.1	E
Phenylsulfate	1500.0	77	34	3.3	I (weak)
Phenylglucuronide	7500.0	106	7	1.0	N

[a] Abbreviations: RS = relative survival; MR = mutant recovery; EX = experimental; CT = control; I = inhibitory; N = none; E = enhancing.

Solvents (ETOH, DMSO)

Ethanol (ETOH) inhibited MC in a dose-dependent fashion at high (10-20 mg/ml) concentrations. ETOH, used extensively as a solvent for MC assay test chemicals, is epidemiologically implicated as a cocarcinogen or tumor promoter in humans (59,62,73,149). Furthermore, because it is surface active, ETOH has been predicted (13) to be a tumor promoter. Hypothetically, we would expect it to suppress MC. Like other anesthetics, ETOH has major effects on cell membranes. ETOH may intercalate between the fatty acids of membrane phospholipids, causing membrane expansion and increased membrane fluidity (20,39,100). These effects alter a number of cellular properties and membrane functions, including membrane-associated enzyme activity and transport. Some ETOH-induced membrane effects may interfere with MC by directly altering gap junction structure. Experimental evidence (16) indicates that ETOH inhibits Na^+K^+-dependent and Ca^{+2}-dependent ATPases which function to maintain normal intercellular Na^+/K^+ balance and low cytoplasmic levels of free calcium (1,17,69). Interestingly, intracellular free calcium mobilization is associated with both inhibition of MC (29,64,66,81,85,95-97) and the stimulation of many events associated with tumor promotion (8,24,30,36,44,57,79,80,143,144).

For comparison, dimethyl sulfoxide (DMSO), another important solvent, induced dose-dependent inhibition of MC between 5 and 20 mg/ml. DMSO was less cytotoxic than ETOH, but a more potent inhibitor of MC. Similar findings with DMSO in the V79 cell assay is reported by Dorman and Boreiko (32). According to one study (118), DMSO is not carcinogenic for mouse skin. DMSO is also reported (110) to strongly inhibit promotion by TPA on mouse skin. Because the tumor-promoting activity of DMSO is not reported, it is unknown if DMSO is a false positive in the MC assay. We note, however, that other promoters such as butylated hydroxytoluene (7,88) and acetic acid (108) also inhibit promotion by TPA (110). Inhibition of TPA-induced promotion by DMSO (a solvent for TPA) may reflect the rapid absorption of DMSO through the skin (28), or its effectiveness as a scavanger of potentially promoting oxygen radicals (31,37,126). DMSO has no effect on the capacity of TPA to inhibit MC in V79 cells (Malcolm and Mills, unpublished results). DMSO induces membrane effects which may cause increases in intracellular free calcium (105,122), and induces differentiation in Friend leukemia cells, further suggesting the cell membrane as a primary site of action (121). DMSO also produces osmotic effects which could inhibit MC by causing cells to round up (32). The potential tumor-promoting properties of DMSO require investigation.

Formaldehyde and Formic Acid

Formaldehyde inhibited MC between 1.3 and 2.5 µg/ml. Formic acid, a principal metabolite, had no effect on MC at all concentrations tested (300 µg/ml or less). Formaldehyde gas is carcinogenic to the upper respiratory tract of rats where it induces squamous cell carcinoma (53). Formaldehyde gas is not carcinogenic in hamsters and is non-promoting, but possibly cocarcinogenic, in animals pretreated with diethylnitrosamine (27). Formaldehyde is neither carcinogenic nor initiating in SENCAR mice, but evidence for promoting effects is inconclusive (113). Formaldehyde is neither initiating nor promoting in a similar study with CD-1 mice (56). *In vitro*, formaldehyde solution is initiating (90) and weakly promoting (38), but, by itself, does not transform (90) C3H10T$\frac{1}{2}$ cells. Our results agree with the C3H10T$\frac{1}{2}$ cell data and predict promoting activity for formaldehyde but not formic acid.

Phenol and Selected Metabolites

Phenol, a weak promoter of tumors on mouse skin (12,138), had no effect on MC at any concentration tested (5-400 µg/ml). Because the skin is an important drug-metabolizing organ (82), seven metabolites of phenol (146) were also tested. Four minor metabolites (1,4-benzoquinone, catechol, hydroxyquinol, and quinol) suppressed MC at moderate (1-3 µg/ml) concentrations (70,71). Phenylsulfate, a major conjugation product (83,146), also inhibited MC, but at high (1-3 mg/ml) concentrations. Phenylglucuronide, another major conjugation product (83,146), was not toxic and had no effect on MC at any concentration (up to 7.5 mg/ml) tested (70). A methylated derivative of catechol, 2-methoxyphenol, enhanced MC in a dose-dependent manner at moderate (20-70 µg/ml) concentrations (70).

Inhibition of MC by five metabolites of phenol indicates that phenol is not an exception to the hypothesis that promoters inhibit MC and demonstrates the need to consider metabolites when testing chemicals. The relative weakness of these metabolites in blocking MC correlates with the weakness of phenol as a promoter (12). The pharmacologic and toxicologic significance of enhanced MC by

2-methoxyphenol requires investigation, particularly regarding antipromoting effects. For example, retinoic acid, a conditional inhibitor of mouse skin tumor promotion (114,139), is known to stimulate an increase in the number of gap junctions between cells (33,58).

At least two metabolites of phenol (catechol and quinol) which inhibit MC in V79 cells are non-promoting in the same assay where phenol shows promoting activity (12). A possible explanation may reside in the observation that promotion on mouse skin is multistage (11,41,109), and that several incomplete (stage) promoters are effective inhibitors of MC. The cation ionophore A23187, 4-O-methyl-TPA, and wounding are stage I promoters (107); wounding is also reported (3,4) to be a complete promoter of skin tumors in CD-1 mice. Mezerein is primarily a stage II promoter, although it has very weak activity as a complete promoter (41,107,109). Hydrogen peroxide is reported to be both a stage I and stage III promoter (107).

Inhibition of MC by A23187 and wounding is probably linked to increases in intracellular free calcium (35,65,95). Inhibition of MC or electrical coupling by hydrogen peroxide (26), 4-O-methyl-TPA (75,131), and mezerein (34,78,132), may also result from increases in intracellular free calcium. Regardless of mechanism, the fact that stage promoters suppress MC may have implications for the non-promoting but MC-inhibiting metabolites of phenol. If these are also stage promoters, exposure to two or more may be necessary for a promoting effect. The fact that mezerein is very weak as a complete promoter (107), but almost as potent an inhibitor of MC as TPA, suggests that inhibition of MC alone is insufficient for tumor promotion.

In summary, our results generally support the hypothesis that tumor promoters suppress MC and demonstrate the importance of considering metabolites when testing this hypothesis. Although there is a good correlation between the tumor-promoting effects of chemicals and their capacity to block MC, the precise role of MC in tumor promotion is unknown. Increased intracellular free calcium seems causally related to both the suppression of MC and the activation of many cellular events associated with tumor promotion. Considering the central and universal role of calcium as a biological switch (1), a connection between such events and intracellular free calcium levels is not surprising. The effective inhibition of MC by stage promoters indicates that suppression of MC alone may be insufficient for tumor promotion. Indeed, the large number of molecular and cellular events involved in the promotion process not only makes it difficult to separate critical from noncritical events, but increases the probability that most of these events will be necessary or facilitating but not sufficient for tumor promotion. The role of MC in tumor promotion and the specificity of suppression of MC as a test endpoint for promoter identification warrant further study.

ACKNOWLEDGEMENTS

This work was supported in part by an EPA Grant to J.E.T. (R811269). We thank Ms. Laurie Parker and Mr. Edward McKenna for expert technical assistance, and Ms. Joan Seites for manuscript preparation.

REFERENCES

1. Alberts, B., Bray, D., Lewis, J., Raff, M., Roberts, K., and Watson, J. D., editors (1983): In: *Molecular Biology of the Cell*, pp. 255-317. Garland Publishing Company, New York.
2. Arffman, E., and Galvind, J. (1971): *Experientia*, 27:1465-1466.
3. Argyris, T. S. (1980): *J. Invest. Dermatol.*, 75:360-362.
4. Argyris, T. S. (1982): In: *Carcinogenesis - A Comprehensive Survey, Vol. 7: Cocarcinogenesis and Biological Effects of Tumor Promoters*, edited by E. Hecker, N. E. Fusenig, W. Kunz, F. Marks, and H. W. Thielmann, pp. 43-48. Raven Press, New York.
5. Armuth, V., and Berenblum, I. (1972): *Cancer Res.*, 32:2259-2262.
6. Aylsworth, C. F., Jone, C., Trosko, J. E., Meites, J., and Welsch, C. W. (1984): *J. Natl. Cancer Inst.*, 72:637-645.
7. Baird, W. M., and Boutwell, R. K. (1971): *Cancer Res.*, 31:1074-1079.
8. Blumberg, P. M. (1980): *CRC Crit. Rev. Toxicol.*, 8:153-234.
9. Bock, F. O., Moore, G. E., and Crouch, S. K. (1964): *Science*, 145:831-833.
10. Bojan, F., Nagy, A., and Herman, K. (1978): *Bull. Environ. Contam. Toxicol.*, 20:573-576.
11. Boutwell, R. K. (1964): *Prog. Exp. Tumor Res.*, 4:207-250.
12. Boutwell, R. K., and Bosch, D. K. (1959): *Cancer Res.*, 19:413-424.
13. Boyland, E. (1983): *Environ. Health Perspect.*, 50:347-350.
14. Bradley, M. O., Bhuyan, B., Francis, M. C., Langenbach, R., Peterson, A., and Huberman, E. (1981): *Mutat Res.*, 87:81-142.
15. Bryan, G. T., and Springberg, P. D. (1966): *Cancer Res.*, 26:105-109.
16. Burke, J. P., Tumbleson, M. E., Seaman, R. N., and Sun, A. Y. (1977) *Res. Commun. Chem. Pathol. Pharmacol.*, 18:569-572.
17. Carafoli, E., and Crompton, M. (1978): *Curr. Topics Membranes Transp.*, 10:151-216.
18. Carroll, K. K., and Khor, H. T. (1970): *Cancer Res.*, 30:2260-2264.
19. Caskey, C. T., and Kruh, G. D. (1979): *Cell*, 16:1-9.
20. Chin, J. H., and Goldstein, D. B. (1976): *Science*, 196:684-685.
21. Clemo, G. R., and Miller, E. W. (1960): *Brit. J. Cancer*, 14:651-656.
22. Cohen, S. M., Murasaki, G., Ellwein, L. B., and Greefield, R. E. (1983): In: *Mechanisms in Tumor Promotion, Vol. 1: Tumor Promotion in Internal Organs*, edited by T. J. Slaga, pp. 131-149. CRC Press, Boca Raton, FL.

23. Colburn, N. H., Former, B. F., Nelson, K. A., and Yuspa, S. H. (1979): *Nature*, 281:589-591.
24. Costa, M., and Nye, J. S. (1978): *Biochem. Biophys. Res. Commun.*, 85:1156-1164.
25. Cox, R. P., Krauss, M. R., Balis, M. E., and Dancis, J. (1970): *Proc. Natl. Acad. Sci. USA*, 67:1573-1579.
26. Cox, R. P., Krauss, M. R., Balis, M. E., and Dancis, J. (1974): *Cell Physiol.*, 84:237-252.
27. Dalby, W. E. (1982): *Toxicology*, 24:9-14.
28. David, N. A. (1972): *Ann. Rev. Pharmacol.*, 16:353-374.
29. Délèze, J., and Loewenstein, W. R. (1976): *J. Membrane Biol.*, 28:71-86.
30. Diamond, L., O'Brien, T. G., and Baird, W. M. (1980): *Adv. Cancer Res.*, 32:1-74.
31. Dorfman, L. M., and Adams, G. E. (1973): *Reactivity of the Hydroxyl Radical in Aqueous Solutions.* U.S. Department of Commerce, National Bureau of Standards. NSRDS-NBS No. 46.
32. Dorman, B. H., and Boreiko, C. J. (1983): *Carcinogenesis*, 4:873-877.
33. Elias, P. M., Grayson, S., Caldwell, T. M., and McNutt, N. S. (1980): *Lab. Invest.*, 42:469-474.
34. Enomoto, T., Sasaki, Y., Shiba, Y., Kanno, Y., and Yamasaki, H. (1981): *Proc. Natl. Acad. Sci. USA*, 78:5628-5632.
35. Flagg-Newton, J., and Loewenstein, W. R. (1979): *J. Membrane Biol.*, 50:65-100.
36. Flavin, D. F., and Kolbye, A. C. (1983): In: *Modulation and Mediation of Cancer by Vitamins*, edited by F. L. Meyskens, pp. 24-38. S. Karger A. G., Basel.
37. Fox, R. B., and Fox, W. K. (1983): *Ann. N.Y. Acad. Sci.*, 411:14-18.
38. Frazelle, J. H., Abernethy, D. J., and Boreiko, C. J. (1983): *Cancer Res.*, 43:3236-3239.
39. Freund, G. (1979): *Cancer Res.*, 39:2899-2901.
40. Fukushima, S., Tatematsu, M., and Takahasi, M. (1974): *Gann*, 65:371-376.
41. Fürstenberger, G., Berry, D. L., Sorg, B., and Marks, F. (1981): *Proc. Natl. Acad. Sci. USA*, 78:7722-7726.
42. Gellhorn, A. (1958): *Cancer Res.*, 18:510-517.
43. Goldstein, B. D., Witz, G., Amoruso, M., Stone, D., and Troll, W. (1981): *Cancer Lett.*, 11:257-262.
44. Haiech, J., and Demaille, J. E. (1983): *Phil. Trans. R. Soc. Lond. B*, 302:91-98.
45. Hartman, T. G., and Rosen, J. D. (1983): *Proc. Natl. Acad. Sci. USA*, 80:5305-5309.
46. Hecker, E., Kubinyi, H., and Bresch, H. (1964): *Angew Chem. Int. Ed.*, 3:747-748.
47. Hiasa, Y., Kitahori, Y., Konishi, N., Enoki, N., Shimoyama, T., and Miyashiro, A. (1984): *J. Natl. Cancer Inst.*, 72:483-488.
48. Hicks, R. M., Wakefield, J. St. J., and Chowaniec, J. (1975): *Chem. Biol. Interact.*, 11:225-233.
49. Hoffmann, D., Hecht, S. S., and Wynder, E. L. (1983): *Environ. Health Perspect.*, 50:247-257.
50. Hoffmann, D., Schmeltz, I., Hecht, S. S., and Wynder, E. L. (1976): In: *Proceedings of the Third World Conference on Smoking*, Vol. 1, pp. 125-145. Department of Health Education and Welfare Publication No. NIH 76-1221, Washington, DC.

51. Hopkins, G. J., West, C. E., and Hard, G. C. (1976): *Lipids*, 11:328-333.
52. Hooper, M. L., and Subak-Sharpe, J. H. (1981): *Int. Rev. Cytol.*, 69:45-104.
53. International Agency for Research on Cancer (1982): *IARC Monographs on the Evaluation of the Carcinogenic Risk of Chemicals to Humans. Some Industrial Chemicals and Dyestuffs*, Vol. 29, pp. 345-389. IARC, Lyon.
54. Jensen, R. K., Sleight, S. D., Goodman, J. I., Aust, S. D., and Trosko, J. E. (1982): *Carcinogenesis*, 3:1183-1186.
55. Kinsella, A. R., and Radman, M. (1978): *Proc. Natl. Acad. Sci. USA*, 75:6149-6153.
56. Krivanek, N. D., Chromey, N. C., and McAlack, J. W. (1983): In: *Formaldehyde Toxicology-Epidemiology-Mechanisms*, edited by J. J. Clary, J. E. Gibson, and R. S. Waritz, pp. 159-171. Marcel Dekker, New York and Basel.
57. Langdon, R. C., Fleckman, P., and McGuire, J. (1984): *J. Cell Physiol.*, 118:39-44.
58. Larsen, W. J. (1977): *Tissue Cell*, 9:373-397.
59. Larsson, L. G., Sandstrom, A., and Westling, P. (1975): *Cancer Res.*, 35:3308-3316.
60. Lawrence, N. J., Parkinson, E. K., and Emmerson, A. (1984): *Carcinogenesis*, 5:419-421.
61. Lee, L. S. (1981) *Proc. Natl. Acad. Sci. USA*, 78:1042-1046.
62. Lieber, C. S., Seitz, H. K., Garro, A. J., and Worner, T. M. (1979): *Cancer Res.*, 39:2863-2886.
63. Liebman, K. C., and Heidelberger, C. (1955): *J. Biol. Chem.*, 216:823-830.
64. Loewenstein, W. R. (1967): *J. Colloid. Interface Sci.*, 15:34-46.
65. Loewenstein, W. R. (1972): *Arch. Intern. Med.*, 129:299-305.
66. Loewenstein, W. R. (1981): *Physiol. Rev.*, 61:829-913.
67. Longnecker, D. S., Roebuck, B. D., Yager, J. D., Lilja, H. S., and Siegmund, B. (1981): *Cancer*, 47:1562-1572.
68. Lucier, G. W., and Hook, G. E. R., editors (1983): *Environ. Health Perspects.*, 50:1-381.
69. MacLennan, D. H., and Campbell, K. P. (1979): *Trends Biochem. Sci.*, 4:148-151.
70. Malcolm, A. R., and Mills, L. J. Presented at the Monsanto Co. Symposium on New Approaches in Toxicity Testing and Their Application to Human Risk Assessment. St. Louis, MO.
71. Malcolm, A. R., Mills, L. J., and McKenna, E. J. (1983): *Ann. N.Y. Acad. Sci.*, 407:448-450.
72. Marchok, A. C., Cone, M. V., and Nettesheim, P. (1975): *Lab. Invest.*, 33:451-460.
73. McCoy, G. D., and Wynder, E. L. (1979): *Cancer Res.*, 39:2844-2850.
74. Mondal, S., Brankow, D. W., and Heidelberger, C. (1976): *Cancer Res.*, 36:2254-2260.
75. Mosser, D. D., and Bols, N. C. (1982): *Carcinogenesis*, 3:1207-1212.
76. Murray, A. W., and Fitzgerald, D. J. (1979): *Biochem. Biophys. Res. Commun.*, 91:395-401.
77. Nettesheim, P., Topping, D. C., and Jamasbi, R. (1981): *Ann. Rev. Pharmacol. Toxicol.*, 21:133-163.
78. Newbold, R. F., and Amos, J. (1981): *Carcinogenesis*, 2:243-249.
79. Nishizuka, Y. (1983): *Phil. Trans. R. Soc. Lond. B*, 302:101-112.
80. Nishizuka, Y. (1984): *Nature*, 308:693-698.

81. Oliveira-Castro, G. M., and Barcinski, M. A. (1974): *Biochem. Biophys. Acta,* 352:338-343.
82. Pannatier, A., Jenner, P., Testa, B., and Etter, J. C. (1978): *Drug Metab. Rev.,* 8:319-343.
83. Parke, D. V., and Williams, R. T. (1953): *Biochemistry,* 55:337-340.
84. Parry, J. M., Parry, E. M., and Barrett, J. C. (1981): *Nature,* 294:263-265.
85. Peracchia, C. (1978): *Nature,* 271:669-671.
86. Peraino, C., Fry, R. J. M., and Staffeldt, E. (1971): *Cancer Res.,* 31:1506-1512.
84. Peraino, C., Fry, R. J. M., Staffeldt, E., and Christopher, J. P. (1975): *Cancer Res.,* 35:2884-2890.
88. Peraino, C., Fry, R. J. M., Staffeldt, E., and Christopher, J. P. (1977): *Food Cosmet. Toxicol.,* 15:93-96.
89. Preston, B. D., Van Miller, J. P., Moore, R. W., and Allen, J. R. (1981): *J. Natl. Cancer Inst.,* 66:509-515.
90. Ragan, D. L., and Boreiko, C. J. (1981): *Cancer Lett.,* 13:325-331.
91. Reddy, B. S. (1983): In: *Mechanisms in Tumor Promotion, Vol. 1: Tumor Promotion in Internal Organs,* edited by T. J. Slaga, pp. 107-129. CRC Press, Boca Raton, FL.
92. Reddy, B. S., Weisburger, J. H., and Wynder, E. L. (1978): In: *Carcinogenesis - A Comprehensive Survey, Vol. 2: Mechanisms of Tumor Promotion and Cocarcinogenesis,* edited by T. J. Slaga, R. K. Boutwell, and A. Sivak, pp. 453-464. Raven Press, New York.
93. Roach, M. K. (1979): In: *Biochemistry and Pharmacology of Ethanol, Vol. 2,* edited by E. Majchrowicz and E. P. Nobel, pp. 67-80. Plenum Press, New York.
94. Roe, F. J. C., Salaman, M. H., and Cohen, J. (1959): *Brit. J. Cancer,* 13:623-633.
95. Rose, B., and Loewenstein, W. R. (1975): *Nature,* 254:250-252.
96. Rose, B., and Loewenstein, W. R. (1976): *J. Membrane Biol.,* 28:87-119.
97. Rose, B., Simpson, I., and Loewenstein, W. R. (1977): *Nature,* 267:625-627.
98. Rous, P., and Kidd, J. G. (1941): *J. Exp. Med.,* 73:365-390.
99. Saffiotti, U., and Shubik, P. (1963): *Natl. Cancer Inst. Monogr.,* 10:489-507.
100. Seeman, P. (1972): *Pharmacol. Rev.,* 24:583-655.
101. Selikoff, I. J., Churg, J., and Hammond, E. C. (1964): *J. Am. Med. Assoc.,* 188:22-26.
102. Selikoff, I. J., Hammond, E. C., and Churg, J. (1968); *J. Am. Med. Assoc.,* 204:104-110.
103. Sellakumar, A. R., Kuschner, M., and Laskin, S. (1975): *Proc. Am. Assoc. Cancer Res.,* 16:57.
104. Setala, H. (1956): *Acta Pathol. Microbiol. Scand., Suppl.,* 115:7-91.
105. Shlafer, M. (1975): *Fed. Proc.,* 34:793.
106. Sivak, A., and Van Duuren, B. L. (1970): *J. Natl. Cancer Inst.,* 44:1091-1097.
107. Slaga, T. J., editor (1983): *Mechanisms of Tumor Promotion, Vol. 1: Tumor Promotion in Internal Organs.* CRC Press, Boca Raton, FL.
108. Slaga, T. J., Bowden, G. T., and Boutwell, R. K. (1975): *J. Natl. Cancer Inst.,* 983-987.
109. Slaga, T. J., Fischer, S. M., Nelson, K., and Gleason, G. L. (1980): *Proc. Natl. Acad. Sci. USA,* 77:3659-3663.
110. Slaga, T. J., Fischer, S. M., Weeks, C. E., and Klein-Szanto, A. J. P. (1981): *Rev. Biochem. Toxicol.,* 3:231-281.
111. Slaga, T. J., Klein-Szanto, A. J. P., Triplett, L. L., Yotti, L. P., and Trosko, J. E. (1981): *Science,* 13:1023-1025.

112. Slaga, T. J., Schribner, J. D., Thompson, S., and Viaje, A. (1976): *J. Natl. Cancer Inst.*, 57:1145-1149.
113. Spangler, F., and Ward., J. M. (1983): In: *Formaldehyde Toxicology-Epidemiology-Mechanisms*, edited by J. J. Clary, J. E. Gibson, and R. S. Waritz, pp. 147-158. Marcel Dekker, New York.
114. Sporn, M. B., Dunlop, N. M., Newlon, D. L., and Smith, J. M. (1976): *Fed. Proc.*, 35:1332-1338.
115. Steele, V. E., Marchok, A. C., and Nettesheim, P. (1980): *Int. J. Cancer*, 26:343-348.
116. Steele, V. E., and Nettesheim, P. (1984): In: *Mechanisms of Tumor Promotion, Vol. 1: Promotion in Internal Organs*, edited by T. J. Slaga, pp. 91-105. CRC Press, Boca Raton, FL.
117. Steele, V. E., Topping, D. C., and Pai, S. B. (1983): *Environ. Health Perspect.*, 50:259-266.
118. Stenback, F., and Garcia, H. (1975): *Ann. N.Y. Acad. Sci.*, 243:209-227.
119. Stinson, S. F., and Donahoe, R. (1980): *Proc. Am. Assoc. Cancer Res.*, 21:122.
120. Sun, A. Y. (1979): In: *Biochemistry and Pharmacology of Ethanol*, Vol. 2, edited by E. Majchrowicz and E. P. Nobel, pp. 81-100. Plenum Press, New York and London.
121. Tapiero, H., Zwingelstein, G., Fourcade, A., and Portoukalian, J. (1983): *Ann. N.Y. Acad. Sci.*, 411:383-388.
122. The, R., and Hasselbach, W. (1977): *Eur. J. Biochem.*, 74:611-621.
123. Theiss, J. C., Arnold, L. J., and Shimkin, M. B. (1980): *Cancer Res.*, 40:4322-4324.
124. Topping, D. C., and Nettesheim, P. (1980): *Cancer Res.*, 40:4352-4355.
125. Topping, D. C., and Nettesheim, P. (1980): *J. Natl. Cancer Inst.*, 65:627-630.
126. Troll, W., Witz, G., Goldstein, B., Stone, D., and Sugimura, T. (1982): In: *Carcinogenesis - A Comprehensive Survey, Vol. 7: Cocarcinogenesis and Biological Effects of Tumor Promoters*, edited by E. Hecker, N. E. Fusenig, W. Kunz, F. Marks, and H. W. Thielmann, pp. 593-597. Raven Press, New York.
127. Trosko, J. E., and Chang, C.-C. (1984): In: *Mechanisms of Tumor Promotion, Vol. 4: Cellular Responses to Tumor Promoters*, edited by T. J. Slaga, pp. 119-145. CRC Press, Boca Raton, FL.
128. Trosko, J. E., Dawson, B., and Chang, C.-C. (1981): *Environ. Health Perspect.*, 37:179-182.
129. Trosko, J. E., Dawson, B., Yotti, L. P., and Chang, C.-C. (1980): *Nature*, 285:109-110.
130. Trosko, J. E., Jone, C., Aylsworth, C., and Tsuchimoto, G. (1982): *Carcinogenesis*, 3:1101-1103.
131. Trosko, J. E., Yotti, L. P., Dawson, B., and Chang, C.-C. (1981): In: *Short-Term Tests for Chemical Carcinogens*, edited by H. F. Stich and R. C. B. San, pp. 420-427. Springer-Verlag, New York.
132. Trosko, J. E., Yotti, L. P., Warren, S. T., Tsushimoto, G., and Chang, C.-C. (1982): In: *Carcinogenesis - A Comprehensive Survey, Vol 7: Cocarcinogenesis and Biological Effects of Tumor Promoters*, edited by E. Hecker, N. E. Fusenig, W. Kunz, F. Marks, and H. W. Thielmann, pp. 565-585. Raven Press, New York.
133. Tsushimoto, G., Asano, S., Trosko, J. E., and Chang, C.-C. (1983): In: *PCB's: Human and Environmental Hazards*, edited by F. D'Imitri and M. Kamrin, pp. 241-252. Ann Arbor Publishing Company, Ann Arbor.

134. Tsushimoto, G., Chang, C.-C., Trosko, J. E., and Matsumura, F. (1983): *Arch. Environ. Contam. Toxicol.*, 12:721-730.
135. U.S. Department of Health, Education and Welfare (1979): *Smoking and Health, A Report of the Surgeon General.* Department of Health Education and Welfare Publication No. (PHS) 79-50066, Washington.
136. Van Duuren, B. L., Orris, L., and Arroyo, E. (1963): *Nature*, 200:1115-1116.
137. Van Duuren, B. L., Sivak, A., and Lagseth, L. (1967): *Brit. J. Cancer*, 21:460-463.
138. Van Duuren, B. L., Witz, G., and Goldschmidt, B. M. (1978): In: *Carcinogenesis - A Comprehensive Survey, Vol. 2: Mechanisms of Tumor Promotion and Cocarcinogenesis*, edited by T. J. Slaga, R. K. Boutwell, and A. Sivak, pp. 491-507. Raven Press, New York.
139. Verma, A. K., Slaga, T. J., Wertz, P. M., Muller, G. C., and Boutwell, R. K. (1980): *Cancer Res.*, 40:2367-2371.
140. Wagner, J. C. (1971): *J. Natl. Cancer Inst.*, 46:i-ix.
141. Ward, J. M., Rice, J. M., Creasia, D., Lynch, P., and Riggs, C. (1983): *Carcinogenesis*, 4:1021-2029.
142. Warren, S. T., Doolittle, D. J., Chang, C.-C., Goodman, J. I., and Trosko, J. E. (1982): *Carcinogenesis*, 3:139-145.
143. Weinstein, I. B., Horowitz, A. D., Mufson, R. A., Fisher, P. B., Ivanovic, V., Greenebaum, E. (1982): In: *Carcinogenesis - A Comprehensive Survey, Vol 7: Cocarcinogenesis and Biological Effects of Tumor Promoters*, edited by E. Hecker, N. E. Fusenig, W. Kunz, F. Marks, and H. W. Thielmann, pp. 599-623. Raven Press, New York.
144. Whitfield, J. F., MacManus, J. P., and Gillan, D. J. (1973): *J. Cell Physiol.*, 82:151-156.
145. Williams, G. M., Telang, S., and Tong, C. (1981): *Cancer Lett.*, 11:339-344.
146. Williams, R. T. (1964): In: *Biochemistry of Phenolic Compounds*, edited by J. B. Harborne, pp. 205-248. Academic Press, New York.
147. Witschi, H. P. (1983): *Environ. Health Perspect.*, 50:267-273.
148. Witschi, H. P., Williamson, D., and Lock, S. (1979): *J. Natl. Cancer Inst.*, 58:301-305.
149. Wynder, E. L., and Fryer, J. H. (1958): *Ann. Intern. Med.*, 49:1106-1128.
150. Wynder, E. L., and Hoffmann, D. (1961): *Cancer*, 14:1306-1315.
151. Wynder, E. L., and Hoffmann, D. (1968): *Science*, 162:862-871.
152. Wynder, E. L., and Hoffmann, D. (1969): *Cancer*, 24:289-301.
153. Yager, J. D. (1983): In: *Mechanisms of Tumor Promotion, Vol. 3: Tumor Promotion and Carcinogenesis In Vitro*, edited by T. J. Slaga, pp. 55-70. CRC Press, Boca Raton, FL.
154. Yotti, L. P., Chang, C.-C., and Trosko, J. E. (1979): *Science*, 206:1089-1091.
155. zur Hausen, H., O'Neill, F. J., Freeze, U. K., and Hecker, E. (1978): *Nature*, 272:373-375.

Carcinogenesis, Vol. 8, edited by M. J. Mass et al.
Raven Press, New York © 1985.

Enhancement and Inhibition of Transformation of Syrian Hamster Embryo Cells

Joseph A. DiPaolo, Jay Doniger, Charles H. Evans,
and Nicolae C. Popescu

*Laboratory of Biology, National Cancer Institute, National Institutes of Health,
Bethesda, Maryland 20205*

Results in various mammalian species with chemicals known to be carcinogenic for experimental animals have often provided the basis for suspecting that they may be carcinogenic for humans, particularly when epidemiologic data is weak or lacking. Tomatis et al. (28) reported positive correlations between induction of liver parenchymal tumors in the mouse and in various organs in the rat and hamster by a variety of carcinogens. Of 58 chemicals analyzed, seven are recognized or suspected to be human carcinogens. The seven produced hepatocarcinomas in mice; of 4 tested in hamster, all were tumorigenic.

The *in vitro* Syrian hamster embryo cell (HEC) transformation model is a rapid, quantitative bioassay that uses diploid cells, (1,3) and compares favorably with both experimental long-term animal studies and epidemiologic data. Similar to human cells, normal HEC senesce; furthermore, spontaneous transformation is a rare event. *In vitro* morphologic transformation is characterized by random crisscrossing and piling up of cells not seen in controls which occurs in a dose-dependent manner. The morphologic transformation frequency can be modulated to elucidate the mechanism of factors responsible for enhancing or inhibiting transformation. Morphologic transformation correlates with tumorigenicity because individually transformed colonies can be isolated, cell lines established, and the formation of tumors demonstrated by injecting the transformed cells into either Syrian hamster or athymic nude mice. In addition, the phenotypic alterations seen *in vitro* that are characteristic for morphologic transformation are similar to those observed when primary tumors induced *in vivo* by carcinogens in hamsters are cultured. Thus, the HEC model for transformation is relevant to the study of the biology of carcinogenesis.

Carcinogenic polycyclic hydrocarbons can induce sarcomas in hamsters after one injection. Six primary subcutaneous tumors induced with a single injection of benzo(a)pyrene or 7,12-dimethylbenz(a)anthracene were analyzed for histopathology, growth *in vitro*, transplantability, and chromosome changes (13). All tumors were fibrosarcomas with varying degrees of differentiation. Cultures from tumors were characterized by rapid growth and increase in acidity of medium followed by rapid degeneration followed by survival of a few cells which produced a population that grew indefinitely *in vitro*. The initial populations were diploid, near diploid, or tetraploid and had acentric chromosome fragments, chromatid rearrangements, and marker chromosomes, but lacked a common karyotypic change; subsequently, heteroploidy increased. The mass cultures were typified by a lack of orientation with occasional piling up of cells. Cloning without an irradiated feeder layer resulted in diverse colonies, some of which were randomly oriented with crisscrossing of filaments. Tumor cells derived from these cultures were transplantable into hamsters. Resultant tumors were more anaplastic than the primary tumors. The results of these studies reinforce the conclusion that *in vitro* induction of transformation that results in neoplasia provides information relevant to carcinogenesis occuring *in vivo*.

A quantitative colony assay approach has made it possible to demonstrate dose-response relationships with a large variety of known organic and inorganic chemical carcinogens, and with ultraviolet irradiation (5). Transformation is inductive and not the result of selection of pre-existing transformed cells (20); furthermore, the carcinogenic action is direct because there is no evidence of viral involvement. The role of the mutation mechanism of chemical carcinogenesis remains less well understood. The transformation frequency is greater than the mutation frequency in HEC and transformation can occur with nonmutagenic chemicals such as bisulfite (7), diethylstilbesterol (2), or asbestos (8,21).

With hamster cells in culture, cocarcinogenesis, promotion, and anticarcinogenesis have also been demonstrated. Studies involving chemical carcinogens and physical carcinogens such as X-rays or ultraviolet irradiation have demonstrated enhancement of the transformation frequency (10,15). The enhancement of the transformation frequency is dependent on the time interval between the two insults; however, enhancement cannot be attributed to either chromosome changes or DNA repair. A noncarcinogen, caffeine, also enhanced the transformation frequency of chemical and physical carcinogen in a time and dose-dependent fashion (17). Caffeine affected the mode of DNA replication in hamster cells (14). It caused an increase in nascent strands of DNA which may be pivotal to increasing the transformation frequency. The transformation frequency can be increased by promoting agents (12) or prevented by using lymphotoxin (18), an immunologic hormone.

This report summarizes some of the carcinogen-target cell interactions involving agents that may be relevant to the etiology of human respiratory cancer. The present data emphasize that the carcinogenic response can be modulated so that either enhancement or inhibition of transformation results.

MATERIAL AND METHODS

Transformation Assay

Secondary HEC were used except as noted. Cells were cultured in Dulbecco's modified Eagle's medium supplemented with 10% fetal bovine serum (referred to as culture medium) and incubated in 10% CO_2 in a humidified atmosphere at 37°. Details of the transformation and cell survival assays have been presented (4). Cells were seeded for cloning (300 cells/60 mm dish). The next day treatment was begun; 12 dishes were used for each experimental point. After incubation for an additional six days to allow growth of colonies, the colonies were fixed with methanol and stained with Giemsa. In nontreated dishes the average number of colonies per dish ranged from 75 to 85. Colonies were examined with a stereoscopic microscope at $10 \times$ to $50 \times$; nontransformed colonies display a regularly oriented arrangement of cells and the transformed colonies are characterized by a random crisscrossed piling of cells not seen in the controls. The transformation frequency was calculated on the basis of the number of surviving colonies.

Chemicals

Stock solutions of chemical carcinogens and 12-O-tetradecanoyl-phorbol-13-acetate (TPA) were first dissolved and then sterilized in acetone. Asbestos fibers (UICC standard references) were sterilized with dry heat (175°) overnight. Chemical stock solutions were made in complete medium, and further dilutions were made just prior to use. Asbestos was suspended in serum and diluted with incomplete medium.

This suspension was diluted with complete medium. Because of the tendency of asbestos to settle rapidly, the suspension required frequent agitation.

Lymphotoxin

Ten ml of mineral oil were injected i.p. into adult male hamsters. Three days later, peritoneal cells were collected aseptically, washed 3 times by centrifugation at 280 × g for 10 min with culture medium RPMI 1640, and plated at a density of 2 × 10^7 cells per 20 ml of RPMI 1640 containing 10 µg of PHA (leukoagglutinin type IV; Sigma Chemical Co., St. Louis, MO) per ml in 100 mm Petri dishes. The peritoneal cells consisted of 60% macrophages, 20% lymphocytes, and 20% polymorphonuclear leukocytes. After 24 hr, the cell-free culture medium was collected, diafiltered against phosphate-buffered saline - 0.1% polyethylene glycol (M_r4000), and concentrated 40-fold with an Amicon diafiltration apparatus containing a 10,000 nominal molecular weight-excluding YM10 membrane (Amicon Corp., Danvers, MA) (26). Each preparation consisted of the concentrated, pooled culture medium after stimulation of cells from 6 animals. The concentrated culture medium from cells cultured in the absence of PHA did not display any lymphotoxin-mediated cytolytic, cytostatic, or anticarcinogenic activities.

Irradiation

UV irradiation was performed with a single 15-watt General Electric germicidal lamp (G15T8) from a distance of 24 cm at a fluence rate of 6.0 J/m^2/sec. Prior to UV irradiation, the medium was removed; the cells were uncovered during irradiation. After irradiation, cells were incubated in complete fresh medium.

Cultures were subjected to X-rays using a Torrex 120 machine (180 rads/min; 100 kV; 5 ma). The cells were covered with 2 ml of phosphate-buffered saline during exposure and the saline replaced by 8 ml of complete medium afterwards.

RESULTS AND DISCUSSION

Results demonstrating the applicability of the HEC model to carcinogenesis, cocarcinogenesis, promotion, and inhibition of transformation were obtained with combinations of agents, many of which may exist in polluted air and thus are relevant to respiratory carcinogenesis. Transformation has been demonstrated with polycyclic aromatic hydrocarbons and with bisulfite (SO_2); cocarcinogenesis with asbestos fibers and benzo(a)pyrene; promoted transformation with a classical noncarcinogen, 12-O-tetradecanoylphorbol-13-acetate (TPA); and inhibition with an immunologic hormone lymphotoxin derived from lymphocytes.

A series of nitrated polycyclic aromatic hydrocarbons were examined because the nitrated derivatives are potent bacterial mutagens while many of the parental compounds such as fluoranthene, chrysens, and pyrene are non-carcinogens that do not transform HEC. This class of polycyclic hydrocarbons is of increasing interest because a number of them are found in cigarette smoke, diesel exhaust, and photocopier fluids. The transforming potential of the nitro derivatives varied from compound to compound. None was as active as benzo(a)pyrene; however, 1,8-dinitropyrene, the most active compound tested, was one order of magnitude less effective than benzo(a)pyrene (6). Because of the dose-dependent transformation frequencies and the ubiquitous distribution of these nitrated compounds, these materials probably have deleterious effects on human health. In general, these compounds induced frame shift mutations, and are active in reductase-deficient bacteria. Because the nitrated compounds are able to stimulate DNA repair synthesis in cultured human cells, there is an implication of a possibility of a reductase activity occurring in mammalian cells that accounts for their ability to transform cells.

Because bisulfite is a food and pharmaceutical additive, and is a ubiquitous air pollutant in the form of SO_2 as a result of decay of organic material and combustion of coal and petroleum, it has been widely studied. Ordinarily, the interaction of carcinogens with DNA appears to be a requirement for the induction of cancer by carcinogens that are also considered mutagens. Bisufite, a chemical that at neutral pH does not induce mutations at two loci in Chinese hamster V-79 cells (22), does induce dose-dependent transformation of HEC at neutral pH that results in tumors when the cells are injected into athymic nude mice (7). Although bisulfite affects DNA metabolism, there is no evidence of bisulfite-induced DNA damage (16). Bisulfite induced no excision repair replication, caused no DNA strand breaks detectable in alkaline sucrose gradients, had no effect on the size distribution of DNA nascent daughter strands, and did not affect excision or post-replication repair of UV-induced damage. However, bisulfite did induce a dose-dependent decrease in the rate of DNA replication per cell, apparently due to a reduction in the number of functioning replicons. The data indicate that bisulfite causes no detectable DNA damage. Permanent transformed lines have evolved as a result of bisulfite treatment of HEC. These transformed lines are being further characterized in terms of chromosome and polypeptide changes.

This symposium has emphasized the hazards of asbestos as a representative of silicate minerals that have extensive commercial use and are major health hazards. Numerous epidemiologic and experimental animal studies have established the cancer-producing potential of asbestos fibers. Until recently, *in vitro* cell studies have dealt primarily with the relative toxicity of different fiber types, and have dealt with attempts to determine the mechanism by which fibers cause deleterious effects. Asbestos has been shown to elicit multiple effects that include suppression of interferon synthesis, induction of chromosome changes, alterations in epithelial organ cultures, and stimulation of macrophages to secrete plasminogen activator (23). Interestingly, when the toxicity of a variety of asbestos fibers was measured using epithelial cells, including those from embryonic human intestine-derived cells, the inhibition of colony growth was ordered in the same fashion as it is for the Syrian HEC. The mechanism of interaction of asbestos with cells is unknown and the site of toxicity is poorly understood. The fibers are insoluble in tissue culture medium but lethality is dependent upon dose. Other evidence, particularly with carcinogenic hydrocarbons, has demonstrated that toxicity and transformation can be separated in HEC. Because transformation of fibroblasts is relevant to carcinogenicity, the effects of asbestos fibers on cloning efficiency and transformation alone and in combination with benzo(a)pyrene was determined. The later combination was selected because the incidence of pulmonary carcinomas among asbestos workers who are also cigarette smokers is 80 to 90 times greater than that of the general population. Studies with hamster cells *in vitro* have provided evidence that both serpentine and amphibole mineral fibers cause transformation (8,21). The four varieties of asbestos fibers tested: crocidolite, anthophylite, amosite, and crysotile, induced a low rate of transformation when suspended in medium with 10% serum (8). Co-exposure to various amounts of suspension, different asbestos fibers, and a constant concentration of benzo(a)pyrene or ultraviolet irradiation, resulted in an enhancement of transformation only with the carcinogenic hydrocarbon. The enhancement was dose-dependent with all fiber species except amosite, which was not dependent on dose. A similar enhancement of morphologic transformation occurred if benzo(a)pyrene was added either 24, 48, or 72 hr after asbestos exposure. The synergism obtained with benzo(a)pyrene suggests that asbestos facilitates the transport of the hydrocarbon to cell sites that are critical for transformation. This situation parallels one that occurs with cigarette smokers. The *in vitro* results suggest that asbestos is both a complete carcinogen as well as a cocarcinogen for transformation - a situation analogous to that observed in humans.

HEC can also be used to investigate specific stages of carcinogenesis such as initiation and promotion (9,12,24) that were first demonstrated on the skin of mice. One day after seeding of cells for colony formation, HEC were exposed to X-irradiation (300 R). Two days later the tumor promoter TPA was added. The transformation frequency increased from 0.1% of the surviving colonies to 7% in a linear fashion as the TPA concentration was increased from 0 to 160 nM. Above this concentration of TPA, the transformation frequency remained at 7%. The increase in transformation frequency was not accompanied by any change in the relative cloning efficiency after exposure to X-rays. Phorbol-12,13-dihexanoate, another tumor promoter active *in vivo*, also increased X-ray-initiated transformation. No increase in transformation was observed with phorbol or with 3 different phorbol ester derivatives that have no tumor promoting activity *in vivo*. Furthermore, when HEC were treated with 80 nM TPA 2 days after X-irradiation, there was a linear increase in the transformation frequency as the dose of X-rays increased from 0 to 350 R.

In another study using N-methyl-N'-nitro-N-nitrosoguanadine (MNNG) as an initiating agent, TPA also significantly increased the absolute number of transformed colonies per dish and the average transformation frequency when the cells were treated with TPA 24, 48, or 72 hr after exposure to MNNG (24). TPA was more effective in enhancing transformation induced with lower MNNG concentrations (0.025, 0.05, and 0.1 µg/ml). Consistent with results derived *in vivo* with relatively high concentrations of carcinogen, TPA had a minimal effect on increasing transformation produced by MNNG at 0.25 µg/ml, which ordinarily induces approximately one transformant per dish. Of three polycyclic hydrocarbons: perylene, benzo(g,h,i)perylene, and benz(a)anthracene, that are weak or noncarcinogenic, only benz(a)anthracene induced a very low transformation frequency; however, after TPA, transformation occurred with all three hydrocarbons. The TPA-enhanced transformation was not accompanied by a change in the level of spontaneous nor induced sister chromatid exchange indicating that neither mitotic recombination nor futher DNA damage is responsible for the enhanced transformation frequency. These results indicate that *in vitro* promotion by phorbol esters is quantitative and mimics *in vivo* promotion.

Increased transformation frequencies occurring after TPA promotion of X-irradiated or UV irradiated diploid HEC can be inhibited at different steps in the process of carcinogenesis by either phytohemagglutinin (PHA) (11) - a naturally occurring mitogen, or by lymphotoxin (LT) - an immunologic hormone (18). Although both compounds interact with the cell surface through glycoproteins, it is hypothesized that the inhibition of transformation occurs as a result of different mechanisms. LT is anticarcinogenic *in vitro* (18) and *in vivo* (24,27), and is active during several stages of carcinogenesis. The anitcarcinogenic activity of LT is irreversible and occurs without inhibiting the growth of normal cells, i.e., it is noncytotoxic (18). The mechanism of action of LT is multifaceted. LT induces the synthesis of large-molecular-weight membrane glycoproteins in normal cells which accompanies an LT-induced state of resistance to carcinogenesis (19).

Sensitivity of HEC to the anticarcinogenic action of hamster LT depends on the stage of transformation, either initiation or promotion. LT was produced by mitogen stimulation of hamster leukocytes and purified by 10,000 MW exclusion ultrafiltration and isoelectric focusing at pH 4.5 - 5.5. LT irreversibly inhibits chemical or irradiation induced *in vitro* morphologic transformation of HEC when added at any point subsequent to carcinogen treatment. Galactose, a specific LT inhibitor, prevented the anticarcinogenic activity of LT, confirming that LT rather than another lymphokine, was responsible for inhibiting transformation (11). Twice as much LT is required to obtain a 50% reduction in TPA promoted transformation than in non-promoted transformation, suggesting a difference in sensitivity of the two stages of transformation to LT. In another study of stages of promoted transformation, a 48 hr LT treatment inhibited transformation when added either immediately before or after X-irradiation, or during TPA exposure.

The degree of sensitivity of different steps in carcinogenesis as the cells undergo the physiologic changes associated with transformation was examined more precisely with 6 hr LT treatments (12). If added for 6 hr., 72 hr before radiation, LT is ineffective, but is effective if added for 6 hr, 48 hr prior to irradiation. Cells became more sensitive to LT as the interval between the LT pulse and carcinogen insult or TPA addition was reduced. When added during the last 6 hr of the experiment, LT was equally inhibitory whether or not TPA was present. LT pretreatment before irradiation and TPA exposure caused a persistent but nonpermanent effect unless fixed by the caricnogen treatment of the cells. Similar results with LT were obtained with nonpromoted transformation. These results indicate that LT induces an anticarcinogenic physiological state in noncarcinogen treated cells that is short lived or transient; the temporal relationship between LT and carcinogen exposure is critical for preventing transformation.

Whereas LT, an immunologic hormone, has a persistent anti-carcinogenic effect, independent of whether added prior to or after TPA, PHA is inhibitory only if added during TPA treatment. Moreover, PHA in conjunction with LT causes additional inhibition of TPA promoted transformation. Thus, PHA and LT affect the biological activity of TPA by diverse mechanisms; LT alters the physiological state of the cell, causing a change in the cellular response to TPA; PHA may either affect the binding of TPA to a critical cellular receptor for promotion or a later step in promotion.

CONCLUSION

Diploid Syrian hamster embryo cells are particularly appropriate for the study of the transformation phenomenon in target cells. *In vitro* morphologic transformation occurs in a dose-dependent manner and is characterized by random crisscrossing and piling of cells; it correlates with tumorigenicity because individually transformed cell colonies can be isolated, cell lines can be developed, and the formation of tumors can be demonstrated after the injection of the transformed cells into either Syrian hamsters or athymic nude mice. HEC can also be used to investigate stages of carcinogenesis, initiation, and promotion.

The susceptibility of normal HEC to transformation by environ-mental carcinogens including asbestos, bisulfite, nitrated non-carcino-genic polycyclic hydrocarbons, and X- or ultraviolet irradiation has made possible the determination of a variety of cell responses as they procede to the neoplastic state. The initiation is usually a heriditary process involving single-hit kinetics and the transformation data indicate there is no measurable threshold response to carcinogens. The promotional aspects of transformaton are readily modulated by environmental factors and have a threshold, as well as a maximal effect.

The results of transformation studies using hamster cells indicate that *in vitro* studies are relevant to carcinogenesis and indicate that the various steps involved can be identified. Therefore, it should be possible to intervene with the various stages or steps leading to neoplasia so that cancer can be prevented.

REFERENCES

1. Barrett, J. C., and Ts'o, P. O. P. (1978): *Proc. Natl. Acad. Sci. USA*, 75:3761-3765.
2. Barrett, J. C., Wong, A., and McLachlan, J. A. (1981): *Science*, 212:1402-1404.
3. Berwald, Y., and Sachs, L. (1965): *J. Natl. Cancer Inst.*, 35:641-661.
4. DiPaolo, J. A. (1980): *J. Natl. Cancer Inst.*, 64:1485-1489.
5. DiPaolo, J. A., and Casto, B. C. (1978): In: *Third Decennial Review Conference: Cell Tissue and Organ Culture. Gene Expression and Regulation in Cultured Cells*, edited by K. Sanford, pp. 245-257. U.S. Government Printing Office, Washington, DC.
6. DiPaolo, J. A., DeMarinis, A. J., Chow, F. L., Garner, R. C., Martin, C. N., and Doniger, J. (1983): *Carcinogenesis*, 4:357-359.
7. DiPaolo, J. A., DeMarinis, A. J., and Doniger, J. (1981): *Cancer Lett.*, 12:203-208.
8. DiPaolo, J. A., DeMarinis, A. J., and Doniger, J. (1982): *Pharmacology*, 27:65-73.
9. DiPaolo, J. A., DeMarinis, A. J., Evans, C. H., and Doniger, J. (1981): *Cancer Lett.*, 12:243-249.
10. DiPaolo, J. A., Donovan, P. J., and Popescu, N. C. (1976): *Radiat. Res.*, 66:310-325.
11. DiPaolo, J. A., Evans, C. H., DeMarinis, A. J., and Doniger, J. (1982): *Int. J. Cancer*, 30:781-786.
12. DiPaolo, J. A., Evans, C. H., DeMarinis, A. J., and Doniger, J. (1984): *Cancer Res.*, 44:1965-1971.
13. DiPaolo, J. A., Nelson, R. L., and Donovan, P. J. (1971): *J. Natl. Cancer Inst.*, 40:171-181.
14. Doniger, J., and DiPaolo, J. A. (1980): *Biophys. J.*, 31:247-254.
15. Doniger, J., and DiPaolo, J. A. (1980): *Cancer Res.*, 40:582-587.
16. Doniger, J., O'Neil, R., and DiPaolo, J. A. (1981): *Carcinogenesis*, 3:27-32.
17. Donovan, P. J., and DiPaolo, J. A. (1974): *Cancer Res.*, 34:2720-2727.
18. Evans, C. H., and DiPaolo, J. A. (1981): *Int. J. Cancer*, 127:45-49.
19. Fuhrer, J. P., and Evans, C. H. (1983): *Cancer Lett.*, 19:283-292.
20. Gart, J. J., DiPaolo, J. A., and Donovan, P. J. (1979): *Cancer Res.*, 39:5069-5075.
21. Hesterberg, T. W., and Barrett, J. C. (1984): *Cancer Res.*, 44:2170-2180.
22. Mallon, R. G., and Rossman, T. G. (1981): *Mutat. Res.*, 88:125-133.
23. Mossman, B., Light, W., and Wei, E. (1983): *Ann. Rev. Pharmacol. Toxicol.*, 23:595-615.
24. Popescu, N. C., Amsbaugh, S. C., and DiPaolo, J. A. (1980): *Proc. Natl. Acad. Sci. USA*, 77:7282-7286.
25. Ransom, J. H., Evans, C. H., and DiPaolo, J. A. (1982): *J. Natl. Cancer Inst.*, 69:741-744.
26. Ransom, J. H., and Evans, C. H. (1983): *Cancer Res.*, 43:5222-5227.
27. Ransom, J. H., Evans, C. H., Jones, A. E., Zoon, R. A., and DiPaolo, J. A. (1983): *Cancer Immunol. Immunother.*, 15:126-130.
28. Tomatis, L., Partensky, C., and Montesano, R. (1973): *Int. J. Cancer*, 12:1-20.

Carcinogenesis, Vol. 8, edited by M. J. Mass et al.
Raven Press, New York © 1985.

Initiation and Promotion in Cultures of C3H10T½ Mouse Embryo Fibroblasts

Craig J. Boreiko

*Department of Genetic Toxicology, Chemical Industry Institute of Toxicology,
Research Triangle Park, North Carolina 27709*

Carcinogenesis in rodent model systems can proceed through multiple stages (10,44,46,52). Although specific genetic alterations seem to be involved in some of these stages (29), carcinogenesis can also be modulated by chemicals which by themselves appear to possess limited mutagenic or carcinogenic activity. Substances commonly referred to as tumor promoters have the ability to enhance (promote) the development of tumors in animals which have been previously exposed to subthreshold concentrations of a chemical carcinogen.

Promotion of carcinogenesis by chemicals has now been observed at numerous different tissue sites in several animal species (44,52). Evidence suggesting that tumor promotion may also play a causal role in the etiology of human neoplasia (50) has resulted in substantial efforts to develop short-term tests for the detection and study of tumor promoters. A variety of *in vitro* model systems have been developed, or are under development, for this purpose (6,45).

The use of *in vitro* systems for the detection of tumor promoters is complicated by practical and theoretical considerations. The effects of a tumor promoter can exhibit marked species and tissue specificity. For this reason it is unlikely that a single system can be used to detect all chemicals capable of promoting *in vivo* carcinogenesis. Furthermore, tumor promoters cause a variety of phenotypic changes in cultured cells (4,5) and there is often uncertainty as to whether the biological endpoint under study in a given assay system is relevant to promotion. Efforts to identify biologically-relevant *in vitro* endpoints are in turn complicated by a limited understanding of the mechanism(s) responsible for *in vivo* promotion.

In an attempt to overcome some of these considerations, efforts have been made to use cell transformation systems for the detection and study of tumor promoters. Cell transformation systems permit study of the ability of chemicals to convert normal cells to a "preneoplastic" state or "preneoplastic" cells to a tumorigenic state (23). Promotion-like enhancement of transformation has been observed in several different model systems (26). Since cell transformation systems appear to mimic central aspects of the carcinogenic process, it is generally assumed that the biological endpoint of enhanced transformation is relevant to multistage carcinogenesis *in vivo*. The C3H10T½ cell transformation system has been the system most extensively studied for this purpose.

C3H10T½ CELL TRANSFORMATION

The C3H10T½ cell transformation system was originally developed in the laboratory of Dr. Charles Heidelberger (42). This cell transformation system employs an immortal cell line of murine fibroblasts, C3H10T½ Cl 8, isolated from the embryos of C3H mice (43). A distinctive feature of this cell line is the strong density-dependent control maintained by the cells over cell division. When C3H10T½ cells are plated into a cell culture dish, they grow to form an evenly staining monolayer across the bottom of the dish and then cease proliferation (Fig. 1a). When cells are plated into a dish and then treated with an effective dose of a chemical carcinogen, some of the cells are transformed and as a result exhibit altered growth control. These transformed cells proliferate after a confluent monolayer has formed until, approximately six weeks after the start of an experiment, densely staining multilayered foci of actively growing transformed cells are evident (Fig. 1b). Foci can be categorized into one of three different morphological types. Cells from two of these focus types, type II and type III, will usually grow to form fibrosarcomas if injected into a suitable host animal.

Initiation and Promotion

Shortly after the development of the C3H10T½ cell transformation system, studies conducted in Heidelberger's laboratory demonstrated that the process of C3H10T½ transformation could proceed through discrete steps analogous to initiation and promotion in mouse skin. Treatment of low density C3H10T½ cultures with ultraviolet radiation (34) or low doses of polycyclic aromatic hydrocarbons (32) was not sufficient to produce significant numbers of transformed foci. Numerous transformed foci developed, however, when carcinogen-treated cultures were subsequently exposed to the tumor promoter 12-O-tetradecanoylphorbol-13-acetate (TPA).

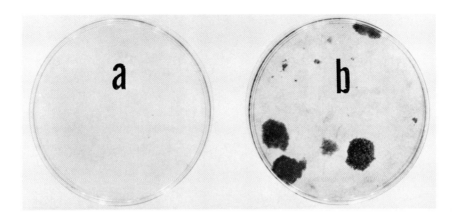

FIG. 1. Representative fixed and stained 60 mm dishes from a C3H10T½ cell transformation assay depicting: (A) The evenly staining cell monolayer which develops in solvent treated controls; (B) The development of transformed foci in a dish treated with 1.0 µg/ml 3-methylcholanthrene.

Initiation and promotion phenomena have now been observed in C3H10T½ cultures treated with a variety of chemicals and radiations (26). In fact, initiation of transformation appears to be the predominant consequence of treatment with many chemical carcinogens (1,9,17,19,41). Treatment with such chemicals will not produce foci unless the cultures are subsequently exposed to a tumor promoter such as TPA. Chemicals observed to function primarily as initiating agents for transformation in the standard C3H10T½ treatment protocols include numerous direct acting mutagens (eg., MNNG, EMS, MMS, ENU, MNU), procarcinogens such as aflatoxin B1, and respiratory carcinogens such as formaldehyde and acetaldehyde.

At this time it is not clear whether mechanistic significance should be attributed to the observation that some chemicals appear to function just as initiating agents for transformation. Many of these compounds are potent complete carcinogens *in vivo*. In addition, some can transform C3H10T½ cells in the absence of promoter treatments if the cultures are synchronized prior to carcinogen exposure (3,38) or altered treatment protocols are employed (37). For these reasons, classification of a chemical as an initiating agent, as opposed to transforming agent, in cell culture is probably best viewed as an arbitrary distinction of primary relevance to the standard C3H10T½ cell transformation system.

Although questions exist concerning the significance of initiation in cell culture for carcinogenesis *in vivo*, the work of several laboratories (26) has demonstrated that multiple aspects of promotion in C3H10T½ cultures mirror key operational features of promotion *in vivo*. For example, the initial work of Mondal and Heidelberger (32,34) showed the following:

1. Treatment with TPA alone did not produce transformation.
2. Transformed focus production resulted when cells were first initiated and then exposed to TPA.
3. Transformation did not result when cultures were first exposed to TPA and then initiated.
4. Promotion could be observed long after initiation. Cells could be initiated, grown to confluence in the absence of TPA, and then replated. Exposure of replated cells to TPA produced transformed foci.

Some of these characteristics have proved to be generalizations. For example, work conducted in this laboratory has indicated that exposure to an initiating agent or a tumor promoter alone is often sufficient to produce foci in up to 10% of the treated cultures. This compares to a "spontaneous" transformation rate of one focus for every 200 to 500 solvent control cultures.

Several other operational similarities exist between initiation and promotion *in vivo* and *in vitro*. In the presence of a constant amount of tumor promoter, the incidence of foci in C3H10T½ cultures will increase as a function of initiating agent concentration until high levels of cytotoxicity are achieved (9,41). In contrast, tumor promoters will exert their effects without overt cytotoxicity and dose response curves typically exhibit a no-effect dose range followed by a rapid rise to a response maxima. This maxima is then followed by a response plateau or a decline in focus formation. Such dose-response relationships are often observed with promoters *in vivo* and are consistent with "all or none" concepts of promoter action.

Studies here have observed this characteristic dose response for a number of structurally-diverse tumor promoters (Fig. 2). Moreover, these studies have found that chemicals active as promoting agents in the C3H10T½ system can be effective at widely different concentrations and can exhibit different levels of intrinsic activity. For example, 2,3,7,8-tetrachlorodibenzo-*p*-dioxin (TCDD), which lacks initiating or transforming activity for C3H10T½ cells (2), will promote focus formation at concentrations as low as 4 pM. A maximal response is attained at 40 pM TCDD. Treatment with TPA requires approximately

10,000-fold higher concentrations to produce a response, but the extent of focus enhancement observed is twice that obtained with TCDD. Mezerein will produce a response at concentrations comparable to TPA, but tends to exhibit a lower level of activity (8). High concentrations of formaldehyde are required to produce a very weak promotional response (18).

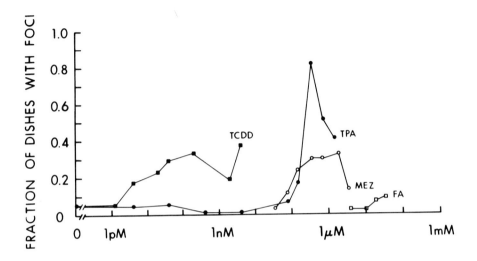

FIG. 2. Composite plot of dose response curves for the promotion of transformation by TCDD (2), TPA (17), mezerein (MEZ; 8), and formaldehyde (FA; 18). Data are plotted as the fraction of initiated dishes which develop foci vs. concentration of the promoting chemical.

The treatment regimen required to produce a response in the C3H10T½ promotion assay with TPA is also similar to that required on mouse skin. Promotion on mouse skin requires weeks or months of repeated promoter applications. In C3H10T½ cultures initiated with X-rays (27) or MNNG (17), multiple exposures to TPA for several weeks are necessary for the enhancement of focus formation. Moreover, exposure of the cells to TPA just at confluence will not promote transformation. Optimal responses are obtained only when cells are exposed during logarithmic growth and confluence (17,27).

Finally, preliminary studies have indicated that the promotion of morphological transformation in C3H10T½ cultures may be a reversible process (7). When cultures were initiated with MNNG and then exposed to TPA for five weeks, many transformed foci developed.

Continued incubation in the presence of TPA caused an increase in both the size and number of foci. When cultures containing foci were supplied medium which did not contain TPA, many of the foci regressed within 7 days. This reversion process was characterized by a rapid (within 24 hr) loss of polar transformed cell morphology and slow detachment of cells from the multilayered areas of the focus to yield a monolayer of morphologically nontransformed cells. Studies conducted *in vivo* have similarly indicated that papillomas on mouse skin (11) and preneoplastic nodules in rat liver (49) can regress upon the termination of promoter treatments.

Response of the System to Mouse Skin Promoters

Over the past several years, a limited data base has been developed which permits evaluation of the specificity of the C3H10T$\frac{1}{2}$ system. The number of chemicals studied to date is relatively small, a probable reflection of the fact that this conceptually simple system is subject to variation produced by a large number of cell culture variables (17). For example, promotion by TPA can exhibit extreme specificity for the lot of fetal bovine serum used to cultivate the cells. Still, the data base is sufficient to ask whether the C3H10T$\frac{1}{2}$ system responds in an appropriate fashion to mouse skin tumor promoters.

A listing of agents studied in the C3H10T$\frac{1}{2}$ system and on mouse skin is presented in Table 1. An indication is included of the nature and strength of the response each agent generates in both systems. Many of the agents listed have been studied using diverse treatment regimens, different animal strains, and often without complete dose response studies. Estimates of the magnitude of response generated by each agent are thus arbitrary designations made for the purposes of this comparison.

The potent mouse skin promoters TPA (17,26) and croton oil (Boreiko, Abernethy and Huband: unpublished results) elicit strong responses in cell culture. Anthralin, TCDD, phorbol didecanoate, and formaldehyde elicit weak to moderate activity in both systems (2,18,21,36,40). 4-α-Phorbol didecanoate is moderately active in cell cultures (32) but is reported to be inactive on mouse skin (22). Phorbol and 4-O-methyl-TPA both lack activity as complete promoters on mouse skin (22) and are inactive in the C3H10T$\frac{1}{2}$ system (8,9,32).

Curiously, mezerein is quite active as a promoter of cell transformation (Fig. 2). Slaga and colleagues (46,47) have observed that while mezerein has only weak promoting activity on mouse skin, it

TABLE 1. Effect of chemicals studied on mouse skin upon the promotion of C3H10T½ cell transformation[a]

Chemical	Effect on mouse skin	Effect in 10T½
Croton oil	+ + + +	+ + + +
TPA	+ + + +	+ + + +
Mezerein	+[b]	+ + +
PDD	+ +	+ +
4-a-PDD	-	+ +
4-O-Me-TPA	-[c]	-
Phorbol	-	-
Anthralin	+ +	+
TCDD	+ +	+ +
Formaldehyde	+	+

[a]Compounds lacking activity in a given system are indicated by a (-). Positive responses are indicated +'s with (+ + + +) being a strong response and (+) weak.
[b]Effective stage II promoter on mouse skin.
[c]Effective stage I promoter on mouse skin.

can effectively enhance tumorigenesis in initiated mice which have been exposed for a limited number of treatments to TPA or 4-O-methyl-TPA. Mezerein has thus been classified as a potent stage II tumor promoter. In this multistage promotion strategy, TPA is in turn viewed as a complete promoter and 4-O-methyl-TPA as a stage I promoter.

This comparison indicates that the C3H10T½ system is sensitive to numerous mouse skin tumor promoters. The observation that mezerein elicits a response in cell culture, but 4-O-methyl-TPA does not, suggests that the C3H10T½ system may have preferential sensitivity to chemicals with stage II promotional activity. Indeed, Slaga and colleagues have suggested (46,47) that stage I of promotion entails the induction of an embryonic phenotype. Since C3H10T½ cells are of embryonic origin, stage II specificity might be expected (46). The response produced by 4-α-phorbol didecanoate in C3H10T½ cells might thus be an indication that this chemical possesses some stage II activity.

However, not all studies are concordant with the view that promotion in C3H10T½ cells reflects only stage II processes. Promotion on mouse skin can be inhibited by a variety of agents and this inhibition can exhibit stage specificity (47). Glucocorticoid hormones will typically inhibit both stage I and stage II promotion. Retinoids appear to inhibit stage II promotion. Both classes of chemicals inhibit promotion in C3H10T$\frac{1}{2}$ cultures (31,35), although some criticism of the retinoid studies has been raised (26). The protease inhibitor TPCK preferentially blocks stage I promotion on mouse skin. While TPCK has not been studied in the C3H10T$\frac{1}{2}$ system, numerous other protease inhibitors will inhibit promotion in these cells (26). Since protease inhibitors inhibit promotion in cell culture, efforts to classify the C3H10T$\frac{1}{2}$ system as possessing only stage II sensitivity may be premature. Additional research will be required to define the relationship between promotion in C3H10T$\frac{1}{2}$ cultures and the different stages of promotion in mouse skin.

Response to Chemicals Active at Sites Other than Mouse Skin

The C3H10T$\frac{1}{2}$ systems has also demonstrated sensitivity to promotion by chemicals which exert activity at sites other than skin (Table 2). Some of the agents tested are chemicals which have carcinogenic effects *in vivo*, but for which little data on tumor promoting activity is available. Only three chemicals of immediate relevance to respiratory tract carcinogenesis have been examined.

TABLE 2. Promoting effects of agents known to have carcinogenic or promoting effects at other tissue sites[a]

Chemical	10T$\frac{1}{2}$ response	Site of *in vivo* activity
Formaldehyde	+	Respiratory tract (rat)
Methanol	-	?
Formic acid	-	?
Acetaldehyde	-	Respiratory tract (hamster)
BHT	+ +	Lung (mouse), bladder (rat)
TCDD	+ +	Liver (rat), multiple other
Saccharin	+ +	Bladder (rat)
DES	+ + +	Vagina, cervix (human), breast (rat)
Estradiol	+ +	Breast, testes? (rodent)
Roussin's red	+ +	Esophageal? (human)
EGF	+ + + +	?

[a](-) indicates a chemical lacks promoting activity. Positive responses are indicated by + with (+) constituting a weak response and (+ + + +) the strongest.

The rodent respiratory carcinogen formaldehyde (21) produces a weak response as a promoter in the C3H10T$\frac{1}{2}$ system (Fig. 1) and is also active as an initiating agent in cell culture (41). Metabolism of formaldehyde to formate, or contamination of commercial formaldehyde preparations by methanol, are not responsible for this promoting effect (18). Whether formaldehyde is capable of promoting carcinogenesis of the respiratory tract is not known. As discussed earlier, formaldehyde possesses weak promoting activity on mouse skin (21).

The structurally related respiratory tract carcinogen acetaldehyde is reported to have promoting activity in hamsters (15). Cell culture studies with acetaldehyde have detected initiating but not promoting activity (1). Finally, butylated hydroxytoluene (BHT) has been reported to be a promoter of transformation (14). BHT can enhance lung adenoma formation in mice (51) and may also promote bladder carcinogenesis in rats (24). However, inhibition of liver carcinogenesis has also been observed (24).

Other agents which exhibit promoting activity in C3H10T$\frac{1}{2}$ cultures include saccharin (33), TCDD (2), Roussin's red (12), diethylstilbestrol (DES; 30), estradiol (28), and epidermal growth factor (16). Four of these chemicals are known or suspected to possess tumor promoting activity. TCDD, in addition to being a promoter on mouse skin (40), is a potent promoter in rat liver (39). Saccharin appears to have enhancing effects upon bladder carcinogenesis in the rat (13,20). DES has been causally associated with cervical and vaginal cancer in humans (25) and appears to be capable of enhancing mammary carcinogenesis in rodents (48). Such enhancement may be a characteristic effect of estrogenic sex hormones (25,48), leading one to suspect that estradiol may have *in vivo* promoting activity.

The carcinogenic and promoting activity of the remaining two agents listed in Table 2 is uncertain. Roussin's red is a nitroso compound found in pickled vegetables in China. Epidemiology studies have suggested that the consumption of pickled vegetables is associated with increased mortality from esophageal cancer (12). Epidermal growth factor has not been fully characterized for tumor promoting activity, but numerous similarities have been noted between its cellular effects and those of TPA (16).

SUMMARY AND CONCLUSIONS

Studies conducted in numerous laboratories have demonstrated that the transformation of C3H10T$\frac{1}{2}$ cells can proceed through discrete stages of initiation and promotion. Indeed, multiple operational aspects of initiation and promotion in this system closely mimic the essential characteristics of initiation and promotion on mouse skin. The sensitivity of this system to the effects of different tumor promoters also appears to parallel that of mouse skin, and there is evidence to suggest that the C3H10T½ system is most sensitive to agents acting as stage II tumor promoters on mouse skin. Sensitivity to compounds active at other tissue sites in rodents and perhaps man has also been observed.

At this time it is difficult to assess the relevance of the C3H10T½ system for the study of agents capable of modulating respiratory carcinogenesis. The process of promotion can possess extreme tissue and species specificity and effects observed in murine fibroblasts of embryonic origin may have little practical bearing upon effects to be anticipated in the tracheal epithelium of the rat or the bronchial epithelium of man. This is not to say that the C3H10T½ system is irrelevant to respiratory carcinogenesis. However, due recognition must be taken of the probable natural limitations of this system for the study of promoters of respiratory carcinogenesis. As the data base for the use of this system is expanded, the relationship between promotion in C3H10T½ cells and the respiratory tract of man and rodents will become better defined. Until such time as this relationship is firmly established, it is perhaps best to regard the C3H10T½ system as an interesting model with which results obtained using respiratory tissue can be compared or contrasted.

REFERENCES

1. Abernethy, D. J., Frazelle, J. H., and Boreiko, C. J. (1983): *Environ. Mutagen.*, 5:419.
2. Abernethy, D. J., Huband, J. C., Greenlee, W. F., and Boreiko, C. J. (1984): *Environ. Mutagen.*, 6:461.
3. Bertram, J. S., and Heidelberger, C. (1974): *Cancer Res.*, 34:526-537.
4. Blumberg, P. (1980): *CRC Crit. Rev. Toxicol.*, 8:153-197.
5. Blumberg, P. (1981): *CRC Crit. Rev. Toxicol.*, 8:199-234.
6. Bohrman, J. S. (1983): *CRC Crit. Rev. Toxicol.*, 11:121-167.
7. Boreiko, C., Abernethy, D., and Frazelle, J. (1983): *Proc. Am. Assoc. Cancer Res.*, 24:99.
8. Boreiko, C. J., and Dorman, B. H. (1984): *Proc. Am. Assoc. Cancer Res.*, 25:143.
9. Boreiko, C. J., Ragan, D. L., Abernethy, D. J., and Frazelle, J. H. (1982): *Carcinogenesis*, 3:391-395.
10. Boutwell, R. K. (1964): *Prog. Exp. Tumor Res.*, 4:207-250.
11. Burns, F. J., Vanderlaan, M., Sivak, A., and Albert, R. E. (1976): *Cancer Res.*, 36:1422-1427.
12. Cheng, S. J., Sala, M., Li, M. H., Courtois, I., and Chouroulinkov, I. (1981): *Carcinogenesis*, 2:313-319.

13. Cohen, S. M., Aria, M., Jacobs, J. B., and Friedell, G. H. (1979): *Cancer Res.*, 39:1207-1217.

14. Djurhuus, R., and Lillehaug, J. R. (1982): *Bull. Environ. Contam. Toxicol.*, 29:115-120.

15. Feron, V. J., Kruysse, A., and Woutersen, R. A. (1982): *Eur. J. Cancer Clin. Oncol.*, 18:13-31.

16. Fisher, P. B., Mufson, A., Weinstein, I. B., and Little, J. B. (1981): *Carcinogenesis*, 2:183-187.

17. Frazelle, J. H., Abernethy, D. J., and Boreiko, C. J. (1983): *Carcinogenesis*, 4:709-715.

18. Frazelle, J. H., Abernethy, D. J., and Boreiko, C. J. (1983): *Cancer Res.*, 43:3236-3239.

19. Frazelle, J. H., Abernethy, D. J., and Boreiko, C. J. (1984): *Environ. Mutagen.* 6:81-89.

20. Fukushima, S., Friedell, G. H., Jacobs, J. B., and Cohen, S. M. (1981): *Cancer Res.*, 41:3100-3103.

21. Griesemer, R., Boreiko, C., de Serres, F. J., Feron, V. J., McCormick, J. J., Swenberg, J. A., Trump, B. F., Upton, A., and Ward, J. (1984): *Environ. Health Perspect.*, in press.

22. Hecker, E. (1978): In: *Carcinogenesis - A Comprehensive Survey, Vol 2: Mechanisms of Tumor Promotion and Cocarcinogenesis*, edited by T. J. Slaga, A. Sivak, R. K. Boutwell, pp. 11-48. Raven Press, New York.

23. Heidelberger, C., Freeman, A. E., Pienta, R. J., Sivak, A., Bertram, J. S., Casto, B. C., Dunkel, V. C., Francis, M. W., Kakunaga, T., Little, J. B., and Schechtman, L. M. (1983): *Mutat. Res.*, 114:283-385.

24. Imaida, K., Fukushima, S., Shirai, T., Ohtani, M., Nakanishi, K., and Ito, N. (1983): *Carcinogenesis*, 4:895-899.

25. International Agency for Research on Cancer (1979): *IARC Monographs on the Evaluation of the Carcinogenic Risk of Chemicals to Humans, Vol. 21, Sex Hormones (II)*. IARC, Lyon.

26. Kennedy, A. R. (1984): In: *Mechanisms of Tumor Promotion, Vol. III*, edited by T. J. Slaga, pp. 13-55. CRC Press, Inc., Boca Raton, FL.

27. Kennedy, A. R., Murphy, G., and Little, J. B. (1980): *Cancer Res.*, 40:1915-1920.

28. Kennedy, A. R., and Weichselbaum, R. R. (1981): *Carcinogenesis*, 2:67-69.

29. Land, H., Parada, L. F., and Weinberg, R. A. (1983): *Science*, 222:771-778.

30. Lillehaug, J. R., and Djurhuus, R. (1982): *Carcinogenesis*, 3:797-799.

31. Miller, R. C., Geard, C. R., Osmak, R. S., Rutledge-Freeman, M., Ong, A., Mason, H., Napholz, A., Perez, N., Harisiadis, L., and Borek, C. (1981): *Cancer Res.*, 41:655-659.

32. Mondal, S., Brankow, D. W., and Heidelberger, C. (1976): *Cancer Res.*, 36:2254-2260.

33. Mondal, S., Brankow, D. W., and Heidelberger, C. (1978): *Science*, 201:1141-1142.

34. Mondal, S., and Heidelberger, C. (1976): *Nature*, 260:710-711.

35. Mondal, S., and Heidelberger, C. (1980): *Proc. Am. Assoc. Cancer Res.*, 21:96.

36. Mondal, S., and Heidelberger, C. (1980): *Cancer Res.*, 40:334-338.

37. Nesnow, S., Garland, H., and Curtis, G. (1982): *Carcinogenesis*, 3:377-380.

38. Oshiro, Y., Balwierz, P. S., and Molinary, S. V. (1981): *Toxicol. Lett.* 9:301-306.

39. Pitot, H. C., Goldsworthy, T., Campbell, H. A., and Poland, A. (1980): *Cancer Res.*, 40:3616-3620.

40. Poland, A., Palen, D., and Glover, E. (1982): *Nature*, 300: 271-273.
41. Ragan, D. L., and Boreiko, C. J. (1981): *Cancer Lett.*, 13:325-331.
42. Reznikoff, C. A., Bertram, J. S., Brankow, D. W., and Heidelberger, C. (1973): *Cancer Res.*, 33:3239-3249.
43. Reznikoff, C. A., Brankow, D. W., and Heidelberger, C. (1973): *Cancer Res.*, 33:3231-3238.
44. Scribner, J. D. and Süss, R. (1978): *Int. Rev. Exp. Pathol.*, 18:137-198.
45. Sivak, A. (1982): *Mutat. Res.*, 98:377-387.
46. Slaga, T. J., Fischer, S. M., Weeks, C. E., Klein-Szanto, A. J. P., and Reiners, J. (1982): *J. Cell. Biochem.*, 18:99-119.
47. Slaga, T. J., Klein-Szanto, A. J. P., Fischer, S. M., Weeks, C. E., Nelson, K., and Major, S. (1980): *Proc. Natl. Acad. Sci. USA*, 77: 2251-2254.
48. Stone, J. P., Holtzman, S., and Shellabarger, C. J. (1980): *Cancer Res.*, 40:3966-3972.
49. Tatematsu, M., Nagamine, Y., and Farber, E. (1983): *Cancer Res.*, 43:5049-5058.
50. Weisburger, J. H., Reddy, B. S., Cohen, L. A., Hill, P., and Wynder, E. L. (1982): In: *Carcinogenesis - A Comprehensive Survey, Vol. 7: Cocarcinogenesis and Biological Effects of Tumor Promoters*, edited by E. Hecker, N. E. Fusenig, W. Kunz, F. Marks, and H. W. Thielmann, pp. 565-585. Raven Press, New York.
51. Witschi, H., and Lock, S. (1978): In: *Carcinogenesis - A Comprehensive Survey, Vol. 2: Mechanisms of Tumor Promotion and Cocarcinogenesis*, edited by T. J. Slaga, A. Sivak, and R. K. Boutwell, pp. 465-474. Raven Press, New York.
52. Yuspa, S. H., Hennings, H., Lichte, U., and Kulesz-Martin, M. (1983): In: *Organ and Species Specificity in Chemical Carcinogenesis*, edited by R. Langenbach, S. Nesnow, and J. M. Rice, pp. 157-171. Plenum Press, New York.

Carcinogenesis, Vol. 8, edited by M. J. Mass et al.
Raven Press, New York © 1985.

Genes and Signal Transduction in Tumor Promotion: Conclusions from Studies with Promoter Resistant Variants of JB-6 Mouse Epidermal Cells

Thomas D. Gindhart, *Yoshiyuki Nakamura, Linda A. Stevens,
*Glenn A. Hegameyer, †Michael W. West, *Bonita M. Smith,
and *Nancy H. Colburn

*Laboratory of Experimental Pathology, National Cancer Institute, *Laboratory of Viral
Carcinogenesis, National Cancer Institute, †Program Resources Inc.,
Frederick, Maryland 21701*

Tumor promoters are noncarcinogenic compounds that cause the development of tumors when applied repeatedly after initiation with a single subthreshold dose of a carcinogen. The phenomenon of two-stage carcinogenesis (initiation followed by promotion) has been studied most thoroughly in mouse skin, where diesters of the tetracyclic diterpene phorbol, are the most potent promoting agents (18,84). A major question in tumor promotion concerns the determination of distinguishing properties of post-initiated cells which allow them to progress irreversibly to transformation in response to tumor promoters.

In the last five years the ability to test directly naked DNA for genes determining the neoplastic phenotype has led to identification of over 20 different genes which appear required to maintain transformation (32,63,92,110). Transfection of calcium phosphate-precipitated DNA from tumor cells into NIH 3T3 mouse embryo cells has provided an assay for transforming genes (oncogenes). Using the same assay, individual genes with transforming activity can be retrieved from plasmid libraries in which the genes of a tumor have been cloned. Recombinant DNA techniques appropriately combined with classic Mendelian genetics can pinpoint molecular changes activating genes for neoplasia. We can expect additional genes determining tumor development to be identified since 80% of tumor cell DNAs fail to transform NIH 3T3 cells and a total of 200 different human genetic disorders predispose to cancer (63,83).

Several specific questions can now be asked regarding the genetic basis of the preneoplastic phenotype: [1] Which gene(s) are altered?

[2] What kinds of alterations produce the preneoplastic phenotype? [3] How do tumor promoters interact with genes determining promotion to produce preneoplastic progression?

This communication summarizes the derivation and properties of an *in vitro* model system for late stage tumor promotion in mouse skin. This model utilizes the JB-6 family of mouse epidermal cell lines developed to address these questions. Genes specifically required for transformation by tumor promoters are discussed, and the signal transduction mechanisms considered most closely linked to the actions of these genes are presented.

METHODS AND MATERIALS

Transformation of JB-6 Cells by Tumor Promoters in Soft Agar

Points requiring special emphasis are given here and in the legend to Table II. JB-6 mouse epidermal cell lines are routinely subcultured weekly without being allowed to remain confluent as previously described (19,22). Exposure to tumor promoters while the cells are suspended in 0.33% agar induces anchorage independent (AI) transformation more efficiently than exposure in monolayer culture (19). Special attention must be given to producing a suspension of single cells, as epidermal cells aggregate more than do fibroblasts. 12-O-tetradecanoylphorbol-13-acetate (TPA) is used as the standard positive control. Colonies of eight or more cells are counted after 14 days (19,22).

The value for each AI colony count for the results presented in Fig. 2 and 6 represents the mean ± one half the range for two separate experiments run in duplicate.

Kreyberg Stain for Keratin

After fixation in glutaraldehyde, cells and colonies in agar layers can be stained for keratin with the Kreyberg stain, listed as "Dane's method" in the A.F.I.P. Manual of Histology.

RESULTS AND DISCUSSION

The JB-6 Cell System

Overall Description, General Properties

The JB-6 mouse epidermal cell line was established from untreated Balb/c primary mouse epidermal cell cultures (Fig. 1). The immortal line was monitored for promotion of neoplastic transformation in response to tumor promoters. JB-6 cells spontaneously acquired promotion sensitivity (the P^+ trait) after 35 serial passages in culture (16,19,31).

Derivation of JB6 Clonal Cell Lines

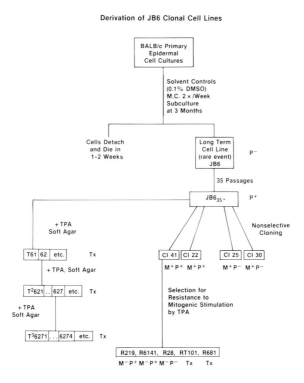

FIG. 1. Derivation of JB-6 clonal cell lines.

The JB-6 cell system is analogous to late or 2nd stage promotion in mouse skin (93,95). Promoters such as TPA, and inhibitors such as fluocinolone acetonide or agents that increase cyclic AMP levels, active in both stages of promotion in mouse skin, are active in JB-6 cells.

Stage II promoters, such as mezerein, and stage II inhibitors such as retinoids, are active in JB-6 cells; a stage I promoter, ionophore A23187, and stage I inhibitors, antipain and leupeptin, are not active in the JB-6 cell system (22,30). Promotion of transformation of JB-6 cells occurs by an induction mechanism rather than by selection of pre-existing transformants (17,19). Up to 40% of P^+ cells can be transformed at one time. This high efficiency is also inconsistent with production of infrequent events, such as chromosomal rearrangements. Tumor promoter-induced anchorage-independent (AI) clonal derivatives remain AI in the absence of promoters (i.e., the promotion event is as irreversible as is neoplastic transformation *in vivo*). Over 90% of transformed (Tx) cells lines derived from induced AI colonies are tumorigenic in syngeneic newborn mice (18,22,31). These transformation endpoints are used to ensure that biochemical events studied in this system are related to tumor cell formation.

Non-selective cloning of the JB-6 cell line after the 35th passage yielded stable clonal derivatives sensitive to (P^+) or resistant to (P^-) promotion of transformation. The capacity for promotion of transformation is specific to the phenotypes of the cell lines, and is not restricted to a particular agent such as TPA. P^+ lines sensitive to one agent are sensitive to others, and P^- lines resist promotion by all agents which promote P^+ lines (22,30). Convergence of pathways of signal transduction common to TPA and other tumor promoters can account for this phenomenon (37,43,58,76,87,104). Selective cloning of P^+ clone 41 for variants resistant to mitogenic stimulation by TPA yielded the R series of clonal cell lines used to dissociate mitogenic stimulation events from promotion of transformation (29). Table 1 summarizes the properties of JB-6 and clonal derivatives.

Several markers demonstrate the epidermal origin of JB-6 cells. They react with a rabbit antiserum specific for an epidermal antigen (16). Trisialoganglioside GT_{1b} (G_T), the major ganglioside of epidermal cells but not fibroblasts, constitutes over 60% of the total gangliosides of JB-6 cells (98,100). The cells also stain positively for keratin with the Kreyberg stain. Histologic study of P^+ JB-6 cells fixed in 0.33% agar also shows the increased nuclear/cytoplasmic ratio (N/C) familiar to pathologists as a marker of dysplastic lesions with malignant potential. The N/C ratio is further increased in tumor cell lines. Growth arrest in suspension culture must involve more than assumption of a round shape because up to 50% of growth arrested, demonstrably viable, single JB-6 cells are morphologically flat and extended in 0.33% agar (Gindhart and Keller, unpublished results).

TABLE 1. JB-6 clonal cell lines and their phenotypes[a]

Cell line	Tumorigenicity	Anchorage dependence	Sensitivity to promotion	Sensitivity to mitogenesis
JB-6$_{35}$-	N	D	P$^-$	M$^+$
JB-6$_{35}$+	N	D	P$^+$	M$^+$
Clone 41	N	D	P$^+$	M$^+$
Clone 22	N	D	P$^+$	M$^+$
Clone 30	N	D	P$^-$	M$^+$
Clone 25	N	D	P$^-$	M$^+$
R 219	N	D	P$^+$	M$^-$
R6141	ND	D	P$^+$	M$^-$
R28	ND	D	P$^-$	M$^-$
RT 101	T	AI	-	-
R 681	ND	AI	-	-
T^{3}6274[b]	T	AI	-	-
T^{3}6271	T	AI	-	-

[a] Tumorigencity was assayed by subcutaneous injection of 1-2 × 10^6 cells into nude mice or neonatal Balb/c mice. Anchorage independence, promotion of neoplastic transformation, and mitogenesis were assayed as described (19,29).
[b] Tumor cell lines T^{3}6274 and T^{3}6271 were derived from P$^+$ JB-6 at passage 60 by three cycles of cloning of AI colonies induced by TPA in soft agar (16). The R lines and other cells lines are described in the text (29).

Abbreviations: N, nontumorigenic; T, tumorigenic; D, anchorage dependent; AI, anchorage independent; P$^+$/P$^-$, sensitive/insensitive to promotion of anchorage independence and tumorigenicity by phorbol esters and nonphorbol tumor promoters; M$^+$/M$^-$, sensitive/insensitive to stimulation of cell division at plateau density by TPA; ND, not determined.

To date only one of the many biochemical changes produced by tumor promoters has consistently been associated with the promotion process and distinguished the P$^+$ from the P$^-$ phenotype. Treatment with TPA reduces net synthesis of G$_T$ by 90% in P$^+$ clones but not in P$^-$ JB-6 lines, primary mouse epidermal cells or epidermal cell lines resistant to induction of terminal differentiation by calcium (100). Promotion of transformation by phorbol esters, mezerein, epidermal growth factor (EGF), or benzoyl peroxide (BZP) is associated with the same effect of GT synthesis (98,100). The reduction in G$_T$ synthesis is related only to promotion, not to mitogenic stimulation. G_T synthesis remains reduced in transformed lines in the absence of promoters and addition of exogenous G_T blocks the induction phase of promotion but not AI growth in the absence of TPA (101). Since genetic drift allows unrelated traits to dissociate in culture (48), retention of tight linkage between the G_T response and the P^+ phenotype during extended serial passages favors a causal role for the G_T response in promotion of JB-6 cells.

Use in Detection of Tumor Promoters

The use of cell culture systems for detection of and mechanism analysis of tumor promoters has been reviewed (26). Established cell lines may more readily detect certain agents because they are already immortalized and resistant to calcium induced terminal differentiation. Immortalization, or escape from senescence, occurs early in establishment of cell lines in culture but can occur late in tumor development in vivo. Genetic changes determining immortality have been distinguished from genes producing the transformed phenotype without escape from senescence (63,75).

Table 2 lists agents tested for promoting activity in JB-6 cells according to class. Agents not previously reported as cited below are marked with an asterisk (*). The standard phorbol diesters show the same order of potency in JB-6 cells as on mouse skin (22). Retinoylphorbol acetate (RPA), a second stage promoter in NMRI mice (42), is a strong promoter for JB-6 cells. Mezerein and teleocidin, strong promoters for JB-6 cells as they are on mouse skin, also bind to the TPA receptor (76).

Polypeptide growth hormones were tested because these are candidates for endogenous tumor promoters in vivo, i.e., physiologic substances thought to stimulate tumor development during the latent period after a full dose of a complete carcinogen (16,18). Although preneoplastic progression of lymphomas in autoimmune mice can be attributed to chronic antigenic stimulation (47), the endogenous promoters of chemically-induced tumors remain unidentified. Platelet derived growth factor (PDGF), arginine vasopressin (AVP), and EGF are mitogenic for different cultured cells while transforming growth factor (TGF) extracted from tumor cell lines reversibly induces AI growth of nontransformed cells (37,53). The protein products of transforming genes, which may be expressed in preneoplastic cells, can activate the same 2nd messenger system as does TPA and endogenous hormones, which is the phosphatidylinositol (PI) pathway (6,7). PDGF and AVP stimulate PI turnover in different cell types, however, the relationship of EGF to the PI pathway appears complex (41,53). The transforming protein of *sis* is nearly identical to PDGF. The "tyrosine-specific protein kinases" of *src* and *ros* have lipid kinase activities which phosphorylate key intermediates of the PI cycle (7,68,103). The transforming protein of type B avian erythroblastosis virus is homologous to the intracellular portion of the EGF receptor (53). Such convergence of pathways at the second messenger level indicates a common distal mechanism of tumor promotion by diverse agents.

EGF promotes JB-6 cells strongly and several TGFs moderately. Type B TGF can promote P^+ cell lines lacking EGF receptors (20). AVP is a moderate promoter for JB-6 cells; it will be discussed more fully below. Polypeptide hormones targeted for epithelial cells such as EGF, EFG-related TGF's and AVP are promoters for JB-6 cells but several mitogens for mesenchymal cells (53), PDGF, thrombin, insulin, multiplication stimulating activity (MSA), and fibroblast growth factor (FGF) are not (Table 2).

Oxidants and free radical generators promote tumors in several animal models and may represent convergence of pathways for promotion by phorbol esters and complete carcinogens (13,14,57,94,96). Benzoyl peroxide (BZP), which promotes a high incidence of carcinomas on mouse skin, is a moderate promoter for JB-6 cells (49,84). Two additions of BZP to soft agar are required to readily detect promotion of JB-6 cells by BZP. Addition of G_T but not retinoic acid inhibits promotion by BZP. H_2O_2, a stage I promoter on mouse skin, has weak but detectable activity with JB-6 cells (30,59). Promotion of JB-6 cells by $NaIO_4$ may be due to oxidant stress or mild oxidation of cell surface sialic acids, which is mitogenic for lymphocytes (99). Hyperbaric oxygen is a promoter of mouse pulmonary adenomas (57). Fifty percent oxygen did not promote JB-6 cells but inhibited AI growth.

Environmental agents are considered an important source of exposure to tumor promoting compounds for humans. Cigarette smoke condensate contains many compounds that could account for weak promotion of JB-6 cells observed with the unfractionated mixture (22). Diethylhexylphthalate (DEHP), a plasticizer found in human blood stored in transfusion bags, a stage II promoter on mouse skin and liver tumor promoter, is a strong promoter for JB-6 cells (39, 109). Induction of peroxisomes, which produce reactive oxygen as a by-product of lipid catabolism, may account for the effectiveness of DEHP as a tumor promoter. Non-specific changes in membrane fluidity have been

TABLE 2. Detection of tumor promoters by JB-6 cells[a]

Class	Positive agents	Negative agents
Phorbol diesters	TPA (0.16-16 nM) PDBZ (16 nM) PDBU (16 nM) RPA (1.6-16 nM)*	Phorbol (1.6 µM) PDA (1.6 µM)
Nonphorbol diterpenes	Mezerein (1.6-16 nM)	
Other plant products	Teleocidin (0.16-16 mM)*	
Polypeptide hormones	EGF (1-50 ng/ml) TGF (5 µg/ml) AVP (1-100 ng/ml)*	PDGF (1 U/ml)* Thrombin (1 ng/ml)* Insulin (0.1 mg/ml) MSA (1-100 ng/ml)* FGF (1-100 ng/ml)*
Oxidants	Benzoyl peroxide (10 nM)* H_2O_2 (10 µM) $NaIO_4$ (0.2 mM)	50% oxygen*
Environmental agents	Cigarette smoke (20 µg/ml) DEHP (0.01%)	Mellitin (1-4 µg/ml)* Capsaicin (0.03-6.5 µM)*
Drugs	Cis-platinum (1 µM) Trans-platinum (17 µM)	Mestranol (1-10 µM)* Norethynodrel (1-10 µM)* Adriamycin (0.2-10 µg/ml)* Colchicine (0.03-3.0 µM)* A23187 (0.1 nM-10 µM)*
Food additives		Sodium saccharin (2-5 mM) Sodium cyclamate (2-5 mM)

*Indicates agents not previously reported as cited in text.
[a] Promotion sensitive (P[+]) JB-6 cells or P[+] clones derived from JB-6, clones 21, 22, 41 or R219 were exposed to agents in 0.33% agar medium containing 10% or 20% fetal bovine serum (17). Duplicate 60 mm Petri dishes are plated for each concentration tested and each agent has been tested in at least two independent experiments. Minimally positive agents induced at least a ten-fold increase in AI colonies over solvent control values of 0-100/10,000 cells. The strongest agents induce over a 100-fold increase. Negative agents fail to induce a significant increase over solvent control values. Where the entire range tested is not shown the lowest effective concentrations are given for the positive agents and the highest concentrations tested for negative agents. Potencies of positive agents relative to TPA and other abbreviations are indicated in the text.

Abbreviations: PDBZ, phorbol-12,13-dibenzoate; PDBU, phorbol-12,13-dibutyrate; PDA, phorbol-12,13-diacetate; RPA, 12-O-retinoylphorbol-13-acetate.

considered of possible importance in tumor promotion (16). Mellitin and capsaicin, the "membrane active" inflammatory agents of bee stings and hot peppers, respectively, lack promoting activity for JB-6 cells. Mellitin activates phospholipase A_2 and is mitogenic for Swiss 3T3 cells (86,90), but fails to activate phospholipase C (PLC) which would activate the PI pathway (6).

Tumor development after drug treatment is a problem of modern medicine. *Cis*-platinum and *trans*-platinum are both weak but detectable promoters for JB-6 cells (30). The promoting effect appears related to heavy metal tumor induction since *trans*-platinum showed the same promoting effect as *cis*-platinum, but lacks anti-cancer activity. Mestranol and norethynodrel, components of oral contraceptives associated with the development of liver tumors in women (46) and rats (115), did not promote JB-6 cells. The cardiotoxicity of adriamycin has been attributed to "membrane activity" unrelated to its anti-cancer effect. Low concentrations of colchicine stimulate DNA synthesis in fibroblasts and colcemid promotes transformation of preneoplastic Syrian hamster embryo cells associated with aneuploidy (35,107). Promotion of JB-6 cells by colchicine was not detected in the standard soft agar assay with the above agents. Some aneuploidy-dependent promotion events have probably already occurred in JB-6 cells in the course of immortalization and colchicine may produce aneuploidy-dependent promotion events in JB-6 cells at a low frequency. Treatment of JB-6 clone 41 with colchicine plus TPA yielded nontransformed cell lines with high hexose uptake rates (33) and a tendency to spontaneously transform with serial passage in culture (unpublished results). The calcium ionophore A23187 is an effective stage I but not stage II promoter on mouse skin. Repeated testing of ionophore A23187 over a wide dose range has failed to detect any promoting effect on JB-6 cells. Food additives of concern as potential tumor promoters in human diet, sodium saccharin and sodium cyclamate, are not promoters for JB-6 cells (100).

P⁻ JB-6 cells serve as promotion-specificity controls when testing agents for promoting activity. They undergo mitogenic stimulation by TPA or EGF but not promotion of transformation (29). None of the agents in Table 2 promote transformation of P⁻ JB-6 cells. P⁻ JB-6 cells are competent for expression of transformation as they can be transformed by viral transforming genes or by tumor promoters if transfected with DNA from P⁺ cell lines (27,100).

Arginine Vasopressin: A Tumor Promoter Associated with Bronchogenic Carcinomas, the Phosphatidylinositol Pathway and Calcium

AVP is produced by human lung tumors, usually bronchogenic carcinomas of the undifferentiated small cell type (38,60). Two physiologic activities of the hormone, the antidiuretic hormone (ADH) effect on renal tubules at low doses and the vasopressor (VP) effect on arterioles at higher doses, are mediated by different second messengers (6). When tumors secrete AVP systemically the clinically familiar Syndrome of Inappropriate ADH (SIADH) is produced by the ADH activity. A general role for AVP in tumor promotion was suggested when AVP was found to be mitogenic for Swiss 3T3 mouse embryo cells by a mechanism common with TPA and bombesin (37,86).

AVP promoted transformation of JB-6 clones 41 and R219 in a dose-dependent fashion at 1.0 to 100 ng/ml. (Results shown in Fig. 2.) AVP may properly be classified as a B-TGF since the effect of AVP appears not to require EGF receptors. Clone R219, which lacks EGF receptors (20), showed a low but definite response to 10 ng/ml of AVP. R219 has binding sites for TGF and can be promoted by TGF or TPA but not by EGF. Promotion by AVP was not affected by retinoic acid (data not shown).

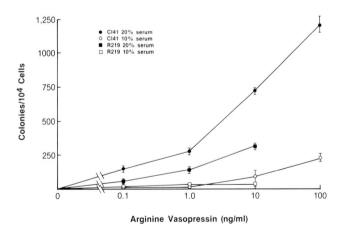

FIG. 2. Arginine vasopressin promotion of JB-6 cell lines clone 41 and R219.

Promotion of transformation by AVP is significant for many reasons. AVP is a well characterized polypeptide hormone, 9 amino acids in length, indispensible for life (M.W. 1,087 daltons, isoelectric point 10.9). AVP should be an endogenous tumor promoter since it is a mitogen and tumor promoter that is always present in plasma and extracellular fluid. Because it is also produced by human tumors AVP should be a model "transforming growth factor" for mechanistic studies. Biologically AVP should be an efficient TGF since 9 amino acids can be coded for by only 27 nucleotides. The clinical incidence of SIADH probably underestimates the number of lung tumors producing AVP (34,38), and as shown here, AVP can promote transformation of preneoplastic cells derived from non-bronchial epithelium such as epidermis.

Recent findings relate tumor promotion by AVP to its VP activity coupled to the PI pathway (6,43,86). Dicker and Rozengurt attributed the mitogenic effect of AVP to its ADH activity which is coupled to adenyl cyclase and Na^+ influx (37). However, in mouse skin, elevators of cyclic AMP block tumor promotion (94), as Forskolin does in JB-6 cells (unpublished results). Forskolin is a strong direct stimulator of adenyl cyclase (45). The VP activity of AVP triggers PI turnover, mobilization of intracellular calcium, and generation of diacylglycerol (DG) but not cyclic AMP (6). DG and TPA bind to and activate the same cellular target, protein kinase C (PKC), a biochemical point of convergence for TPA and at least a dozen hormones, neurotransmitters, inflammatory factors (6,7,76,87) and possibly transforming gene products (68,103). Increased PI turnover found in cells transformed either chemically or by viruses (68) suggests that the PI cycle is a common pivot point for transformation by a wide variety of agents.

Use of AVP as a model agent for analysis of mechanisms of promotion and transformation by polypeptide growth factors offers many practical advantages. It is a completely defined peptide synthesized commercially in large batches. It is inexpensive and consistently available. The hundreds of structural analogs synthesized to modify the ADH and VP activities should facilitate analysis of structure-activity relationships relevant to tumor promotion. Potentially antipromoting, blocking analogs already exist. Biologically active radiolabeled forms can confirm actual concentrations and half-life of AVP under various culture conditions. AVP is simple and clearly linked to human cancer as well as current major developments in basic physiology. These features recommend AVP as a valuable agent for mechanism studies of tumor promotion in many experimental systems, especially in respiratory carcinogenesis.

Genetic Basis of Promotion in JB-6 Cell Lines

The genetic basis of the capacity of P^+ JB-6 cell lines to transform when treated with tumor promoters has been analyzed by DNA transfection (27,28) and subsequent gene cloning (Lerman, unpublished results). In transfection experiments, one takes DNA from cells possessing a trait of interest and attempts to transfer the trait to cells lacking it (Fig. 3). If transfer is successful with whole cellular DNA, a genetic basis for the trait can be presumed and one can survey DNAs from pertinent sources for the gene(s), compare them according to restriction endonuclease sensitivity, identify cells permissive for expression of the gene(s), and probe active DNAs for genes already cloned and considered relevant to the trait. The transfection assay is then used to isolate the genes cloned in plasmids by testing the plasmid DNAs for biological activity (69).

**Mouse Epidermal JB-6 Cell DNA From a Promotable Donor
Is Transfected Into a Nonpromotable Recipient**

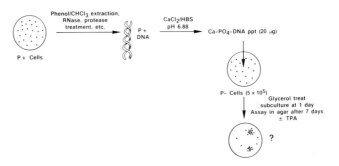

FIG. 3. Technique of DNA transfection.

Cell fusion studies with P^+ and P^- cell lines showed that promotion sensitivity was determined by a dominant gene and so could potentially be transferred from P^+ to P^- cells by transfection of DNA (28). Transfection of naked DNA from P^+ to P^- cell lines by the calcium phosphate co-precipitation method did transfer the P^+ trait. Transfection of DNA (20 μg) from P^+ clones into P^- clone 30 or P^- clone

25 produced transfection-dependent induction of AI colonies by TPA at a frequency of 200-400 colonies/10^5 cells. Transfection of P^- cells with DNA from P^+ cells (P^+ DNA) did not produce transformation (Tx) in the absence of TPA. Transfection of P^- cells with pertinent control DNAs does not produce the P^+ trait. Important negative controls include calcium phosphate precipitates alone, DNA from salmon sperm, P^- cells, *E. coli* and plasmids used for gene cloning. Digestion of P^+ DNA with some but not all restriction endonucleases prior to transfection eliminated the P^+ activity (25). P^- JB-6 cells can express the transfected P^+ trait but NIH 3T3 cells (27) do not. Transfection of P^- clones with DNA from tumor cell lines derived from JB-6 by TPA treatment also conferred promotion responsiveness (24,25). The genes determining promotion in P^+ JB-6 cells have been called *pro* for promotogenes, in analogy with oncogenes (25).

Transfection of DNA from the tumor cell lines did not transform P^- cells or NIH 3T3 cells in the absence of TPA. Reasoning that *pro* genes may also be required for maintenance of transformation, tumor cell DNA was transfected instead into P^+ cells which were tested for AI growth without induction by TPA. JB-6 P^+cell recipients but not NIH 3T3 or JB-6 P^- cells allowed detection of transforming gene (Tx) activity in DNA from tumor cell lines (23,25).

The Tx activity differs from the P^+ activity according to pattern of inactivation by restriction enzymes (25). Bam HI inactivated P^+ activity of DNA from either P^+ or tumor cells, but not tumor cell Tx activity. Bgl II inactivated Tx activity but had no effect on P^+ activity (25). These findings are summarized in Table 3.

P^+ DNA from a P^+ JB-6 cell line has been cloned (Lerman et al., Laboratory of Experimental Pathology, National Cancer Institute, unpublished results). Usually, genomic DNA libraries are screened with a specific cDNA probe to obtain the genomic DNA form of a gene previously isolated from another source. This simplifies selecting the few plasmids of interest out of 250,000 but presumes that the previously isolated gene is the one relevant to the biological endpoint. To ensure selection of genes determining P^+ activity, the library was repeatedly subdivided and individual pools screened for P^+ activity in the transfection assay. This search routine of sib selection led to screening of individual plasmids after six cycles of selection. Individual active plasmids conferred the P^+ trait in the transfection assay with much greater specific activity than uncloned whole P^+ DNA (24).

P^+ cell lines derived by transfection of cloned *pro* genes into P^- clone 30 have been established. Their phenotypes are being compared

TABLE 3. Genetic basis of promotion of JB-6 cells: Findings with transfection of genomic DNA[a]

	Phenotypic trait			
	P[+]		Tx	
Feature	From:	To:	From:	To:
Can be transfected	P[+] JB-6	P[-] JB-6	Tx JB-6	P[+] JB-6
	Tx JB-6	P[-] JB-6		Not P[-] JB-6
		Not NIH 3T3		Not NIH 3T3
Not inactivated by	Bgl II		Bam HI	

[a] DNA transfections, testing of transfectants and restriction endonuclease digestion were performed as described (23,25,27). See Fig. 3.

Abbreviations: P[+], promotion sensitive; Tx, tumor cell phenotype.

with the parental P[+] phenotype to determine if the individual cloned genes can account for all the differences between the P[-] and P[+] phenotypes. P[+] transfectants derived from either whole cell P[+] DNA (27) or cloned P[+] genes are like parental P[+] cell lines (Colburn et al., unpublished results).

Possible functions for *pro* gene products can be ruled in or out on the basis of these data and previous studies (24). They should involve *trans*-acting gene regulation and their absence should not impair the viability of P[-] cells. They are probably not receptors for TPA, EGF, transferrin, or insulin; mitogenic response mediators; mediators of total DNA methylation (10); or heat shock protein 80 (50). The *pro* gene products appear unrelated to 11 common viral oncogenes. Candidates for *pro* gene products include: 1) an inducible neuraminidase that decreases net G_T synthesis; 2) a PI pathway-linked calcium binding protein or a substrate for PKC; 3) an adenyl cyclase inhibitor; 4) an inducible inhibitor of SOD or other oxidant defenses; 5) an inducible ornithine decarboxylase; 6) a growth factor or growth factor receptor; 7) a nuclear matrix or chromatin protein.

Three different functions appear to be genetically determined in promotion of transformation of JB-6 cells. These involve one or more genes required for induction of transformation by tumor promoters, genes maintaining transformation, and an immortalizing genetic change in all JB-6 cells that permits expression of *pro* genes. Products of *pro* genes may be present at some basal level in P^+ cells or their production be completely dependent on TPA treatment. Unexpressed transforming genes must be present in P^- cells as well as P^+ cells since TPA can transform P^- cells after addition of *pro* genes which do not by themselves transform JB-6 cells.

Signal Transduction: PKC Substrates, a Heat Stress Protein and Oxidant Stress in Tumor Promotion

How do the products of *pro* genes permit TPA to activate transforming genes in P^+ JB-6 cells? Possible mechanisms should take into account available information about how tumor promoters produce effects on cells. Since the receptor for TPA is a calcium and phopholipid dependent protein kinase, PKC, phosphorylation of a substrate for PKC should mediate the first step in promotion by TPA (15,58,76). Transduction of TPA signals in P^- and P^+ cells should depend on PKC substrates but many other factors could account for the P^- phenotype. PKC substrates marking dedifferentiation in leukemias (54) and normal developmental stages in brain (106) suggest that PKC substrates may be oncofetal proteins. Different PKC substrates in variant EL-4 thymoma cells resistant to induction of interleukin-2 by TPA suggest that PKC substrates can account for differential responses to TPA related to tumor promotion (62).

Phosphorylation of a nuclear transcriptional regulator by PKC would be the most direct mechanism for gene regulation by TPA. Gene activation by TPA in a 5' promoter sequence-specific fashion associated with phosphorylation of a nonhistone chromatin protein has been reported (73,104). Products of *pro* genes could determine the P^+ phenotype very efficiently this way but direct transcriptional regulation in eukaryotes is reversible in most cases (63), and promotion of transformation of JB-6 cells is irreversible. Mitogenic stimulation after the induction phase of promotion could "lock in" such a change during new synthesis of DNA.

Phosphorylation of non-nuclear substrates for PKC should also regulate gene expression but indirectly. Protein substrates for PKC identified in cell-free systems associated with indirect gene regulation include: receptors for EGF and acetylcholine (1,41); signal transduction enzymes such as the PI lipid kinase B-50 (2); cytoskeletal components (76); and regulatory components of ribosomes such as eIF_2 (36,76), and the 90K subunit of the heme controlled inhibitor of protein synthesis (36). How site specific phosphorylation affects functions of substrates for PKC has been studied with B-50 (2); tyrosine hydroxylase (52); and the EGF receptor (41). TPA treatment of intact cells also affects phosphoproteins other than substrates for PKC. Phosphorylation on tyrosine of receptors for insulin and somatomedin stimulated by TPA in intact cells may reflect physiologic events (76). TPA-stimulated phosphorylation of transferrin receptors appears to represent exaggerated desensitization of hormone receptors (70). PKC does appear to function as a normal negative feedback loop of the PI pathway (2) also able to inhibit other signal transduction mechanisms such as cyclic AMP generation by adenyl cyclase and tyrosine phosphorylation by EGF receptors (41,42). *Pro* genes could determine the promotion response by changing ultimate effects of unregulated phosphorylation of regulatory proteins by PKC.

Metabolic stresses also alter gene expression indirectly as during induction of tolerance to anoxia or glucose deprivation (3). TPA mimics a second messenger but drives processes normally controlled by hormones in the direct persistent fashion of metabolic stresses which require gene regulation instead of receptor down regulation for adaptive tolerance. TPA activates PKC by substituting for diacylglycerol (DG) from hormonally stimulated PI breakdown (76). Metabolism of DG allows limited hormone-dependent activation of PKC but the effect of TPA is direct and persistent. Unbalanced stimulation of a two-branched second messenger system can account for actual metabolic stresses produced by TPA, augmented by the persistence of the TPA effect. Since hormonally stimulated DG is coordinated with calcium mobilization, isolated activation of PKC by TPA creates unbalanced, incomplete, hormone-like effects (1,58). Phosphorylation of three of ten proteins affected by AVP in hepatocytes is stimulated by TPA while ionophore A23187 affects the other seven in a complementary fashion (43). AVP stimulates glycogenolysis in hepatocytes, but TPA generally disrupts glucose utilization (4,14) and stimulates hexose uptake (33). PKC synergizes with calcium dependent processes for short terms and appears to down-modulate them over time which can lead to hormone-independent efflux of calcium in response to TPA (97). Achieving equilibrium under anaerobic metabolism, if possible, is characterized by broad gene switching which can be irreversible.

Stresses evoke post-transcriptional modes of gene regulation exceptional in adult life but important during early embryonic development (5,42,113). Central control is exerted by simple metabolites and autoregulated signal molecules generated internally.

In viral infections selective mRNA translation mediated by interferon's oligoisoadenylate (2'-5')pppApApA is coordinated with phosphorylation of ribosomal eIF_2, a PKC substrate (85). *Pro* gene products and TPA could operate in some parallel fetal arrangement to trigger an irreversible transformation event under stress conditions.

P⁻ and P⁺ JB-6 cells have equivalent numbers of TPA receptors (21), PKC enzyme activity (unpublished results), and shut-off of procollagen sysnthesis, which occurs at the pretranslational level (26). TPA does not produce detectable changes in total cytosine methylation of DNA in JB-6 cells (10), and processes dependent on cyclic AMP or glucocorticoids antagonize promotion in JB-6 cells.

Substrates for PKC were studied in P⁻ and P⁺ JB-6 cells by incubating cell fractions under PKC reaction conditions (61) and analyzing the reaction products by sodium dodecylsulfate polyacrylamide gel electrophoresis (results in Fig. 4). Cytosol (C), 100,000 x g pellet (M) or equal amounts of both (C + M) from JB-6 clone 41 were incubated without or with activation of PKC by addition of phospholipids (PL–, PL +). The cytosol contains PKC enzyme activity but few substrates (C lanes). The pellet contains little enzyme activity (M lanes), but substrates for PKC in the pellet become apparent when mixed with cytosol (C + M lanes). Figure 4 shows two endogenous substrates for PKC with apparent molecular weights of 34,000 daltons (pp34) and 37,000 daltons (pp37). An 80,000 dalton phosphoprotein in the pellet (pp80) is not a PKC substrate (M and C + M lanes in Fig. 5). To date comparison of P⁻ and P⁺ JB-6 cell fractions has not indicated a PKC substrate indispensible for promotion. The same 12 substrates for PKC have been found in P⁻, P⁺, and Tx JB-6 cell lines (unpublished result). Substrates for protein kinases detected in cell free studies are not necessarily substrates in intact cells and vice-versa.

Phosphoprotein patterns of P⁻, P⁺, and Tx cells were studied with and without TPA treatment in search of PKC substrate differences not detected in the cell free studies. A phosphoprotein affected by both TPA treatment and transformation was also sought in the metabolically labeled cells. Such a phosphoprotein would indicate a process linking TPA treatment to transformation and, if also a PKC substrate, should be one involved in promotion of transformation.

Two-dimensional (2-D) gels revealed an acidic 80,000 dalton phosphoprotein (pp80) which was most abundant in P⁻ cell lines, less in P⁺ cell lines and nearly undetectable in tumor cell lines (50). TPA increased pp80 2-3 fold in P⁻ and P⁺ cell lines, but not tumor cell lines. The time course was biphasic with a maximum at five hr and returned

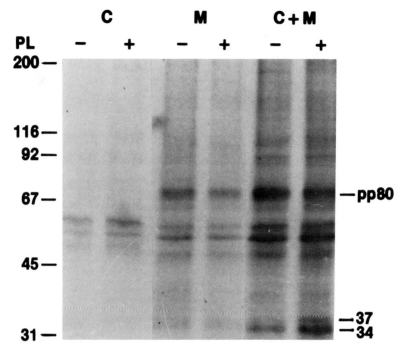

FIG. 4. Endogenous substrates for protein kinase C (PKC) in subcellular fractions of JB-6 clone 41 cells.

to baseline by 24 hr.   More pp80 was associated with resistance to transformation in P$^-$ cell lines while progressive reduction in pp80 correlated with capacity for transformation in P$^+$ cell lines and with tranformation in tumor cell lines.

Cell-free studies have shown that pp80 is in the particulate fraction and that it is not a PKC substrate (Fig. 5). The tumor cell lines produce very little pp80 to phosphorylate (unpublished results). Protein pp80 does appear to mark a mechanism inhibiting transformation by TPA which is defective in the tumor cell lines.

By all criteria tested to date pp80 is identical to the mammalian heat stress protein hsp 80 (111,114). The defining property of heat stress proteins is preferential synthesis during heat stress.   Heat stressing JB-6 clone 41 cells at 42° increased ^{32}P-labeled-pp80 as much as did TPA (50). Silver-stained parallel 2-D gels (Fig. 5) have shown that TPA (middle panel) or heat stress (right panel) also increased the amount of pp80 protein. Dotted circles mark pp80's position and the "a" marks Actin's position for reference.   Gels were loaded with 45 μg

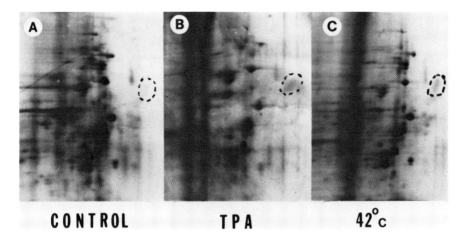

FIG. 5. Effects of TPA and heat stress on the amount of pp80 protein in JB-6 clone 41 cells.

protein equivalent to 5×10^5 cells. Figure 6 shows the effect of hyperthermia on promotion of JB-6 clone 41 cells by TPA. Elevation of temperature by 1.5° reduced AI colony induction by TPA about 50% (solid circles) and induced no AI colonies by itself (open circles). No AI colonies formed at 40° without or with TPA. Some of these large effects of modest hyperthermia may be due to long exposure but activation of stress responses by heat affects more than hsp 80.

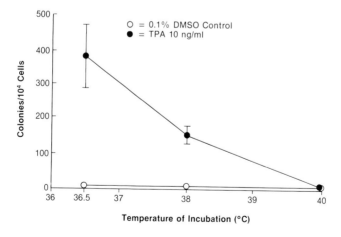

FIG. 6. Effect of heat stress on promotion of JB-6 clone 41 cells by TPA.

An apparently identical phosphoprotein, "80K", is stimulated in 3T3 cells by TPA with a similar biphasic time course (87). Phospholipase C itself or mitogens activating the PI pathway PDGF, AVP, bombesin stimulate "80K", but not EGF, cyclic AMP, insulin or phospholipase A_2, which all fail to activate PI breakdown. EGF and cyclic AMP also fail to enhance pp80 in JB-6 cells (unpublished results). The "80K" of 3T3 cells, which are P-, and pp80 both appear to be hsp 80.

Hsp 80 appears specifically related to glucose utilization and intracellular calcium. Calcium stress from ionophore A23187 and glucose deprivation increase hsps 80 and 100 but not the other hsps (114). Hsps 80 and 100 have high contents of acidic amino acids similar to known calcium binding proteins (64). The role of calcium in glucose utilization has been reviewed (15). Heat and TPA both alter glucose utilization and calcium sequestration, either by inhibiting sialic acid dependent microsomal calcium binding (82) or by inhibition of the microsomal calcium ATPase (56). Hormonal stimulation of "80K" is associated with PI turnover (87). Decreased pp80 in tumor cells may represent a late-stage AI calcium resistant phenotype (Smith et al., unpublished results).

Stresses elicit pre-emptive regulation of basic processes, temporary growth arrest, stress proteins and loss of normal control of gene expression. The high molecular weight heat stress proteins have been implicated in maintenance of normal cell cycle arrest (55). Stimulation of a stress protein by TPA in JB-6 cells and loss of the same protein in neoplastic derivatives link promotion and transformation directly to stress responses and an abnormal mechanism of gene regulation in preneoplasia. *Trans*-acting transcriptional activation of hsp genes dependent on a heat stress-enhanced protein has been described (80). Preferential processing of transcripts from exceptional eukaryotic genes lacking introns such as the hsp genes also occurs during heat stress (81). Non-hsp genes inserted adjacent to the 5' promoter region sequence of an hsp gene can be strongly activated by heat stress (66). Selective sequestration of mRNAs in a translatable form is a normal fetal mode of gene regulation restricting synthesis of hsps 80 and 100 during sustained stress (111,114) but also of keratin in tumors (113). These all suggest ways stress-driven mechanisms could be redirected to activate transforming genes.

Heat creates multiple forms of stress, principally anaerobic metabolism and oxidant stress (3,14,71,105). Induction of tolerance to sustained heat stress is a differentiation event demanding gene switching under error-prone conditions. Selective expression of genes for at least seven heat stress proteins occurs during disaggregation of nuclear ribonucleoprotein particles and polyribosomes, altered phosphorylation of ribosomal proteins, and binding of preexisting hsps to the nuclear matrix (3,81).

Active regulation of gene expression in stress responses can involve signal molecules generated by partially inactivated enzymes. Heat or oxidant stress induce a thermostable lysyl tRNA synthetase in bacterial strains while repressing synthesis of the temperature sensitive enzyme usually present (9,65). Oxidation of sulfhydryl groups inhibits tRNA synthetase function but the enzyme steadily produces diadenosine tetraphosphate (ApppA) which is followed by induction of the temperature resistant form of the enzyme. ApppA can bind to DNA polymerase α and poly(ADP-ribose)synthetase (108). A more familiar "alarmone" in mammals controlled by interferon activates a specific endonuclease (85). Targets for oxidant stress in mammalian cells include the microsomal calcium pump and glucocorticoid receptors, regulatory molecules also sensitive to modest oxidation (36,51,56,72,79,102).

The possibility that oxidant stress in preneoplastic cells directly mediates promotion by TPA is supported by many observed effects of TPA either producing or reflecting intracellular oxidant overload (4,14,57,96). Extracellular reactive metabolites of oxygen have been shown to mediate several promotion relevant effects of TPA including suppression of natural killer cell lysis of tumor cells (88,89) and production of chromosomal breaks (13,14,57). Superoxide anion is primarily implicated in promotion by TPA, while lipid hydroperoxides and hydroxyl radicals appear secondary. SOD activity or antioxidants inhibit TPA promotion in diverse systems including mouse skin and JB-6 cells (57,74,96). A free radical generator which promotes JB-6 cells (BZP in Table 2) is a more general tumor promoter on mouse skin than TPA (84). TPA decreases SOD in mouse skin, and human fibroblasts (57,96). Sialic acids, of which G_T contains three, are especially sensitive to oxidation (82,99). TPA affects many other processes similarly in P^- and P^+ JB-6 cells but reduces SOD more in P^+ cells and G_T only in P^+ cells (25). *Pro* genes may affect oxidant stress responses, specifically.

Other observations independently link stress responses and carcinogenesis. Several oncogenic viruses either induce or otherwise become associated with hsps (65,105). Carcinogens or promoting agents which have been tested induce hsp synthesis. Examples include arsenic, cadmium, other heavy metals, hydroquinones, ionophore

A23187, H_2O_2, ethanol, and TPA (3,12,105). DNA repair and stress responses are linked in mutants of Drosophila selected for defective thermotolerance found to have defective postreplication DNA repair, increased sensitivity to mutagens and abnormal heterochromatin condensation (44). Binding of hsps to the nuclear matrix and frequent apparent lethality of homozygous deletions of hsp loci also indicate that intact stress responses are required for normal chromatin function (91).

Heat stress immediately arrests cell cycle progression in normal cells and induces oxidant defenses later. Mechanisms effecting these changes must operate incompletely in tumor cells since growth proceeds despite the common presence of anaerobic metabolism, an inducer of the heat stress response, and lowered oxidant defenses prevail (40,77,105). Depleting oxidant defenses produces aneuploidy by disrupting mitotic spindles (3,71). However, escape from metabolic stress-induced growth arrest may account for AI growth of tumor cells and selective retention of other stress responses would produce dedifferentiation by inhibiting synthesis of differentiated cell products (12,81,113).

Synthesis of subsets of hsps during stages of embryonic development identify hsps as fetal proteins and associate increased hsp production with fetal phenotypes as early as the zygote (5,8). Special control of hsp synthesis in dividing spermatocytes is suggested by a unique inability to produce the major hsp in response to heat (11) in the presence of marked thermal sensitivity. Heat stress is a stage-specific teratogen (12). Oxidant drug-induced teratogenesis and hormonally induced arrest of embryonic differentiation are both asssociated with unscheduled hsp synthesis in Drosophila (8,12). PDGF-like transforming gene products in tumor cells may do the same since PDGF has been reported to induce synthesis of hsps in cultured endothelial cells and of "80K" in embryonic Swiss 3T3 cells (87,112).

Action through fetal rather than adult regulatory mechanisms is an aspect of tumor promotion by TPA matching the fetal genes and phenotypes associated with neoplasia. These trans-acting mechanisms control growth and differentiation in response to internal metabolic signals and their own feedback loops autonomous of external signals. These features are common to neoplasia, embryonic development, stress responses, and TPA effects, but not differentiated adult states. Pro gene-dependent activation of transforming genes may mark a fetal mode of gene regulation generally involved in neoplasia.

CONCLUSION

The late stage preneoplastic phenotype of JB-6 cell lines allows study of tumor promoters and their mechanisms using irreversible transformation as the endpoint. Genes of at least two different types are required for promotion of transformation of JB-6 cells. *Pro* genes determine sensitivity to transformation by tumor promoters but do not produce transformation alone. Transforming gene activity detected by DNA transfection can transform P^+ JB-6 cells in the absence of tumor promoters. Both types of genes can be expressed in JB-6 mouse epidermal cells but not in NIH 3T3 fibroblasts and appear unrelated to 11 common viral oncogenes (Lerman, unpublished results).

How *pro* genes determine transformation of P^+ JB-6 cells by tumor promoters remains to be determined. Activation of the PI pathway, PKC and reactive oxygen generation are the signal transduction mechanisms most clearly linked to their actions. Identification of the *pro* gene products, their normal function, their distributions in mouse and human tissues and alterations in preneoplasia is planned. Oxidant stress can link *trans*-acting stress driven mechanisms regulating genes to tumor promotion. Study of interactions between carcinogens and stress responses promises additional insights into mechanisms of transformation as the "Heat Shock Protein" turn out to be normal fetal proteins, transcriptional regulators, nuclear matrix binding proteins, tRNA synthetases, free radical defenses and candidates for G_o maintenance factors.

ACKNOWLEDGEMENTS

We thank Ms. Jean Keller for excellent Kreyberg stains; Ms. J. L. Radford and Mrs. Beverly Bales for super typing of this manuscript; and Dr. Umberto Saffiotti for stimulating discussions.

REFERENCES

1. Albert, K. A., Wu, W. C.-S., Nairn, A. C., and Greengard, P. (1984): *Proc. Natl. Acad. Sci. USA*, 81:3622-3625.
2. Aloyo, V. J., Zwiers, H., and Gispen, W. H. (1983): *J. Neurochem.*, 41:649-653.
3. Ashburner, M. (1982): In: *Heat Shock from Bacteria to Man*, edited by M J. Schlesinger, M. Ashburner, and A. Tissieres, pp. 1-9. Cold Spring Harbor Laboratory, New York.

4. Backer, J. M., Boersig, M. R., and Weinstein, I. B. (1982): *Biochem. Biophys. Res. Commun.*, 105:855-860.
5. Bensaude, O., Babinet, C., Morange, M., and Jacob, F. (1983): *Nature*, 305:331-333.
6. Berridge, M. J. (1984): *J. Biochem.*, 220:345-360.
7. Berridge, M. J. (1984): *Biotechnology*, 2:541-547.
8. Bienz, M. (1984): *Proc. Natl. Acad. Sci. USA*, 81:3138-3142.
9. Bochner, B. R., Lee, P. C., Wilson, S. W., Cutler, C. W., and Ames, B. N. (1984): *Cell*, 37:225-232.
10. Bondy, G. P., and Denhardt, D. T. (1983): *Carcinogenesis*, 4:1599-1603.
11. Bonner, J. J., Parks, C., Parker-Thornburg, J., Mortin, M. A., and Pelham, H. R. B. (1984): *Cell*, 37:979-991.
12. Buzin, C. H., and Bournias-Vardiabasis, N. (1984): *Proc. Natl. Acad. Sci. USA*, 81:4075-4079.
13. Cerutti, P. A. (1984): In: *Comparison of Mechanisms of Carcinogenesis by Radiation and Chemical Agents*, edited by D. Longfellow and O. F. Nygaard, in press. Academic Press, New York.
14. Cerutti, P. A., Emerit, I., and Amstad, P. (1983): In: *Proteins in Oncogenesis*, edited by I. B. Weinstein and H. J. Vogel, pp. 55-67. Academic Press, New York.
15. Cohen,, P. (1982): *Nature*, 296:613-620.
16. Colburn, N. H. (1979): In: *Neoplastic Transformation in Differentiated Epithelial Cell Systems In Vitro*, edited by L. M. Franks and C. B. Wigley, pp. 113-134. Academic Press, New York.
17. Colburn, N. H. (1980): *Carcinogenesis* 1:951-954.
18. Colburn, N. H. (1980): In: *Carcinogenesis - A Comprehensive Survey, Vol. 5: Modifiers of Carcinogenesis*, edited by T. J. Slaga, pp. 33-56. Raven Press, New York.
19. Colburn, N. H., Former, B. F., Nelson, K. A., and Yuspa, S. H. (1979): *Nature*, 282:589-591.
20. Colburn, N. H., and Gindhart, T. D. (1981): *Biochem. Biophys. Res. Commun.*, 102:799-807.
21. Colburn, N. H., Gindhart, T. D., Dalal, B., and Hegamyer, G. A. (1983): In: *Organ and Species Specificity in Chemical Carcinogenesis*, edited by R. Langenbach, S. Nesnow, and J. M. Rice, pp. 189-200. Plenum Publishing Corporation, New York.
22. Colburn, N. H., Kohler, B. A., and Nelson, K. J. (1980): *Teratogen. Carcinogen. Mutagen.*, 1:87-96.
23. Colburn, N. H., Lerman, M. I., Hegamyer, G. A., and Gindhart, T. D. (1984): *Mol. Cell. Biol.*, in press.
24. Colburn, N. H., Lerman, M. I., Hegamyer, G. A., Wendel, E., and Gindhart, T. D. (1984): In: *Genes and Cancer*, edited by J. M. Bishop, M. Greaves, and J. D. Rowley, in press. Alan R. Liss, New York.
25. Colburn, N. H., Lerman, M. I., Srinivas, L., Nakamura, Y., and Gindhart, T. D. (1984): In: *Cellular Interactions by Environmental Tumor Promoters*, edited by H. Fujiki and T. Sugimura, in press. Japan Scientific Societies Press, Tokyo.
26. Colburn, N. H., Srinivas, L.,Hegamyer, G. A., Dion, L. D., Wendel, E. J., Cohen, M., and Gindhart, T. D. (1984): In: *The Role of Cocarcinogens and Promoters in Human Experimental Carcinogenesis*, edited by M. Borzsonyi, H. Yamasaki, and E. Hecker, in press. International Agency for Research on Cancer Scientific Publications, Lyon.

27. Colburn, N. H., Talmadge, C. B., and Gindhart, T. D. (1983): *Mol. Cell. Biol.*, 3:1182-1186.
28. Colburn, N. H., Talmadge, C. B., and Gindhart, T. D. (1983): *Prog. Nucleic Acid Res. Mol. Biol.*, 29:107-110.
29. Colburn, N. H., Wendel, E. J., and Abruzzo, G. (1981): *Proc. Natl. Acad. Sci. USA*, 78:6912-6916.
30. Colburn, N. H., Wendel, E. J., and Srinivas, L. (1982): *J. Cell Biochem.*, 18:261-270.
31. Colburn, N. H., Vorder-Bruegge, W. F., Bates, J. R., Gray, R. H., Rossen, J. D., Kelsey, W. H., and Shimada, T. (1978): *Cancer Res.*, 38:624-634.
32. Cooper, G. M. (1982): *Science*, 218:801-806.
33. Copley, M. P., Gindhart, T. D., and Colburn, N. H. (1983): *J. Cell. Physiol.*, 114:173-178.
34. Christy, N. P. (1975): In: *Textbook of Medicine*, edited by P. B. Beeson and W. McDermatt, pp. 1804. W. B. Sanders Company, Philadelphia.
35. Crossin, K. L., Carney, D. H. (1981): *Cell*, 23:61-71.
36. DeHaro, C., DeHerreros, A. G., and Ochoa, S. (1983): *Proc. Natl. Acad. Sci. USA*, 80:6843-6847.
37. Dicker, P., and Rozengurt, E. (1980): *Nature*, 287:607-612.
38. Dingman, J. F., and Thorn, G. W. (1974): In: *Harrison's Principles of Internal Medicine*, edited by M. M. Wintrobe, G. W. Thorn, R. D. Adams, E. Braunwald, K. J. Isselbacher, and R. G. Petersdorf, pp. 456-465. McGraw-Hill Book Company, New York.
39. Diwan, B., Ward, J. M., Colburn, N. H., Spangler, F., Creasia, D., Lynch, P. and Rice, J. M. (1983): *Proc. Am. Assoc. Cancer Res.*, 24:105.
40. Fernandez-Pol., J. A., Hamilton, P. D., and Klos, D. J., (1982): *Cancer Res.*, 42:609-617.
41. Friedman, B. A., Frackelton, A. R., Jr., Ross, A. H., Connors, J. M., Fujiki, H., Sugimura, T., and Rosner, M. R. (1984): *Proc. Natl. Acad. Sci. USA*, 81:3034-3038.
42. Furstenberger, G., and Marks, F. (1983): *J. Invest. Dermatol.*, 81:157s-161s.
43. Garrison, J. C., Johnson, D. E., and Campanile, C. P. (1984): *J. Biol. Chem.*, 259:3283-3292.
44. Gatti, M., Smith, D. A., and Baker, B. S. (1983): *Science*, 221:83-85.
45. Gilman, A. G. (1984): *Cell*, 36:577-579.
46. Gindhart, T. D. (1978): *Ann. Clin. Lab. Sci.*, 8:443-446.
47. Gindhart, T. D., and Greenspan, J. S. (1980): *Am. J. Pathol.*, 99:805-808.
48. Gindhart, T. D., Pettingill, O., Cate, C., and Sorenson, G. (1980): *Ann. Clin. Lab. Sci.* 10:320-326.
49. Gindhart, T. D., Srinivas, L., and Colburn, N. H. (1984): *Carcinogenesis*, in press.
50. Gindhart, T. D., Stevens, L., and Copley, M. P. (1984): *Carcinogenesis*, 5:1115-1121.
51. Grippo, J. F., Tienrungroj, W., Dahmer, M. K., Housley, P. R., and Pratt, W. B. (1983): *J. Biol. Chem.*, 258:13658-13664.
52. Haycock, J. W., Bennett, W. F., George, R. J., and Waymire, J. C. (1982): *J. Biol. Chem.*, 257:13699-13782.
53. Heldin, C., and Westermark, B. (1984): *Cell*, 37:9-20.
54. Helfman, D. M., Barnes, K. C., Kinkade, J. M., Jr., Volger, W. R., Shoji, M., and Kuo, J. F. (1983): *Cancer Res.*, 43:2955-2961.
55. Iida, H., and Yahara, I. (1984): *J. Cell Biol.*, 99:199-207.

56. Jones, D. P., Thor, H., Smith, M. T., Jewell, S. A., and Orrenius, S. (1983): *J. Biol. Chem.*, 258:6390-6393.
57. Kensler, T. W., and Trush, M. A. (1984): In: *Superoxide Dismutase*, edited by L. W. Oberley, in press.
58. Kikkawa, U., Kaibuchi K., Castagna, M., Yamanishi, J., Sano, K., Tanaka, Y., Miyake, R., Takai, Y., and Nishizuka, Y. (1984): In: *Advances in Cyclic Nucleotide and Protein Phosphorylation Research*, edited by P. Greengard, pp. 437-442. Raven Press, New York.
59. Klein-Szanto, A. J. P., and Slaga, T. J. (1982): *J. Invest. Dermatol.*, 79:30-34.
60. Kondo, Y., Mizumoto, Y., Katayama, S., Murase, T., Yamaji, T., Ohsawa, N., and Kosaka, K. (1981): *Cancer Res.*, 41:1545-1548.
61. Kraft, A. S., Anderson, W. B., Cooper, H. L., and Sando, J. J. (1982): *J. Biol. Chem.*, 257:13193-13196.
62. Kramer, C. M., and Sando, J. J. (1984): *Proc. Am. Assoc. Cancer Res.*, 25:149.
63. Land, H., Parada, L. F., and Weinberg, R. A. (1983): *Science*, 222:771-778.
64. Lee, A. S., Bell, J., and Ting, J. (1984): *J. Biol. Chem.*, 259:4616-4621.
65. Lee, P. C., Bochner, B. R., and Ames, B. N. (1983): *Proc. Natl. Acad Sci. USA*, 80:7496-7500.
66. Lis, J. T., Simon, J. A., and Sutton, C. A. (1983): *Cell*, 35:403-410.
67. Luna, L. G., editor (1968): *Manual of Histologic Staining Methods of the Armed Forces Institute of Pathology*. McGraw-Hill, New York.
68. Macara, I. G., Marinetti, G. V., and Balduzzi, P. C. (1984): *Proc. Natl. Acad. Sci. USA*, 81:2728-2732.
69. Maniatis, T., Fritsch, E. F., and Sambrook, J. (1982): *Molecular Cloning: A Laboratory Manual*. Cold Spring Harbor Laboratory Publications, New York.
70. May, W. S., Jacobs, S., and Cuatrecasas, P. (1984): *Proc. Natl. Acad. Sci. USA*, 81:2016-2020.
71. Mitchell, J. B., Russo, A., Kinsella, T. J., and Glatstein, E. (1983): *Cancer Res.*, 43:987-991.
72. Murad, F., Mittal C. K., Arnold, W. P., Katsuki, S., and Kirmura, H. (1978): In: *Advances in Cyclic Nucleotide Research*, edited by W. J. George and L. J. Ignarro, pp. 145-158. Raven Press, New York.
73. Murdoch, G. H., Franco, R., Evans, R. M., and Rosenfeld, M. G. (1983): *J. Biol. Chem.*, 258:15329-15335.
74. Nakamura, Y., Gindhart, T. D., and Colburn, N. H. (1984): *Proc. Am. Assoc. Cancer Res.*, 25:139.
75. Newbold, R. F., Overell, R. W., and Connell, J. R. (1982): *Nature*, 299:633-635.
76. Nishizuka, Y. (1984): *Nature*, 308:693-698.
77. Oberley, L. W., and Buettner, G. R. (1979): *Cancer Res.*, 39:1141-1149.
78. Okayama, H., and Berg, P. (1983): *Mol. Cell. Biol.*, 3:280-289.
79. Oliver, J. M., Albertini, D. F., and Berlin, R. D. (1976): *J. Cell Biol.*, 71:921-932.
80. Parker, C. S., and Topol, J. (1984): *Cell*, 37:273-283.
81. Pederson, T. (1983): *J. Cell Biol.*, 97:1321-1326.
82. Pierce, G. N., Kutryk, M. B. J., and Dhalla, N. S. (1983): *Proc. Natl. Acad. Sci. USA*, 80:5412-5416.
83. Purtilo, D., Paquin,, L., and Gindhart, T. D. (1978): *Am. J. Pathol.* 91:607-688.
84. Reiners, J. J., Nesnow, S., and Slaga, T. J. (1984): *Carcinogenesis*, 5:301-307.
85. Revel, M. (1979): In: *Interferon 1979*, edited by I. Gresser, pp. 102-163. Academic Press, New York.

86. Rozengurt, E., Legg, A., and Pettican, P. (1979): *Proc. Natl. Acad. Sci. USA*, 76:1284-1287.
87. Rozengurt, E., Rodriguez-Pena, M., and Smith, K. A. (1983): *Proc. Natl. Acad. Sci. USA*, 80:7244-7248.
88. Seaman, W. S., Gindhart, T. D., Blackman, M. A., Dalal, B., Talal, N., and Werb, Z. (1981): *J. Clin. Invest.* 67:1324-1333.
89. Seaman, W. S., Gindhart, T. D., Balckman, M. A., Dalal, B., Talal, N., and Werb, Z. (1982): *J. Clin. Invest.* 67:876-888.
90. Shier, W. T. (1979): *Proc. Natl. Acad. Sci. USA*, 76:195-199.
91. Sinibaldi, R. M., and Morris, P. W. (1981): *J. Biol. Chem.*, 256:10735-10738.
92. Slamon, D. J., DeKernion, J. B., Verma, I. M., and Cline, M. J. (1984): *Science*, 224:256-262.
93. Slaga, T. J., Fisher, S. M., Nelson, K., and Gleason, G. E. (1980); *Proc. Natl. Acad. Sci. USA*, 77:3659-3663.
94. Slaga, T. J., Fisher, S. M., Weeks, C. E., Klein-Szanto, A. J. P., and Reiners, J. (1982); *J. Cell. Biochem.*, 18:99-119.
95. Slaga, T. J., Klein-Szanto, A. J. P., Fisher, S. M., Weeks, C. E., Nelson, K., and Major, S. (1980): *Proc. Natl. Acad. Sci. USA*, 77:2251-2254.
96. Slaga, T. J., Solanki, V., and Logani, M. (1983): In: *Radioprotectors and Anticarcinogens*, edited by O. F. Nygaard, and M. G. Simic, pp. 471-485. Academic Press, New York.
97. Smith, B. M., Warner, W., and Carchman, R. A. (1984): *Cell Calcium*, submitted.
98. Srinivas, L., and Colburn, N. H. (1982): *J. Natl. Cancer Inst.*, 68:469-473.
99. Srinivas, L., and Colburn, N. H. (1984): *Carcinogenesis*, 5:515-519.
100. Srinivas, L., and Colburn, N. H. (1984): *Cancer Res.*, 44:1510-1514.
101. Srinivas, L., Gindhart, T. D., and Colburn, N. H. (1982): *Proc. Natl. Acad. Sci. USA*, 79:4988-4991.
102. Staehelin, L. A., and Arntzen, C. J. (1983): *J. Cell Biol.*, 97:1327-1337.
103. Sugimoto, Y., Whitman, M., Cantley, L. C., and Erikson, R. L. (1984): *Proc. Natl. Acad. Sci. USA*, 81:2117-2121.
104. Supowit, S. C., Potter, E., Evans, R. M., and Rosenfeld, M. G. (1984): *Proc. Natl. Acad. Sci. USA*, 81:2975-2979.
105. Thomas, G. P., Welch, W. J., Mathews, M. B., and Feramisco, J. R. (1982): *Cold Spring Harbor Symp. Quant. Biol.*, 46:985-996.
106. Turner, R. S., Raynor, R. L., Mazzei, G. J., Girard, P. R., and Kuo, J. F. (1984): *Proc. Natl. Acad. Sci. USA*, 81:3143-3147.
107. Tsutsui, T. Maizumi, H., and Barrett, J. C. (1984): *Carcinogenesis*, 5:89-93.
108. Varshavsky, A. (1983): *Cell*, 43:711-712.
109. Ward, J. M., Rice, J. M., Creasia, D., Lynch, P., and Riggs, C. (1983): *Carcinogenesis*, 4:1021-1029.
110. Weinberg, R. A. (1983): *Sci. Am.*, 249:126-138.
111. Welch, W. J., Garels, J. I., Thomas, G. P., Lin, J. J.-C., and Feramisco, J. R. (1983): *J. Biol. Chem.*, 258:7102-7111.
112. White, F. P., and Hightower, L. E. (1981): *J. Cell Biol.*, 91:160a.
113. Winter, H., and Schweizer, J. (1983): *Proc. Natl. Acad. Sci. USA*, 80:6480-6484.
114. Wu, F. S., Park, Y. C., Roufa, D., and Martonosi, A. (1981): *J. Biol. Chem.*, 256:5309-5312.
115. Yager, J. D., and Yager, R. (1980): *Cancer Res.*, 40:3680-3685.

Carcinogenesis, Vol. 8, edited by M. J. Mass et al.
Raven Press, New York © 1985.

Cellular Mechanisms for Tumor Promotion and Enhancement

Jill C. Pelling and Thomas J. Slaga

*Science Park—Research Division, The University of Texas System Cancer Center,
Smithville, Texas 78957*

The multistage nature of chemical carcinogenesis has been demonstrated in a number of tissues and systems, including the skin, liver, bladder, respiratory system, colon, esophagus, stomach, mammary gland, pancreas, and cells in culture (67,68,73,87,133). A wide variety of tumor promoting or enhancing agents have been identified, such as diterpenes, fatty acids, peroxides, indole alkaloids, polyacetates, polychlorinated biphenyls, butylated hydroxytoluene (BHT), anthralin, chrysarobin, phenols, dioxins, phenobarbital, hormones, bile acids, oral contraceptives, and diet (Table 1). Presently, no common mechanism has been found for these diverse promoting and enhancing agents, except that they bring about the expansion of the initiated cells in a target tissue through their effects on cell proliferation and differentiation. In addition, it is now becoming quite evident that the process of tumor promotion may involve the interaction and cooperation of endogenous factors as well as exogenous (environmental) factors, including chemical promoting agents, radiation, viruses, and diet. While the mechanism of promotion is still not understood at the molecular level, extensive progress has been made in recent years in the elucidation of the cellular and molecular events which accompany tumor promotion. It is the cellular and molecular basis for tumor promotion which is the subject of this review.

MULTI-STEP MODELS FOR CARCINOGENESIS IN VARIOUS ORGAN SYSTEMS

Among the various *in vivo* systems for which multistage models of initiation and promotion have been established, those of the liver and bladder are probably the most thoroughly characterized, with the exception of the skin, which will be discussed in a separate section.

TABLE 1. Summary of promoting and/or enhancing agents in various organ systems

Promoter/Enhancer	Tissue/Organ
Saccharin, tryptophan	Bladder
Hormones, fatty diet, phorbol	Mammary gland
Bile acids, fatty diet, high cholesterol diet	Colon
Phorbol, BHT	Lung
Diet, alcohol, smoking	Esophagus
Diet, smoking	Pancreas
Phorbol esters	Rat tracheal cell and organ culture
Phorbol esters, saccharin	Mouse cell culture
DDT, BHT, polychlorinated biphenyls, TCDD, phenobarbital, phorbol, thioacetamide, α-hexachlorocyclohexane	Liver

The multi-step nature of hepatocarcinogenesis was first predicted by studies of Farber and others (31) suggesting that the hyperplastic nodule was a preneoplastic lesion of hepatocellular carcinoma. These preneoplastic nodules were further characterized by Goldfarb and Zak (36), who demonstrated that the nodules were deficient in glucose-6-phosphatase, a feature of many hepatocellular carcinomas. Subsequently, the work of Teebor and Becker (102) demonstrated that many of these nodules induced by 2-acetylaminofluorene (AAF) regressed following removal of the carcinogen from the diet. Later studies by Farber et al., however, showed that the cells within a hyperplastic nodule expressed a new antigen which, upon nodular regression and remodeling, was retained by the cells (32). A second type of preneoplastic lesion, the enzyme altered focus, was identified following injections of diethylnitrosamine (DEN) into rats (34). Rabes et al. (69) showed that such foci could be identified by a deficiency in canalicular triphosphatase activity and β-glucuronidase, and by an increased thymidine labeling index.

Peraino and coworkers were the first to demonstrate promotion during hepatocarcinogenesis, by feeding rats AAF for 18 days followed by diets containing 0.05% phenobarbital at various times for up to 30 days following AAF (64). Animals fed phenobarbital developed hepatic tumors within 180 days after AAF, while only 20% of animals receiving AAF alone developed tumors. Other systems demonstrating promotion in the liver (or multi-step hepatocarcinogenesis) have been described as well (66,67,79,83,99). In addition to phenobarbital, other agents have been shown to possess promoting activity, including DDT, BHT, polychlorinated biphenyls, and estradiol (67). Recently Pitot and coworkers have demonstrated that TCDD is also a potent liver promoter following DEN treatment (67). The promoting capabilities of diet are also under study, notably the feeding of a choline-deficient, low methionine diet, or dietary orotic acid.

In addition to the liver, two-stage carcinogenesis has been demonstrated in the bladder as well. Several lines of evidence have pointed to the possible promotional role of tryptophan in bladder carcinogenesis. A classic experiment by Dunning et al. showed that feeding D,L-tryptophan combined with AAF produced a high incidence of bladder cancer in rats (30). No bladder tumors were produced by administration of D,L-tryptophan or AAF alone (30). Radomski and coworkers have observed a similar promoting effect of D,L-tryptophan in 2-naphthylamine-induced bladder tumors in Beagle dogs (71). The ability of saccharin to promote has been demonstrated in rats initiated by vesicular administration of N-methyl-N-nitrosourea (41).

In the colon, the promoting effect of sodium lithocholate, cholesterol, cholesterol epoxide, and cholesterol triol has been studied in conventional and germ-free rats (74). Sodium lithocholate, but not the cholesterols were found to have a promoting effect in N-methyl-N'-nitro-N-nitrosoguanidine-induced carcinogenesis (74). Other studies have demonstrated that cholic acid and chenodeoxycholic acid act as colon tumor promoters in conventional rats, whereas deoxycholic acid acts as a colon tumor promoter in both germ-free and conventional rats (75).

Promotion of mammary carcinogenesis and the leukemogenic action by phorbol has been observed in virgin female Wistar rats (5). This is in contrast to the inactivity of phorbol as a skin tumor promoter (38). In addition, phorbol proved to be active as a promoter for liver and lung carcinogenesis when administered systemically in AKR mice (4).

Although promotion has now been demonstrated in numerous organ systems, much of our present knowledge about the cellular and molecular events involved in tumor promotion is derived from studies in mouse skin (67,86,87,110). The two-stage model of skin carcinogenesis is characterized by the sequential application of a subcarcinogenic dose of a direct-acting or indirect-acting carcinogen (initiation stage) followed by repetitive treatment with a noncarcinogenic promoting agent (promotion stage). Papillomas occur after a relatively short latency period of 9-15 weeks, with carcinomas appearing as long as a year later. The repetitive application of the promoter without initiation usually does not give rise to tumors or produces only a few (85). Furthermore, a dose response effect has been demonstrated using 12-O-tetradecanoylphorbol-13-acetate (TPA) as the promoter (92).

An important characteristic of the two-stage carcinogenesis model in mouse skin is the irreversible nature of the initiation step. A lapse of up to one year between application of the initiating agent and the beginning of promotion treatment results in a tumor response approaching that observed when promotion begins one week following initiation (13). Promotion, on the other hand, is reversible at least in early states, requiring a certain frequency of application in order to induce tumors (13).

At the molecular level, the initiation step has been portrayed as an irreversible step occurring in the target cell population, presumably brought about by genetic damage resulting from the interaction of a chemical carcinogen with a critical target macromolecule. In support of this model are studies showing a strong correlation between the carcinogenic potency of many chemical carcinogens and their relative mutagenic activities (14,85,93). The promotional state is hypothesized to result in the selection and amplification of these "initiated" target cells. It is now becoming apparent, however, that these models of initiation and promotion are oversimplified. Current evidence suggests that the genetic damage occurring during initiation may be much more complex, with gene rearrangements and/or amplifications resulting in the realignment of previously quiescent genetic information with new genetic promoters and enhancers (11,17,111). Promotion would subsequently result in selection and amplification of those cells containing newly arranged genetic promoters (51,115).

A large number of diverse agents have been shown to possess tumor promoting activity in mouse skin, as shown in Table 2. The phorbol esters, and in particular TPA, are the most potent of the skin tumor promoters identified thus far (91). Another agent, dihydroteleocidin B is a potent tumor promoter not belonging to the phorbol ester class (35,100). Chrysarobin and anthralin have also been shown to possess promoting activity (106). Recent studies indicate the benzo(e)pyrene has moderate activity as a tumor promoter (94). Benzoyl peroxide as well as lauroyl peroxide and decanoyl peroxide are good promoters, perhaps by means of their ability to generate free radicals (96); evidence indicates that benzoyl peroxide may possess broader spectrum promoting activity than TPA in several strains and stocks of mice, and perhaps in humans (86).

TABLE 2. Skin tumor promoting agents

Promoters	Potency
Croton oil	Strong
Certain phorbol esters in croton oil	Strong
Some synthetic phorbol esters	Strong
Certain euphorbia latices	Strong
7-Bromomethylbenz(a)anthracene	Strong
Indole alkaloids (teleocidin and lyngbyatoxin)	Strong
Polyacetates (aplysiatoxin)	Strong
Chrysarobin and anthralin	Moderate
Extracts of unburned tobacco	Moderate
Tobacco smoke condensate	Moderate
1-Fluoro-2,4-dinitrobenzene	Moderate
Benzo(e)pyrene	Moderate
Benzoyl peroxide	Moderate
Lauroyl peroxide	Moderate
Certain fatty acids and fatty acid methyl esters	Weak
Certain long-change alkanes	Weak
A number of phenolic compounds	Weak
Surface active agents (sodium laurylsulfate, Tween 60)	Weak
Citrus oils	Weak
Iodoacetic acid	Weak

The skin tumor promoters listed in Table 2 are not mutagenic themselves, and are believed to elicit their promotional effects in skin chiefly by bringing about important epigenetic changes in the epidermal cells exposed to these agents, although genetic events may be involved as well. The phorbol esters, as well as other promoting agents, induce numerous and diverse phenotypic changes in skin (summarized in Table 3). In general, promoters cause inflammation and hyperplasia (92), they inhibit differentiation (72), and they have been found to induce transient mimicry of the neoplastic phenotype causing cells to regain a basal or embryonic cell type (Table 3). Many of the major effects brought about by promoters in the phorbol ester class are the result of alterations to the cell membrane (86), including inhibition of cell-cell communication (116), phospholipid turnover (77), and altered cell morphology (29,77). These effects are now believed to be the result of activation of protein kinase C (PKC), the putative TPA receptor (discussed further below). TPA, one of the most potent promoters, acts to lower histidase activity (21), an enzyme which is low or absent in epidermal tumors. Ornithine decarboxylase (ODC), which is transiently induced by TPA (59), is elevated in epidermal papillomas and carcinomas. TPA also increases polyamine and prostaglandin synthesis, protease activity, cyclic AMP-independent protein kinase, and induces dark basal keratinocytes, a response found in wound healing (52,60,103). Skin tumor promoters cause a decrease in epidermal superoxide and catalase activities as well as a decrease in the number of glucocorticoid receptors and a decreased response of G_1 chalone in adult skin (24,98). The changes induced by teleocidin and the phorbol esters apparently are mediated through their interaction with specific receptors, whereas many of the other promoters do not act through this receptor mechanism and may involve free radical mechanism. Of the observed phorbol ester-related effects on the epidermis, the induction of epidermal cell proliferation, ornithine decarboxylase activity, and dark basal keratinocytes have the best correlation with potency of promoting activity (52,60,97).

INHIBITORS OF PROMOTION

The wide variety of effects elicited in epidermis by tumor promoters makes it difficult to determine which of the many responses induced are essential in promotion. For this reason, a number of inhibitors and modifiers of skin tumor promotion have been very useful in elucidating which of the cellular and molecular events induced by

TABLE 3. Summary of morphological and biochemical responses of mouse skin to phorbol ester and other tumor promoters

1.	Induction of inflammation and hyperplasia
2.	Increase in DNA, RNA and protein synthesis
3.	An initial increase in keratinization followed by a decrease
4.	Increase in phospholipid synthesis
5.	Increase in prostaglandin synthesis
6.	Increase in histone synthesis and phosphorylation
7.	Increase in ornithine decarboxylase activity followed by increase in polyamines
8.	Increase in histidine and DOPA decarboxylase activity
9.	Decrease in the isoproterenol stimulation of cyclic AMP
10.	Decrease in the number of dexamethasone receptors
11.	Decrease in superoxide dismutase and catalase
12.	Induction of embryonic state in adult skin
13.	Induction of dark cells (primitive stem cells)
14.	Induction of embryonic proteins in adult skin
15.	Induction of morphological changes in adult skin resembling papillomas, carcinomas and embryonic skin
16.	Decrease in histidase activity
17.	Increase in protease activity
18.	Decrease in response of G_1 chalone in adult skin
19.	Increase in cyclic AMP independent protein kinase in adult skin resembling tumors and embryonic skin
20.	Interaction with receptor and/or activation of protein kinase C

promoters are important in the skin promotion process. In general, the majority of known inhibitors of skin tumor promotion are agents that inhibit promoter-induced hyperplasia, dark basal keratinocytes, ODC activity and polyamine levels, and prostaglandins (33,92). Also active as inhibitors of promotion are various antioxidants, vitamin derivatives, cyclic nucleotides, and protease inhibitors (10,108). Table 4 lists a number of inhibitors of TPA-induced skin tumor promotion. The anti-inflammatory steroids, including cortisol, dexamethasone, and fluocinolone acetonide (FA) are effective inhibitors of TPA-induced tumor promotion (9,92). FA counteracts the cellular proliferation induced by TPA, and repetitive treatments of 0.01 µg of FA almost completely inhibit skin tumorigenesis (81). Also active as potent inhibitors of promotion are the retinoids, which may act to counteract tumor promotion by inhibiting phorbol ester-induced ODC activity in the mouse epidermis (108). In addition, Weeks et al. have demonstrated a synergistic effect when retinoids and FA are used together to inhibit TPA-induced skin tumor promotion (109).

Another class of agents which inhibit phorbol ester-induced skin tumor promotion are the protease inhibitors, including tosyl lysine chloromethyl ketone (TLCK), tosyl arginine methyl ester (TAME), tosyl phenylalanine chloromethyl ketone (TPCK), antipain, and leupeptin (95). Cyclic nucleotides, phosphodiesterase inhibitors, acetic acid, and dimethylsulfoxide have also been shown to possess promotion inhibiting capacities (53,54,89). The inhibitory effect of bacillus Calmette-Guerin (BCG) vaccination on skin tumor promotion has been reported by Schinitsky and coworkers (80). The polyribonucleotide polyribocytidylic acid (poly I:C) can inhibit carcinogenesis as well as tumor promotion (36), by virtue of its inhibitory effect on promoter- and carcinogen-induced cell proliferation.

Studies by Fischer et al. have shown that certain lipoxygenase and prostaglandin synthesis inhibitors, thromboxane synthesis inhibitors, and phospholipase A2 inhibitors also inhibit skin tumor promotion, indicating that the arachidonic acid metabolic pathways may be crucial in the promotion process (33). Arachidonic acid itself is also inhibitory when used in high doses (33). The role of polyamines in promotion may also be important, since DFMO, an inhibitor of polyamine synthesis, is also capable of inhibiting tumor promotion (92). Free radical scavengers such as butylated hydroxyanisole (BHA), BHT, disulfiram, and parahydroxyanisole are potent inhibitors of skin tumor promotion, supporting the role of free radicals in the mechanism of tumor promotion (88).

MOLECULAR AND CELLULAR MECHANISMS OF TUMOR PROMOTION

A great deal of information on the mechanisms involved in tumor promotion now exists at the molecular level. Various molecular models for tumor promotion have been suggested, including [1] membrane changes and activation of PKC, the putative TPA receptor (58), [2] promotion via growth factors which possess mitogenic control over cell

TABLE 4. Summary of inhibitors of phorbol ester skin tumor promotion[a]

1.	Anti-inflammatory steroids; cortisol, dexamethasone and FA
2.	Retinoids
3.	Combination of retinoids and anti-inflammatory agents
4.	Protease inhibitors: tosyl lysine chloromethyl ketone (TLCK); tosyl arginine methyl ester (TAME); tosyl phenylalanine chloromethyl ketone (TPCK); antipain and leupeptin
5.	Cyclic nucleotides
6.	Phosphodiesterase inhibitors; isobutylmethylxanthine
7.	Dimethylsulfoxide (DMSO)
8.	Butyrate, acetic acid
9.	Bacillus Calmette-Guerin (BCG)
10.	Polyriboinosinic: polyribocytidylic acid (poly I:C)
11.	Prostaglandin synthesis inhibitors 5,8,11,14-eicosatetraynoic acid (ETYA) and phenidone
12.	Thromboxane synthetase inhibitors; imidazolacetophenone (R022-3581) and imidazolphenone (R022-3582).
13.	Phospholipase A_2 inhibitor: dibromoacetophenone
14.	Arachidonic acid
15.	Polyamine synthesis inhibitor (difluoromethylornithine)
16.	Histamine[b]
17.	Diphenhydramine (H_1 receptor inhibitor)[b]
18.	BHA and BHT[b]
19.	Disulfiram and parahydroxyanisole[b]
20.	Vitamin E and C[b]
21.	Selenium[b]
22.	Anti-androgen cyproterone acetate (CPA)[b]

[a]See review by Slaga et al. (92) for individual references.
[b]Slaga et al., unpublished results.

proliferation and cell differentiation (40), and [3] promotion via various genetic effects, including free radical generation, activation of endogenous viruses, activation of oncogene expression, and gene rearrangements and alterations in gene expression.

Studies in a number of cell culture systems indicate that the primary action of tumor promoters such as the phorbol esters occurs at the cell surface (12,39). Table 5 summarizes many of the membrane-associated events caused by exposure of cell cultures to phorbol ester tumor promoters, including increased membrane fluidity, increased uptake of 2-deoxyglucose, [^{32}P], and [^{86}Rb$^+$], and altered Na$^+$/K$^+$ ATPase. Phorbol esters also inhibit binding of EGF to cellular receptors, presumably via induced membrane changes, as reported by Lee and Weinstein (54), Magun et al. (55) and others (15). Increased phospholipid synthesis (77) and turnover as well as prostaglandin synthesis are also observed (61). TPA is also reported to inhibit cell-cell communication (116) and produce altered cell morphology and cell adhesion (29).

TABLE 5. Summary of membrane changes caused by phorbol ester tumor promoters in various cell culture systems

1. Increased membrane fluidity
2. Increased uptake of various nutrients and ions
3. Altered Na$^+$/K$^+$ ATPase
4. Inhibition of EGF binding
5. Interaction with membrane receptor (Protein kinase C)
6. Synergistic interaction with growth factors
7. Increased phospholipid synthesis
8. Increased prostaglandins
9. Inhibition of cell-cell communication
10. Altered cell morphology
11. Altered cell adhesion
12. Increased pinocytosis
13. Altered fucose glycopeptides
14. Decreased LETS protein
15. Uncoupling of β-adrenergic receptors
16. Decrease in acetylcholine receptor

Recent studies by Nishizuka and coworkers indicate that PKC, which acts in signal transduction at the cell membrane, is also a target for phorbol esters (58). PKC is widely distributed in tissues and organs of mammals and other organisms (49) and has broad substrate specificity, phosphorylating serine and threonine residues of many endogenous proteins when tested *in vitro*. PKC is activated by diacylglycerol which is transiently produced in the membrane by inositol phospholipid turnover in response to extracellular signals (58). Kinetic studies have demonstrated that low levels of diacylglycerol can markedly increase the affinity of PKC for calcium, resulting in activation of enzyme. In addition, signal-induced breakdown of inositol phospholipids simultaneously mobilizes calcium, thereby resulting in a synergistic response which elicits the full physiological effect (114).

Extensive evidence now exists that PKC is a target for phorbol esters. Castagna and coworkers (16) as well as Yamanishi et al. (114) report that tumor promoters directly activate PKC *in vitro* and *in vivo*. In addition, there is also a good correlation between the relative tumor promoting ability of various phorbol esters and their capacity for activating PKC, since studies with various phorbol derivatives indicate that strong tumor promoters like TPA are more potent activators of PKC than weak promoters like phorbol (114). TPA, which has a diacylglycerol-like structure, is able to substitute for diacylglycerol at low concentrations, and like diacylglycerol, TPA markedly increases the affinity of PKC for calcium, resulting in complete activation of the enzyme in the absence of calcium mobilization (114). As further support that PKC is the receptor for TPA, it has been demonstrated that the distribution of PKC among various tissues is similar to that of the phorbol ester binding sites (6,84). Furthermore, Niedel and coworkers have observed that the phorbol diester receptor copurifies with PKC in studies of rat brain membranes solubilized by divalent cation chelation in the absence of detergents (57).

Other types of tumor promoters may also act through PKC. Recently Fujiki and Sugimura reported that dihydroteleocidin B, which is structurally unrelated to the phorbol esters, is equipotent with TPA as a tumor promoter in mouse skin (35) and can inhibit the specific binding of phorbol ester [3H]phorbol dibutyrate to membrane-associated receptors with a potency similar to that of TPA (105). Aplysiatoxin, another non-phorbol type promoter, also exhibited equivalent activity with TPA in inhibiting TPA binding to a receptor (42). Another promoter capable of activating PKC is mezerein, a second stage promoter which does not resemble diacylglycerol in structure. Jaken and coworkers (46) have reported that mezerein interacts with the major phorbol dibutyrate receptor to increase prostaglandin E2 production and to decrease the binding of epidermal growth factor (EGF). The above results provide compelling evidence that a variety of tumor promoters have as their receptor the membrane-localized PKC, and the location of this receptor protein in the cell membrane places it in an ideal environment for mediating many of the cellular and molecular events associated with growth and proliferation control in the tumor promotion process. Since the biological substrates of PKC are as yet unknown, the varied effects of promoter binding will depend in part on the acceptor proteins phosphorylated by PKC in different tissues. Further investigation into the role of protein phosphorylation in external signal transduction may ultimately demonstrate that normal growth/proliferation control and tumor promotion involve similar mechanisms requiring activation of membrane-associated kinases.

Another mechanism by which promoting agents may act is through their impact on cell differentiation. During carcinogenesis in the liver for example, intercellular transfer of growth factors and/or differentiation regulating factors could be involved in inhibiting the growth of initiated cells in altered foci. Liver tumor promoting agents may suppress intercellular communication, thus releasing cells in foci for development into neoplasms (112). In the Chinese hamster V79 cell system, Trosko et al. have shown that a variety of non-phorbol ester promoters can inhibit intercellular communication (104). Mechanisms involving the promotional role of effects on differentation have been proposed in the skin as well, and tumor promoters can either inhibit or stimulate differentation of epidermal cells in culture under different circumstances. For example, Klein-Szanto and coworkers have reported that phorbol esters induce an increase in the number of dark basal keratinocytes in adult skin which normally contains low numbers of dark cells compared to embryonic skin and papillomas and carcinomas (52,73). Earlier studies by Raick demonstrated the induction in basal cells of certain morphological characteristics similar to embryonic and neoplastic cells (72). In contrast, Reiners and Slaga have reported that tumor promoters encourage terminal differentiation in a subpopulation of basal cells and, in addition, the rate of differentiation of these committed cells is accelerated (76). Furthermore, Yuspa and coworkers have observed that initiated mouse epidermis contains cells that no longer undergo terminal differentiation upon exposure to high levels of calcium (117,118). These findings are of critical interest in that they suggest the existence of specific cell populations in initiated skin which may possess varying capacities for differentiation versus cellular expansion. Morris and Slaga have attempted to characterize various subpopulations of epidermal cells in culture, in order to delineate the various fates of cells in the basal layer following exposure of the skin to an initiating dose of carcinogen (56).

Altered patterns of differentiation have also been demonstrated with the phorbol esters in other cell culture systems, providing further evidence that effects on differentiation or changes in the balance between cell proliferation and cell differentiation may have important roles in tumor promotion. A list of effects which promoting agents have on cellular differentiation in culture is presented in Table 6. TPA inhibits the terminal differentiation of Friend erythroleukemia cells (26), neuroblastoma cells and adipose cells (26,45), while stimulating differentiation in cultures of human myeloid leukemia cells and human melanoma cells (43,44). Related to these findings are studies by Craig and Bloch, in which TPA was shown to induce differentiation in human myeloblastic leukemia cells, accompanied by a decline in c-*myb* oncogene expression (23). Similarly, Campisi and coworkers have demonstrated that expression of Ki-*ras* is cell-cycle dependent in transformed Balb/C 3T3 cells whereas the levels of c-*myc* RNA in quiescent and transformed cells are nearly the same (18). The specific functions of these oncogene products and their possible role in tumor promotion still remain to be established, however.

TABLE 6. Effects of phorbol ester tumor promoters on differentiation in various cell culture systems

1.	Stimulation and inhibition of differentiation in epidermal cells in culture
2.	Inhibition of terminal differentiation of Friend erythroleukemia cells
3.	Inhibition of differentiation of neuroblastoma cells
4.	Inhibition of differentiation of adipose cells
5.	Stimulation of terminal differentiation of human myeloid leukemia cells
6.	Stimulation of differentiation of human melanoma cells

Also important in maintaining the balance between cell proliferation and differentiation are agents classified as growth factors. The control of proliferation in normal diploid cells in culture is controlled by exogenous growth factors (40). In the absence of proper mitogens, cells leave the cell cycle and become reversibly arrested in the G_1/G_0 phase. Thus, transformed cells have a relaxed cell cycle and may be capable of traversing the cell cycle in the absence of exogenous growth factors. A number of laboratories have provided evidence that growth factor independence and autonomous growth of transformed cells may be due to the constitutive expression of any of the controlling elements along the normal mitogenic pathway, including the growth factor itself, the membrane receptor for the growth factor which communicates the extracellular signal, or the intracellular signal cascade, which results in initiation of DNA synthesis and cell division, as reviewed by Heldin and Westermark (40). Experiments by DeLarco and Todaro, for example, describe the growth factor TGF (transforming growth factor), which is endogenously produced by Moloney murine sarcoma virus transformed cells, thereby blocking EGF receptors on the cells (25). These observations have led to the development of the autocrine secretion hypothesis, in which transformed cells synthesize, release, and respond to their own growth factor thereby overriding normal controls of cellular proliferation.

It is now becoming clear that these constitutively expressed factors can be coded by oncogenes, or alternatively, their expression may be controlled by oncogenes. In the case of platelet derived growth factor (PDGF) for example, its amino acid sequence closely corresponds to the predicted amino acid sequence of the *sis* oncogene, the simian sarcoma virus transforming gene product, P28-*sis* (28,47). Furthermore, P28-*sis* has been shown to undergo a series of processing steps including dimer formation and proteolytic digestion to yield molecules which structurally and immunologically resemble biologically active PDGF, a potent mitogen for cells of connective tissue origin (3). Studies by Downward et al. (27) have established a structural relationship between a growth factor receptor and an oncogene, by demonstrating that the EGF receptor has a close amino acid homology with gp65-*erbB*, the transforming protein of avian erythroblastosis virus (27). Recently, it has been reported that PKC can phosphorylate the EGF receptor (20). The EGF receptor can also undergo autophosphorylation of tyrosine residues which is an uncommon site of phosphorylation in the cell (82), and is associated with cell proliferation and transformation of certain retroviruses. Since promoters like TPA can also cause a decrease in binding of EGF to its receptor (55), further investigation of the relationship between promoting agents and growth factors may clarify the role of tyrosine kinase activity and effects of growth factors on cell proliferation control.

Another family of oncogenes, exemplified by c-*myc*, may be involved in the mechanism by which growth factor- or promoter-induced mitogenic signals are transmitted from the receptor into the cell. Studies by Kelly et al. (48) have shown that addition of PDGF to stationary Balb/C 3T3 cells induces a significant increase in the expression of c-*myc* RNA, as do mitogens added to mouse lymphocytes. Enhanced expression of c-*myc* RNA in association with amplification of the c-*myc* gene has been described in the HL-60 human cell line (22). Little is known at present about the function of *myc*, although it has been suggested that an altered c-*myc* gene encodes an immortalization function whose expression is contingent on coordinate expression of an altered c-*ras* gene (53). Since the *myc* product has been associated with the cell nucleus (1), it may play an important role in regulating the expression of the genetic cascade controlling cell proliferation. Pfeifer-Ohlsson and coworkers have studied the spatial and temporal pattern of c-*myc* in developing human placenta (65). Their results indicate that the abundance of the *myc* transcript in placenta parallels the proliferative activity of the cytotrophoblastic component. Little is known at present about the effects of various tumor promoters in the c-*myc* oncogene. Studies currently underway in a number of laboratories may help to elucidate the relationship between effects of promoting agents on cell proliferation/differentiation and the functional roles which this family of oncogenes plays in tumor promotion.

While many of the morphological and biochemical effects of tumor promoters are classified as epigenetic in nature, studies in a number of laboratories suggest that tumor promoters may be capable of bringing about genetic effects as well. Several of the areas in which tumor promoters may induce genetic effects are listed in Table 7. Promoting agents such as benzoyl peroxide are capable of spontaneously producing free radicals which then may induce genetic effects through DNA damage. Other promoters such as TPA and teleocidin may give rise to free radicals and elicit a clastogenic effect, as reviewed by Cerutti et al. (19). Investigations designed to evaluate the effects of promoters on DNA and chromatin have established that promoters may also be capable of inducing damage at a more complex genetic level such as sister chromatid exchange and aneuploidy (50,62). TPA was shown to bring about gene amplification in studies demonstrating increased incidence of methotrexate resistance in mouse cells (107). Promoting agents such as TPA may also be able to induce gene rearrangements which subsequently result in the realignment of genetic promoters and enhancing sequences with previously quiescent information (11,111).

Exposure to TPA can also turn on endogenous viruses which may exert important influences during promotion. TPA effectively induces replication of Epstein-Barr virus DNA integrated into the cell genome of lymphoid cells (119). Experiments by Amtmann and coworkers have demonstrated that TPA treatment markedly increases the papilloma viral DNA content of skin cells from *mastomys natalensis*, a rat-like

TABLE 7. Summary of genetic effects caused by phorbol ester tumor promoters in various cell culture systems

1. Generation of free radical formation
2. Induction of sister chromatid exchange
3. Induction of mitotic aneuploidy in yeast
4. Induction of gene amplification/gene rearrangements
5. Activation of endogenous viruses
6. Activation of oncogene expression

animal which possesses endogenous papilloma virus DNA molecules in episomal form (2). Induction of papillomas, which normally occurred after one year, developed much sooner in animals treated with TPA (2).

The discovery by Balmain and coworkers, that the Ha-*ras* oncogene is activated in mouse skin tumors induced by dimethyl-benz(a)anthracene (DMBA) and TPA promotion has generated extensive interest in discerning the role of various oncogenes in multistage carcinogenesis and the effects of various promoting agents in altering oncogene expression (7,8). Balmain found that a percentage of papillomas and carcinomas screened contained elevated levels of Ha-*ras* transcripts compared with normal mouse epidermis. Furthermore, the tumor DNA was capable of malignantly transforming NIH 3T3 cells in DNA transfection studies (7). Ha-*ras* oncogene activation has also been demonstrated in mammary carcinomas induced in rats by N-methyl-N-nitrosourea (101), and in the T24 human bladder cacinoma cell line (78). Studies in our laboratory (63) indicate that initiation alone or repetitive TPA treatments are insufficient to turn on the expression of the Ha-*ras* oncogene in adult SENCAR mouse epidermis (Table 8). Initiation followed by either one or six weeks of TPA treatment also failed to activate Ha-*ras* expression. Like Balmain, we observed elevated levels of Ha-*ras* RNA in a percentage of papillomas and carcinomas tested. We are currently performing a time course analysis to establish whether oncogene activation occurs prior to papilloma development, or during a later stage of tumor progression. Studies are also underway to evaluate whether sequential or concurrent activation of other oncogenes occurs in mouse skin during the initiation/promotion two-stage model of tumorigenesis (63). However, it still remains to be determined whether oncogene activation plays a role in multi-step carcinogenesis in mouse skin.

TABLE 8. Induction of oncogene expression at various stages of two-stage carcinogenesis *in vivo*[a]

Treatment of Epidermis[b]	Expression of Ha-*ras* RNA[c]
Untreated	−
TPA only	−
Initiation only	−
Initiation, 1 × TPA	−
Initiation, 12 × TPA	−
Papillomas (8/17)	+
Carcinomas (2/3)	+

[a] Pelling et al., unpublished.
[b] Groups of 20-40 adult SENCAR mice were treated with acetone or initiating doses of DMBA or benzo(a)pyrene diolepoxide, followed by 2 µg of TPA, as indicated.
[c] Total RNA or polyadenylated RNA was purified from mouse skin or tumors, as described by Balmain and Pragnell (113). RNA samples were analyzed by Northern blot hybridization to a [32P]-nick-translated Ha-*ras* cDNA probe. Minus signs (−) indicate low (barely detectable) levels of hybridization density on autoradiograms. Plus signs (+) indicate 5-20 fold increases in hybridization density.

MULTISTAGE TUMOR PROMOTION

The continuing characterization of various inhibitors and modifiers of tumor promotion in mouse skin has led to the discovery that promotion can be operationally and mechanistically divided into at least two stages. The observation that mezerein was effective in inducing many of the phenotypic changes in skin but was a weak tumor promoter compared with TPA, allowed the promotion stage of the two-stage model of carcinogenesis to be further subdivided into two distinct stages of promotion (90). In this model, TPA is given for two weeks (stage I) after initiation, followed by 18 weeks of mezerein treatment (stage II). This regimen produced significant numbers of tumors, compared to the protocol in which TPA was not followed by mezerein, producing no tumor response. Both stages I and II showed a good dose-response relationship. Table 9 summarizes the important features of first and second stages of promotion. In addition to TPA, 4-O-methyl-TPA, calcium ionophore, and hydrogen peroxide have been identified as stage I promoters (92). Since these agents have been shown to increase the number of dark basal keratinocytes, it has been hypothesized that this subpopulation of cells may represent a stem cell population in epidermis which is critical to the first stage of promotion. Other factors which apparently are important to stage I promotion are PGE_2, a stage I enhancer, and FA, TPCK and vitamin E which all inhibit stage I. Since dark basal keratinocytes are normally present in low numbers in normal epidermis, but are present in higher numbers in papillomas and carcinomas (52), these cells may be a critical target cell population for initiation. Subsequently, during stage I promotion, this cell population may be selected for and amplified, possibly via effects induced by activated oncogene products and specific growth factors, resulting in enhanced proliferation of particular cells responding to the autocrine secretion hypothesis described previously. The second stage of promotion (illustrated schematically in Fig. 1) is characterized by maintained levels of cell proliferation and is initially reversible, becoming irreversible later on. Mezerein and 12-deoxyphorbol-13-2,4,6-decatrienoate (DP-tri D) have been classified as stage II promoters (92). Stage II promotion can be inhibited by FA, retinoic acid, difluoromethylornithine (DFMO), BHA, and vitamins E and C, which may counteract ODC induction (92,95). Results of studies with these inhibitors indicate that the important events of stage II promotion are epidermal cell proliferation and polyamines, as summarized in Fig. 1.

SUMMARY

The concepts of tumor promotion discussed in this chapter demonstrate the complexity of the tumor promotion process, and illustrate the difficulty of determining which events are mechanistically important to promotion, and which ones are the result, or by-product of promotion. A number of possible mechanisms of promotion, both epigenetic and genetic, have been described on a molecular level. However, it should be stressed that none of these mechanisms is mutually exclusive; indeed, the enormous complexity of tumor promotion suggests that several of the mechanisms discussed above may very well be interrelated. The effects on epidermal differentiation, for example, may turn out to be the result of altered expression of a particular oncogene whose product is actually a growth factor able to select for and amplify certain subpopulations of cells. Furthermore, the multiple steps which may occur at the molecular level, perhaps by way of sequential gene activation, serve to mirror the multiple stages which now delineate carcinogenesis in mouse skin.

TABLE 9. Characteristics of the first and second stages of tumor promotion

---

Stage I

1. A good dose response exists for TPA and 12-deoxyphorbol-decanoate as stage I promoters

2. The nonpromoting agents, calcium ionophore A23187, 4-O-methyl-TPA, hydrogen peroxide and wounding can act as stage I promoters

3. Only one application of stage I promoter is necessary

4. Prostaglandins are important since PGE_2 can enhance stage I by TPA

5. Partially irreversible

   a) Four to six weeks can separate first and second stages of promotion without a decrease in tumor response

   b) There is a 80% decrease in tumor response if 10 weeks separate stage I and II of promotion

6. Increase in the numer of dark basal keratinocytes (stem cells) are important. This occurs by directly stimulating existing dark cells to divide, converting some basal cells to dark cells, and by increasing the differentiation of some basal cells and differentiated cells

7. Decrease in glucocorticoid receptors by TPA may facilitate proliferation of dark cells

Stage II

1. A good dose response exists for mezerein as a stage II promoter

2. The nonpromoting agent 12-deoxyphorbol-13-2,4,6-decatrienoate can act as stage II promoter

3. Multiple applications are required

4. Reversible for relatively long period but later becomes irreversible

5. Polyamines are important since putrescine can enhance stage II by mezerein

6. Most of the biochemical events shown to be important in promotion occur in this stage

7. Mezerein can maintain dark cell proliferation and decrease in glucocorticoid receptors but can not induce these events by itself

---

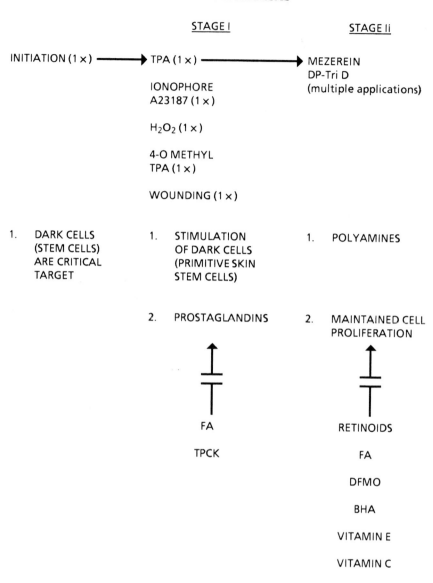

FIG 1. Two-stage promotion.

REFERENCES

1. Abrams, H. D., Rohrschneider, L. R., and Eisenman, R. H. (1982): *Cell*, 29:427-439.
2. Amtmann, E., Volm, M., and Wayss, K. (1984): *Nature*, 308:291-292.
3. Antoniades, H. N., Scher, C. D., and Stiles, C. D. (1979): *Proc. Natl. Acad. Sci. USA*, 76:1809-1813.
4. Armuth, V., and Berenblum, I. (1972): *Cancer Res.*, 32:2259-2262.
5. Armuth, V., and Berenblum, I. (1974): *Cancer Res.*, 34:2704-2707.
6. Ashendel, C. L., Staller, J. M., and Boutwell, R. K. (1983): *Biochem. Biophys. Res. Commun.*, 11:340-345.
7. Balmain, A., and Pragnell, I. B. (1983): *Nature*, 303:72-74.
8. Balmain, A., Ramsden, M., Bowden, G. T.,and Smith, J. (1984): *Nature*, 307:658-660
9. Belman, S., and Troll, W. (1972): *Cancer Res.*, 32:450-454.
10. Belman, S., and Troll, W. (1978): In: *Carcinogenesis-A Comprehensive Survey, Vol. 2: Mechanisms of Tumor Promotion and Carcinogenesis*, edited by T. J. Slaga, A. Sivak, and R. K. Boutwell, pp. 117-134. Raven Press, New York.
11. Bishop, J. M. (1983): *Ann. Rev. Biochem.*, 52:301-354.
12. Blumberg, P. M. (1981): *CRC Crit. Rev. Toxicol.*, 8:199-234.
13. Boutwell, R. K. (1964): *Prog. Exp. Tumor Res.*, 4:207-250.
14. Brookes, P., and Lawley, P. D. (1964): *Nature*, 202:781-784.
15. Brown, K. D., Dicker, P., and Rozengurt, E. (1979): *Biophys. Biochem. Res. Commun.*, 86:1037-1043.
16. Castagna, M., Takai, Y., Kaibuchi, K., Sano, K., Kikkawa, U., and Nishizuka, Y. (1982): *J. Biol. Chem.*, 257:7847-7851.
17. Cairns, J. (1981): *Nature*, 289:353-357.
18. Campisi, J., Gray, H. E., Pardee, A. B., Dean, W. M., and Sonenshein, G. E. (1984): *Cell*, 36:241-247.
19. Cerutti, P., Emerit, I., and Amstad, P. (1983): In: *Proc. of P. and S. Biomedical Sciences Symposium*, edited by I. B. Weinstein, and H. Vogel. Academic Press, New York.
20. Cochett, C., Gill, G. N., Meisenholder, J., Cooper, J. A., and Hunter, T. (1984): *J. Biol. Chem.*, 259:2553-2558.
21. Colburn, N. H., Lau, S., and Head, R. (1975): *Cancer Res.*, 35:3154-3159.
22. Collins, S., and Groudine, M. (1982): *Nature*, 298:679-681.
23. Craig, R. W., and Bloch, A. (1984): *Cancer Res.*, 44:442-446.
24. Davidson, K. A., and Slaga, T. J. (1982): *J. Invest. Dermatol.*, 79:378-383.
25. DeLarco, J. E., and Todaro, G. J. (1978): *Proc. Natl. Acad. Sci. USA*, 75:4001-4005.
26. Diamond, L., O'Brien, T., and Rovera, G. (1978): In: *Carcinogenesis-A Comprehensive Survey, Vol. 2: Mechanisms of Tumor Promotion and Carcinogenesis*, edited by T. J. Slaga, A. Sivak, and R. K. Boutwell, pp. 335-341. Raven Press, New York.
27. Downward, J., Yarden, Y., Mayes, E., Scrace, G., Totty, N., Stockwell, P., Ullrich, A., Schessinger, J., and Waterfield, M. D. (1984): *Nature*, 307:521-527.
28. Doolittle, R. F., Hunkapiller, M. W., Hood, L. E., Devare, S. G., Robbins, K., Aaronson, S. A., and Antoniades, H. N. (1983): *Science*, 221:275-277.
29. Driedeger, P. E., and Blumberg, P. M. (1977): *Cancer Res.*, 37:3257-3265.

30. Dunning, W. F., Curtis, M. R., and Maun, M. E. (1950): *Cancer Res.*, 10:454-459.
31. Farber, E., and Ichinose, H. (1959): *Acta Unio Inter. Contra Cancrum*, 15:152-153.
32. Farber, E. (1976): In: *Hepatocellular Carcinoma*, edited by K. Okuda and R. L. Peters, pp. 3-22. John Wiley and Sons, New York.
33. Fischer, S. M., Gleason, G. L., Hardin, L. G., Bohrman, J. S., and Slaga, T. J. (1980): *Carcinogenesis*, 1:245-248.
34. Friedrich-Freksa, S. H., Gossner, W., and Bonner, P. (1969): *Z. Krebsforsch.*, 72:226-239.
35. Fujiki, H., Mori, M., Nakayosu, M., Terada, M., Sugimura, T., and Moore, R. E. (1981): *Proc. Natl. Acad. Sci. USA*, 78:3872-3876.
36. Gelboin, H. F., and Levy, H. B. (1970): *Science*, 205-207.
37. Goldfarb, S., and Zak, F. G. (1961): *J. Am. Med. Assoc.*, 178:729-731.
38. Hecker, E. (1968): *Cancer Res.*, 28:2338-2349.
39. Hecker, E. (1971): In: *Methods in Cancer Research, Vol. 6*, edited by H. Busch, pp. 439-484. Academic Press, New York and London.
40. Heldin, C.-H., and Westermark, B. (1984): *Cell*, 37:9-20.
41. Hicks, R. M., Wakefield, J. St. J., and Chowanic, J. (1973): *Nature*, 243:347-349.
42. Horowitz, A. D., Fujiki, H., Weinstein, I. B., Jeffrey, A., Okui, E., Moore, R. E., and Sugimura, T. (1983): *Cancer Res.*, 43:1529-1535.
43. Huberman, E., and Callaham, M. F. (1979): *Proc. Natl. Acad. Sci. USA*, 79:1293-1297.
44. Huberman, E., Heckman, C., and Langenbach, R. (1979): *Cancer Res.*, 39:2618-2624.
45. Ishii, D. N., Fibach, E., Yamasaki, H., and Weinstein, I. B. (1978): *Science*, 200:556-559.
46. Jaken, S., Shupnik, M. A., Blumberg, P. M., and Tashijian, A. H. (1983): *Cancer Res.*, 43:11-14.
47. Johnsson, A., Heldin, C.-H., Westermark, B., and Wasteson, A. (1982): *Biochem. Biophys. Res. Commun.*, 104:66-74.
48. Kelly, K., Cochran, B. H., Stiles, C. D., and Leder, P. (1983): *Cell*, 35:603-610.
49. Kikkawa, U., Rakai, Y., Mankuchi, R., Inohara, S., and Nishizuka, Y. (1982): *J. Biol. Chem.*, 257:13341-13348.
50. Kinsella, A. R., and Radman, M. (1978): *Proc. Natl. Acad. Sci. USA*, 75:6149-6153.
51. Klein, G. (1981): *Nature*, 294:313-317.
52. Klein-Szanto, A. J. P., Major, S. M., and Slaga, T. J. (1980): *Carcinogenesis*, 1:399-406.
53. Land, H., Parada, L. F., and Weinberg., R. A. (1983): *Nature*, 304:596-602.
54. Lee, L.-S., and Weinstein, I. B. (1979): *Proc. Natl. Acad. Sci. USA*, 76:5168-5172.
55. Magun, B. E., Matrisian, L. M., and Bowden, G. T. (1980): *J. Biol. Chem.*, 255:6373-6381.
56. Morris, R., and Slaga, T. J., unpublished.
57. Niedel, J. E., Kuhn, L. F., and Vandenbach, G. R. (1983): *Proc. Natl. Acad. Sci. USA*, 80:36-40.
58. Nishizuka, Y. (1984): *Nature*, 308:693-698.
59. O'Brien, T. G. (1976): *Cancer Res.*, 36:2644-2653.

60. O'Brien, T. G., Simsiman, R. C., and Boutwell, R. K. (1975): *Cancer Res.*, 35:1662-1670.
61. Ohuchi, K., and Levine, L. (1978): *J. Biol. Chem.*, 253:483-4790.
62. Parry, J. M., Parry, E. M., and Barrett, J. C. (1981): *Nature*, 294:263-265.
63. Pelling, J. C., Nairn, R. S., Hixson, D. C., and Slaga, T. J., unpublished.
64. Peraino, C., Fry, R. J. M., Staffedt, E., and Kisielishki, W. E. (1973): *Cancer Res.*, 33:2701-2708.
65. Pfeifer-Ohlsson, S., Goustin, A. S., Rydnert, J., Wahlstrom, T., Bjersing, L., Stehelin, D., and Ohlsson, R. (1984): *Cell*, 38:585-596.
66. Pitot, H.C., Barsness., L., Goldsworthy, T., and Kitagawa, T. (1978): *Nature*, 271:456-458.
67. Pitot, H. C., and Sirica, A. E. (1980): *Biochim. Biophys. Acta*, 605:191-215.
68. Purnell, D. M. (1978): *Am. J. Pathol.*, 93:311-324.
69. Rabes, H. M., Scholze, P., and Jantsch, B. (1972): *Cancer Res.*, 32:2577-2586.
70. Radomski, J. L., Krischer, C., and Krischer, K. N. (1978): *J. Natl. Cancer. Inst.*, 60:327-333.
71. Radomski, J. L., Radomski, T., and MacDonald, W. E. (1977): *J. Natl. Cancer Inst.*, 58:1831-1834.
72. Raick, A. N. (1973): *Cancer Res.*, 33:269-286.
73. Raick, A. N. (1974): *Cancer Res.*, 34:920-926.
74. Reddy, B. S., and Watanabe, K. (1979): *Cancer Res.*, 39:1521-1524.
75. Reddy, B. S., Weisburger, J. H., and Wynder, E. L. (1978): In: *Carcinogenesis - A Comprehensive Survey, Vol. 2: Mechanisms of Tumor Promotion and Cocarcinogenesis*, edited by T. J. Slaga, A. Sivak, and R. K. Boutwell, pp. 453-464. Raven Press, New York.
76. Reiners, J. J., and Slaga, T. J. (1983): *Cell*, 32:247-255.
77. Rohrschneider, L. R., O'Brien, D. H., and Boutwell, R. K. (1972): *Biochim. Biophys. Acta*, 280:57-70.
78. Santos, E., Reddy, E. P., Pulciani, S., Feldmann, R. J., and Barbacid, M. (1983): *Proc. Natl. Acad. Sci. USA*, 80:4679-4683.
79. Scherer, E., and Emmelot, P. (1975): *Eur. J. Cancer*, 11:689-696.
80. Schinitsky, M. R., Hyman, L. R., Blazkovec, H. A., and Burkholder, P. M. (1973): *Cancer Res.*, 33:659-663.
81. Schwarz, J. A., Viaje, A., Slaga, T. J., Yuspa, S. H., Hennings, H., and Lichti, U. (1977): *Chem. Biol. Interact.*, 17:331-347.
82. Sefton, B. M., Hunter, T., Beemon, K., and Eckhart, W. (1980): *Cell*, 20:807-816.
83. Shinozuka, H., and Lombardi, B. (1980): *Cancer Res.*, 40:3846-3849.
84. Shoyab, M., and Todaro, G. J. (1980): *Nature*, 388:451-455.
85. Slaga, T. J. (1980): In: *Modifiers of Chemical Carcinogenesis*, edited by T. J. Slaga, pp. 243-262. Raven Press, New York.
86. Slaga, T. J. (1983): In: *Cancer Surveys, Advances and Prospects in Clinical, Epidermiological and Laboratory Oncology*, edited by T. J. Slaga, and R. Montesano, Vol. 2, Number 4, pp. 595-612. Oxford University Press, Oxford.
87. Slaga, T. J. (1983): *Environ. Health Perspect.*, 50:3-14.
88. Slaga, T. J., unpublished.
89. Slaga, T. J., Bowden, G. T., and Boutwell, R. K. (1975): *J. Natl. Cancer Inst.*, 55:983-987.
90. Slaga, T. J., Fischer, S. M., Nelson, K., and Gleason, G. L. (1980): *Proc. Natl. Acad. Sci. USA*, 77:3659-3663.

91. Slaga, T. J., Fischer, S. M., Triplett, L. L., and Nesnow, S. (1982): *J. Environ. Pathol. Toxicol.*, 4:1025-1041.
92. Slaga, T. J., Fischer, S. M., Weeks, C. E., and Klein-Szanto, A. J. P. (1981): In: *Reviews in Biochemical Toxicology, Vol. 3*, edited by E. Hodgson, J. Bend, and R. M. Philpot, pp. 231-281. Elsevier North-Holland, Inc., New York.
93. Slaga, T. J., Fischer, S. M., Weeks, C. E., Klein-Szanto, A. J. P., and Reiners, J. (1982): *J. Cell. Biochem.*, 18:99-119.
94. Slaga, T. J., Jecker, L., Bracken, W. M., and Weeks, C. E. (1979): *Cancer Lett.*, 7:51-59.
95. Slaga, T. J., Klein-Szanto, A. J. P., Fischer, S. M., Weeks, C. E., Nelson, K., and Major, S. (1980): *Proc. Natl. Acad. Sci. USA*, 77:22510-2254.
96. Slaga, T. J., Klein-Szanto, A. J. P., Triplett, L. L., Yotti, L. P., and Trosko, J. E. (1981): *Science*, 13:1023-1025.
97. Slaga, T. J., Scribner, J. D., Thompson, S., and Viaje, A. (1974): *J. Natl. Cancer Inst.*, 52:1611-1618.
98. Solanki, V., Rann, R. S., and Slaga, T. J. (1981): *Carcinogenesis*, 2:1141-1146.
99. Solt, D., and Farber, E. (1976): *Nature*, 263:701-703.
100. Sugimura, R. (1982): *Cancer*, 49:1970-1984.
101. Sukumar, S., Notario, V., Martin-Zanca, D., and Barbacid, M. (1983): *Nature*, 306:658-661.
102. Teebor, G. W., and Becker, F. F. (1971): *Cancer Res.*, 31:1-6.
103. Troll, W., Meyn, M. W., and Rossman, T. G. (1978): In: *Carcinogenesis - A Comprehensive Survey, Vol. 2: Mechanisms of Tumor Promotion and Cocarcinogenesis*, edited by T. J. Slaga, A. Sivak, and R. K. Boutwell, pp. 301-312. Raven Press, New York.
104. Trosko, J. E., Yotti, L. P., Warren, S. T., Tsushimoto, G., and Chang, C. C. (1982): In: *Carcinogenesis - A Comprehenisve Survey, Vol. 7: Cocarcinogenesis and Biological Effects of Tumor Promoters*, edited by E. Hecker, W. Kunz, N. E. Fusenig, F. Marks, and H. W. Thielmann, pp. 565-586. Raven Press, New York.
105. Umezawa, K., Weinstein, I. B., Horowitz, A., Fujiki, H., Matsushima, T., and Sugimura, T. (1981): *Nature*, 290:411-413.
106. Van Duuren, B. L., and Goldschmidt, B. M. (1978): In: *Carcinogenesis - A Comprehensive Survey, Vol. 2: Mechanisms of Tumor Promotion and Cocarcinogenesis*, edited by T. J. Slaga, A. Sivak, and R. K. Boutwell, pp. 491-507. Raven Press, New York.
107. Varshavsky, A. (1981): *Cell*, 25:561-572.
108. Verma, A. K., Rice, H. M., Shapas, B. G., and Boutwell, R. K. (1978): *Cancer Res.*, 38:793-801.
109. Weeks, C. E., Slaga, T. J., Hennings, H., Gleason, G. L., and Bracken, W. M. (1979): *J. Natl. Cancer Inst.*, 63:401-406.
110. Weinstein, I. B. (1981): *J. Supramol. Struct. Cell. Biochem.*, 17:99-120.
111. Weinstein, I. B., Yamasaki, H., Wigler, M., Lee, L.-S., Fisher, P. B., Jeffrey, A., and Grunberger, D. (1983): In: *Carcinogens: Identification and Mechanisms of Action*, edited by A. C. Griffin and R. Shaw, Raven Press, New York.
112. Williams, G. M. (1983): *Environ. Health Perspect.*, 50:177-183.
113. Witschi, P., Williamson, D., and Lock, S. (1977): *J. Natl. Cancer Inst.*, 58:301-310.
114. Yamanishi, J., Takai, Y., Kaibuchi, K., Sano, K., Castagna, M., and Nishizuka, Y. (1983): *Biochem. Biophys. Res. Commun.*, 112:778-786.

115. Yaniv, M. (1982): *Nature*, 297:17-18.
116. Yotti, L. P., Chang, C. C., and Trosko, J. E. (1979): *Science*, 206:1089-1091.
117. Yuspa, S. H., Hennings, H., Kulecz-Martin, M., and Lichti, U. (1982): In: *Carcinogenesis - A Comprehensive Survey, Vol. 7: Cocarcinogenesis and Biological Effects of Tumor Promoters*, edited by E. Hecker, N. Kunz, N. E., Fusenig, F. Marks, and H. W. Thielmann, pp. 217-230. Raven Press, New York.
118. Yuspa, S. H., and Morgan, D. L. (1981): *Nature*, 293:72-74.
119. Zur Hausen, H., Bornkamm, G. W., Schmidt, R., and Hecker, E. (1979): *Proc. Natl. Acad. Sci. USA*, 76:782-785.

Carcinogenesis, Vol. 8, edited by M. J. Mass et al.
Raven Press, New York © 1985.

Mechanisms of Multistage Chemical Carcinogenesis and Their Relevance to Respiratory Tract Cancer

I. Bernard Weinstein, John Arcoleo, Michael Lambert,
Wendy Hsiao, Sebastiano Gattoni-Celli, Alan M. Jeffrey,
and Paul Kirschmeier

*Division of Environmental Sciences and Cancer Center, Institute of Cancer Research, Columbia
University, New York, New York 10032*

The concepts of tumor promotion and multistage carcinogenesis were developed largely from studies on mouse skin, and more recently from rat liver. There is good reason to believe, however, that these concepts also apply to causation of cancers of the respiratory tract, both in experimental animals and in humans. An understanding of the mechanisms by which cigarette smoking and other environmental (i.e., exogenous) factors influence the incidence of cancers of the respiratory tract must, therefore, be concerned with multifactor interactions and a multistage process. In this paper we will review recent studies at the biochemical and molecular levels related to the mechanisms of action of the carcinogen benzo(a)pyrene, (BP), the phorbol ester tumor promoters and related compounds. We will emphasize the concept that chemical and radiation carcinogenesis involve changes in multiple cellular genes (including oncogenes) and that these changes occur through a variety of molecular mechanisms. We trust that this review will stimulate studies to determine whether these findings and concepts are relevant to the very important problem of human respiratory tract cancer and its prevention.

INITIATING CARCINOGENS, GENE AMPLIFICATION, AND CHEMICAL-VIRAL SYNERGY

It is now well established that a variety of chemical carcinogens, including chemicals that can induce lung cancer, act, at least in part, by yielding highly reactive intermediates that bind covalently to cellular DNA (71). This, and other findngs, have led to the concept that they act by producing mutations in somatic cells. We would caution, however, that carcinogenesis probably involves much more complex changes in DNA structure than simple point mutations at sites of carcinogen-induced DNA damage. Supporting evidence includes: the high apparent frequency of the initiation process, the long latent period in carcinogenesis, and the accumulating evidence that cellular oncogenes in tumors can display various types of structural changes.

We have demonstrated that the carcinogen BP and its activated derivative BP-7,8-dihydrodiol-9,10-oxide (BPDE) induce a marked increase in the asynchronous replication of polyoma virus DNA (44,45). Furthermore, this effect does not require direct carcinogen damage to the polyoma DNA, since we can induce viral DNA replication by fusing normal cells previously exposed to BPDE to the polyoma-transformed cells (44). In recent studies utilizing recombinant DNA constructs in which either the bacterial drug resistance gene *gpt* or the mammalian dihydrofolate reductase gene *dhfr* were linked to the polyoma DNA, we have found that when cells carrying these constructs were exposed to BPDE, then the latter genes also underwent asynchronous replication (45). These findings, and other evidence (44,45,47) suggest that carcinogen-induced damage to cellular DNA can induce the formation of a *trans*-acting factor that can induce the asynchronous replication and amplification of specific genes. This phenomenon may be relevant to the finding of amplified oncogenes, amplified genes related to drug resistance, and other amplified DNA sequences in tumors.

We would also stress the fact that certain human tumors may result from synergistic interations between DNA viruses and environmental chemicals (23,71,74). Possible examples include: an interaction between hepatitis B virus and aflatoxin in liver cancer causation, and papilloma virus and cigarette smoking in cervical cancer causation. Perhaps chemicals exert a synergistic effect by altering the replication and/or state of integration of viral DNAs. Certain tumor promoters can enhance the replication of Epstein-Barr virus (EBV), and also enhance EBV-induced lymphocyte transformation. This, and other findings, have suggested a synergistic interaction between tumor promoters and EBV in the causation of nasopharyngeal cancer in Southern China (32,38). Other cases of chemical-viral synergy may play an important role in human cancer causation, acting either alone or in combination with direct effects of environmental chemicals on cellular genes (71,74). This subject warrants further consideration in studies on the causation of certain forms of lung cancer.

TUMOR PROMOTERS

Inductive Effects and Activation of Protein Kinase C

In contrast to initating carcinogens and complete carcinogens, the potent tumor promoter 12-O-tetradecanoylphorbol-13-acetate (TPA), and related compounds, do not produce direct damage to cellular DNA. There is now extensive evidence that their primary effects relate to changes in membrane structure and function (32,35,71), and that these effects may be mediated by the ability of these compounds to bind to and enhance the activity of the phospholipid-dependent enzyme protein kinase C (PKC) (7,12,55,72).

We have recently studied the effects of various types of tumor promoters on the activity of PKC *in vitro* (1). The enzyme was partially purified from bovine brain and displayed a high dependence on added phospholipid and Ca^{2+}. Other details of the assay are described in Fig. 1. A striking finding is that maximum stimulation (>10 fold) of PKC activity by TPA occurs in the presence of phospholipid, but in the absence of added Ca^{2+} (Fig. 1). In effect, nanomolar concentrations of TPA substitute for millimolar concentrations of added Ca^{2+}, and the two agents are not synergistic. Biologically active analogs of TPA such as phorbol dibutyrate (PDBu), 12-O-hexadecanoyl-16-hydroxyphorbol-13-acetate (HHPA) (38), and mezerein were also effective activators of PKC, as were the chemically unrelated tumor promoters teleocidin and aplysiatoxin (67), when tested at nanomolar concentrations in the absence of added Ca^{2+} (Table 1). On the other hand, the biologically inactive compounds phorbol and 4-α-phorbol-12,13-didecanoate (4αPDD) did not affect PKC activity in the absence of Ca^{2+} (Table 1). These and additional results are consistent with our previously proposed stereochemical model (Fig. 2 and ref. 36,73) in which the structurally similar hydrophilic domains of certain diterpenes, teleocidin, and aplysiatoxin interact specifically with a protein receptor (in this case PKC apoenzyme), while their less specific hydrophobic domains interact with phospholipid, thus forming an enzymatically active ternary complex. In intact cells these tumor promoters might bind first to lipid domains in cell membranes thus inducing changes in lipid structure which enhance binding to and activation of PKC. This sequence could explain the finding that when intact cells are exposed to TPA there appears to be a migration of the cytosolic apoenzyme to the membrane fraction (42) The ability of tumor promoters to substitute for added Ca^{2+} in the activation of PKC may also be of significance in terms of their action in intact cells. There is previous evidence that TPA lowers the Ca^{2+} requirement for the growth of certain cell types in cell culture (71).

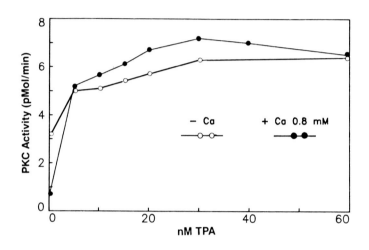

FIG. 1. Effect of TPA on PKC activity in the presence or absence of Ca^{2+}. Assays were done with a partially purified preparation of bovine brain PKC. The 0.2 ml assay system contained: 2.5 nmoles $[^{32}P]ATP$ (2×10^6 cpm), 24 µg PKC extract, 2.0 µg brain phosphatidylserine (Sigma), 40 µg histone (Sigma IIIS), 25 mM PIPES buffer (pH 6.5), 10 mM $MgCl_2$, 200 µM EGTA, 200 µM EDTA, 1 mM 2-mercapto-ethanol, and either 0 or 0.8 mM $CaCl_2$. The reaction was incubated at 30° for 10 min, terminated by spotting a 75 µl aliquot onto 6.25 cm^2 pieces of P81 paper (Whatman), and the papers were washed in 1 liter of water. The radioactivity on the paper was counted in a scintillation counter in 6 ml of Hydroflour (National Diagnostics). For additional details see text and ref. 1.

Several findings suggest that there may be heterogeneity (or subclasses) of receptors for phorbol esters and related tumor promoters. Scatchard analyses of $[^3H]PDBu$-receptor binding to intact cells are consistent with at least two classes of binding sites (35). Although the compound mezerein is quite potent with respect to certain biologic effects including activation of PKC (1), it competes less well than TPA in inhibiting $[^3H]PDBu$-receptor binding, and also is much weaker than TPA as a complete tumor promoter on mouse skin (19,32). Therefore,

TABLE 1. Effects of various tumor promoters on PKC activity in the absence and presence of added Ca^{2+}

	Without Ca^{2+}	With Ca^{2+}
Experiment 1		
Control	0.65	3.60
TPA	4.29	3.60
Teleocidin	4.45	4.20
PDBu	2.49	3.55
Phorbol	0.83	3.25
4-α-PDD	0.68	3.75
Experiment 2		
Control	0.5	19.0
Aplysiatoxin	12.2	21.9
Debromoaplysiatoxin	14.4	22.2
Lyngbyatoxin A	12.0	20.9
Anhydrodebromoaplysiatoxin	2.1	20.5
Experiment 3		
Control	0.8	1.56
TPA	2.17	2.18
Mezerein	2.33	2.33
HHPA	2.19	2.11
HHPA 13,20-diacetate	0.72	1.63
HHPA 1,2-dihydro, 20-deoxy	0.63	1.29

Values are expressed as pMol/min of ^{32}P incorporated into histone. All compounds were tested at 100 nM in the absence and presence of added Ca^{2+} (0.8 mM), but always in the presence of added phospholipid. For additional details see Fig. 1 and ref. 1.

some cell types may have a subset of receptors that discriminate between TPA and mezerein. Differential effects of aplysiatoxin and debromoaplysiatoxin (36,67) are also consistent with receptor heterogeneity. In a study with C3H10T½ cells we found that the dose response curves for TPA, PDBu, and teleocidin inhibition of the binding of [^{3}H]PDBu to high affinity receptors were quite different than those obtained when the same compounds were tested for their ability to alter membrane lipid fluidity in the same cells, as measured with fluorescence polarization probes (69). Receptor heterogeneity could contribute to the tissue specificity and pleiotropic effects of these compounds. The basis for this heterogeneity is not known but it could involve the following mechanisms: 1) heterogeneity of PKCs; 2) variations in lipid domains associated with PKC; and 3) interactions

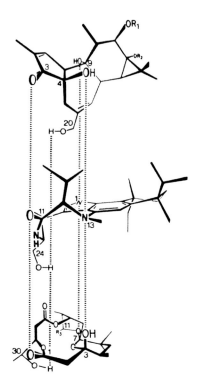

FIG. 2. Perspective drawings of TPA (top), dihydroteleocidin B (middle), and aplysiatoxin (bottom). The dotted lines connect heteroatoms whose spatial positions might correspond with one another, and represent residues that could interact with protein kinase C (PKC) apoenzyme. The hydrophobic R_1 residue on TPA (myristate), the hydrophobic ring system on the right side of dihydro-teleocidin B, and the phenolic side chain of aplysiatoxin might interact with the phospholipid cofactor for PKC. The stereochemistries of dihydroteleocidin B and aplysiatoxin were chosen arbitrarily to maximize their similarity to TPA. Further studies are required to establish their actual stereochemistries. For additional details see 73.

of tumor promoters with other lipid-modulated enzymes, in addition to protein kinase C.

Certain hormones and growth factors induce the turnover of polyphosphatidyl inositol, which can generate transient increases in diacylglycerol and inositol triphosphate (55). The former compound could activate PKC and the latter could act as a second messenger to cause the release of intracellular Ca^{2+} (11,55). Thus, a number of factors, including alterations in dietary lipids (71,74), might indirectly mimic the action of the phorbol ester tumor promoters and thus play a role in multistage carcinogenesis. Recent studies indicating that pp60*v-src* (66) and p68*v-ros* (51) can phosphorylate phosphatidyl inositol, and other lipids, suggest that these oncogene products could also produce effects similar to those of the tumor promoters. Although the idea that diacylglycerol is an endogenous analog of certain tumor promoters is an attractive one, we should stress that TPA and related compounds are about 10^4 times more potent than DAG in activating PKC (12,55), and also in competing for high affinity binding sites (7). Perhaps this is because diacylglycerol lacks the hydrophilic residues so characteristic of the potent tumor promoters (Fig. 2). Furthermore, the chemical structures of mezerein, telocidin, and aplysiatoxin do not display any resemblance to diacylglycerol, and yet these compounds are potent activators of PKC (1). It would seem worthwhile, therefore, to search for more complex amphiphilic cellular lipids as possible endogenous analogs of these tumor promoters.

A fundamental area for future research is the identification of specific cellular proteins phosphorylated by PKC, particularly those that are critical to the process of tumor promotion. A related question is whether or not the multiple effects of tumor promoters represent a simple linear cascade of events. The circuitry may be quite complex. For example tumor promoters induce phospholipid turnover (53) which may be associated with the release of diacylglycerol, itself an activator of PKC (55); and alterations in ion flux (i.e., Ca^{2+}) (71) could also further modulate protein kinase and phospholipid activities. Recent studies indicate that treatment of cells with TPA can alter the state of phosphorylation of epidermal growth factor (EGF) receptor (14,39), and also the receptors for insulin and somatomedin C (40). These effects are presumably mediated via activation of PKC and could explain the fact that TPA treatment leads to an indirect inhibition of EGF-receptor (48) and insulin-receptor binding (40). Other recently identified potential targets for phosphorylation by PKC, that may be relevant to tumor promotion, include the ribosomal S6 protein (49), the cytoskeletal protein vinculin (76) and a retinoid binding protein (17). Furthermore, even though PKC does not phosphorylate tyrosine residues, the exposure of cells to TPA can also enhance the phosphorylation of tyrosine residues on a 43K protein, the same protein which is a target for the action of pp60^{v-src} (5,27). It appears, therefore, that in addition to its effect on PKC, TPA can enhance, either directly or indirectly, the activity of a cellular tyrosine-specific protein kinase.

The above results should encourage studies on the possible role of membrane changes, altered phospholipid turnover, altered protein kinase activity, and changes in growth factors and their receptors in lung cancer causation. In a sense, these parameters may serve as markers of the action of tumor promoters in the lung.

Irreversible Effects and Synergy with Oncogenes

Although our research group has stressed the membrane and cytoplasmic effects of tumor promoters, other investigators have provided evidence that the phorbol ester tumor promoters can also produce chromosomal aberrations and DNA damage, perhaps via activated forms of oxygen (21,32). These effects, however, are most prominent in inflammatory cells and may reflect the specialized responses (i.e., oxidative burst) of these cells to various activators. Furthermore, certain effects of TPA can be seen in the absence of detectable DNA damage (26). We would also stress that since the process of tumor promotion on mouse skin is often reversible (3), it seems unlikely that the early events during tumor promotion involve DNA damage and chromosomal aberrations. It is possible, of course, that with prolonged exposure to TPA, chromosomal changes might occur and contribute to the process of tumor progression, particularly since chromosomal anomalies are more prominent during the late rather than the early stages of carcinogenesis.

A related question is whether tumor promoters act entirely via inductive or hormone-like effects, thus mediating clonal expansion of previously mutated cells, or whether they can themselves produce stable and heritable changes in cell phenotype. Although most of the pleiotropic effects produced by tumor promoters in cell culture are dependent upon the continuous presence of the promoter (71), there are a few examples in which the action of tumor promoters is associated with irreversible effects. These include: 1) the enhancement of cell transformation induced by certain oncogenic viruses, including adenovirus, EB virus, SV40 virus, and polyoma virus (23,32); 2) the enhancement of anchorage independent growth of either adenovirus transformed rat fibroblasts (24) or of certain murine epidermal cell lines (15); and 3) enhancement of the outgrowth of cell variants displaying amplified genes for dihydrofolate reductase (2) or metallothionein (30). In addition, the papillomas and carcinomas induced by initiation and promotion on mouse skin can become autonomous with respect to the promoter (3).

We have carried out a series of experiments to see if tumor promoters might interact synergistically with oncogenes to enhance stable cell transformation (74, Hsiao, W., Gattoni-Celli, S. and Weinstein, I.B., *Science*, in press). We have found that when C3H10T$\frac{1}{2}$ cells are transfected with the cloned human bladder cancer *c-ras*[H] oncogene, growth of the cells in the presence of TPA or teleocidin, but not phorbol, enhances the number of transformed foci obtained at least tenfold (Table 2). In addition, in the presence of the tumor promoter the foci appear earlier and they are larger. Parallel transfection studies with the drug resistance gene *gpt* indicate that TPA does not enhance, and even tends to inhibit, the number of *gpt*[+] colonies obtained (Table 2). Thus, the enhancement of foci obtained with the transfected oncogene does not appear to be a generalized effect of tumor promoters on the transfection process *per se*. Time course studies with teleocidin support this conclusion. Thus, it is possible that tumor promoters can act synergistically with cellular oncogenes during multistage carcinogenesis. We presume that they do so by activating the expression of other cellular genes and are currently attempting to identify these genes.

TABLE 2. Transfection frequencies obtained with pT24 and psSV2-*gpt* plasmid DNAs in C3H10T$\frac{1}{2}$ cells in the absences and presence of TPA

	gpt[+] colonies	T24 transformed foci
Without TPA	313	6
With 100 ng/ml TPA	82	92

Cells transfected with pSV2-*gpt* DNA were scored for *gpt*[+] colonies as previously described (52); cells transfected with the T24 plasmid containing the mutated human bladder cancer *c-ras*[H] oncogene (28), were scored for morphologically transformed foci. Where indicated, TPA (100 ng/ml) was present throughout the transfection and subsequent growth stages. Values represent colonies or foci per plate. Similar results were obtained with teleocidin but phorbol was inactive. The presence of integrated human *c-ras*[H] oncogene in the transformed cells was confirmed by Southern blot analysis (Hsiao, W.-L. W., Gattoni-Celli, S., and Weinstein, I. B., *Science*, in press).

Recent studies indicate that DNA damaging agents are more effective than tumor promoters in enhancing the progression of papillomas to carcinomas on mouse skin (33). This suggests that the evolution of a fully malignant tumor during multistage carcinogenesis may involve more than one cycle of damage to DNA, rather than a simple linear sequence of DNA damage induced by the initiator and subsequent non-genomic effects induced by the promoters. For example, since cigarettes contain both carcinogens and promoters, the chronic cigarette smoker is repeatedly exposed to both types of compounds. It also seems likely that tumor progression involves rather extensive genomic changes including gene amplification (58) and gross chromosomal abnormalities. This is, however, a highly speculative area since even less is known about the mechanism of tumor progression than about the earlier stages of initiation and promotion. In future studies, it will be important to focus on this question because at a clinical level the major therapeutic challenges presented by lung cancer, and other tumors, are related to invasion and metastasis, aspects of the tumor phenotype that probably result from the process of tumor progression.

CELLULAR GENES INVOLVED IN MULTISTAGE CARCINOGENESIS

The complexity of multistage caricnogenesis predicts that the evolution and maintenance of malignant cancer cells involves changes in multiple types of cellular genes (71,73). Indeed, there is accumulating evidence that tumors, including human lung cancers, display a wide variety of alterations in the state of integration and/or expression of several cellular oncogenes (4,16,20,25,31,57,58,70), as well as alterations in the expression of cellular sequences analogous to the long terminal repeat (LTR) sequences of retroviruses (41). DNA transfection studies also indicate that the conversion of normal cells to tumor cells requires the action of at least two oncogenes (46,54,59). Furthermore, since only about 20% of human tumors examined yield DNA which is active in the NIH 3T3 transformation assay (16,70) it is possible that in the majority of human tumors the tumor phenotype is a complex function of multigene interactions, both positive and negative (for supporting evidence see 13,64,65).

We discovered that murine cells transformed by chemical carcinogens or radiation express constitutively a series of poly A$^+$ RNAs that contain murine leukemia virus LTR-like sequences (41). Carcinogen-transformed murine cells also express RNAs homologous to endogenous VL30 (34), and intracisternal (IAP) (43) sequences, both of which are moderately repetitive retrovirus-like sequences present in the mouse genome. These findings have led us to suggest that carcinogenesis involves a disturbance in mechanisms controlling the function of multiple classes of cellular DNA enhancer sequences. Table 3 summarizes evidence that tumor cells display rather widespread disturbances in the control of gene expression and differentiation. In terms of targets for the action of chemical carcinogenesis it is worth noting that, although there are about 18 known cellular oncogenes, the normal mouse genome contains over 1200 copies of various types of LTR-sequences per haploid genome. The structural resemblance of LTRs to known transposable elements (6,63,68), their ability to enhance the transcription of a variety of genes (6,68), and the phenomena of viral LTR-promoter-insertion (31,56), and of insertion-mutation by endogenous intracisternal A-particle sequences (25,43,57,62), indicate the capacity of LTRs to act as mobile elements. Thus these elements, and other transcriptional enhancer sequences yet to be identified, constitute a major repertoire for potential aberrations in the control of gene expression during the course of chemical carcinogenesis. The switch-on in transcription of retrovirus-like sequences may, in part, be related to alterations in the state of methylation of cytidine residues in DNA, which are often associated with carcinogen action and tumor formation (9,37,50,77). Furthermore, since endogenous retrovirus-like sequences can also code for reverse transcriptase, once their expression is switched on, the RNA transcripts might undergo reverse transcription and the resulting DNA copies might then be reinserted into foreign sites in the genome, thus producing insertion mutations and further abnormalities in gene expression. There is evidence that analgous mechanisms might be involved in gene transposition by the *copia* element of Drosophila (60,63). Thus, an epigenetic event (i.e. activaiton of transcription of endogenous retrovirus-like elements) could lead to a stable genetic event. We are currently examining whether this postulated mechanism plays a role in tumor promotion or progression.

Finally, we would stress that although we have speculated about several qualitatively different mechanisms to explain the actions of carcinogens and tumor promoters, these mechanisms need not be mutually exclusive because of the complexity of the process of multistage carcinogenesis and the pervasive phenomenon of tumor heterogeneity.

TABLE 3. Types of genes expressed aberrantly in carcinogen and radiation transformed cells

1.	MLV-like LTR sequences (41)
2.	MLV *ENV* genes (8,22,41)
3.	VL30 sequences (18)
4.	A particle sequences (43)
5.	Multigene "TS DNA" Family (29)
6.	"Set 1" repetitive element, Qa/T1a MHC antigen (10)
7.	Fetal genes and inappropriate differentiation genes (71)

SUMMARY

The evolution of a fully malignant tumor is a multistep process resulting from the action of multiple factors, both environmental and endogenous, and involves alterations in the function of multiple cellular genes. Chemical carcinogens that initiate this process appear to do so by damaging cellular DNA. In addition to producing simple point mutations, this damage appears to induce the synthesis of a *trans*-acting factor that can induce asynchronous DNA replication. This response may result in gene amplification and/or gene rearrangement. This phenomenon may also play a role in synergistic interactions between chemicals and viruses in the causation of certain cancers. The primary target of the tumor promoters TPA, teleocidin, and aplysiatoxin appears to be cell membranes. All three of these agents act, at least in part by, enhancing the activity of the phospholipid-dependent enzyme PKC. We have proposed a stereochemical model to explain the interaction of these amphiphilic compounds with the PKC system. We have found that TPA and teleocidin markedly enhance the transformation of C3H10T$\frac{1}{2}$ mouse fibroblasts when these cells are transfected with the cloned *H-ras* human bladder cancer oncogene. Thus, tumor promoters can act synergistically with an activated oncogene to enhance cell transformation. Furthermore, carcinogen-transformed rodent cells display aberrations in the expression of various endogenous retrovirus-related sequences. Activation of some of these sequences may lead to insertion mutations and further aberrations in gene expression. These findings are discussed in terms of a multistep model that involves progressive changes in cellular oncogenes and aberrations in the function of DNA transcription enhancer sequences. It will be of interest to determine to what extent these concepts apply to the etiology of cancers of the respiratory tract.

ACKNOWLEDGEMENTS

This research was supported by DHS, NCI Grants CA 021111 and CA 26056, funding from the National Foundation for Cancer Research, and funds from the Dupont Company, and the Alma Toorock Memorial for Cancer Research. We thank Dr. Y. Ito for providing the HHPA compounds, Dr. R. E. Moore for the aplysiatoxin and Dr. H. Fujiki for the teleocidin. We are grateful to G. Vande Woude for providing *c-mos* probes. We thank John Mack for the art work shown in Fig. 2, and Evelyn Emeric for assistance in preparing this manuscript.

This paper is based on a similar paper presented by Weinstein, I. B. et al. at a Nobel Conference "Molecular Biology of Tumor Cells," Raven Press, in press, 1984.

REFERENCES

1. Arcoleo, J., and Weinstein, I. B. (1984): *Proc. Am. Assoc. Cancer Res.*, 25:142.
2. Barsoum, J., and Varshavsky, A. (1983): *Proc. Natl. Acad. Sci. USA*, 80:5330-5334.
3. Berenblum, I. (1982): In: *Cancer: A Comprehensive Treatise, Vol 1*, edited by F. F. Becker, pp 451-472. Plenum Publishing Corp., New York.
4. Bishop, J. M. (1983): *Cell*, 32:1018-1020.
5. Bishop, R., Martinez, R., Nakamura, K. D., and Weber, M. J. (1983): *Biochem. Biophys. Res. Commun.*, 115:536-543.
6. Blair, D. G., Oskarsson, M., Wood, T. G., McClements, W. L., Fischinger, P. J., and Vande Woude, G. F. (1981): *Science*, 212:941-943.
7. Blumberg, P. M., Jaken, S., Konig, B., Sharkey, N. E., Leach, K. L., Jeng, A. Y. and Yeh, E. (1984): *Biochem. Pharmacol.*, 33:933-940.
8. Boccara, M., Souyri, M., Magarian, C., Stavnezer, E., and Fleissner, E. (1983): *J. Virol.*, 43:102-109.
9. Boehm, T. L. J., and Drahovsky, D. (1983): *J. Natl. Cancer Inst.*, 71:429-434.
10. Brickell,M., Latchman, S., Murphy, W., and Rigby, W. J. (1983): *Nature*, 306:756-760.
11. Burgess, G. M., Godfrey, P. P., McKinney, J. S., Berridge, M. J., Irvine, R. F., and Putney, J. W. (1984): *Nature*, 309:63-66.
12. Castagna, M., Takai, U., Kaibuchi, K., Sano, K., Kikkawa, U., and Nishizuka, Y. (1982): *J. Biol. Chem.*, 257:7847-7851.
13. Cavenee, W. K., Dryja, T. P., Phillips, R. A., Benedict, W. F., Bodbout, R., Gallie, B. L., Murphree, A. L, Strong, L. C., and White, R. L. (1983): *Nature*, 305:779-784.
14. Cochet, C., Gill, G. N., Meisenhelder, J., Cooper, J. A., and Hunter, T. (1984): *J. Biol. Chem.*, 259:2553-2558.
15. Colburn, N. H., Former, B. F., Nelson, K. A., and Yuspa, S. H. (1979): *Nature*, 281:589-591.
16. Cooper, G. M. (1982): *Science*, 218:801-806.
17. Cope, F. O., Staller, J. M., Mahsem, R. A., and Boutwell, R. K. (1984): *Biochem. Biophys. Res. Commun.*, 120:593-601.

18. Courtney, M. G., Schmidt, L. J., and Getz, M. J. (1982): *Cancer Res.*, 42:569-576.
19. Delclos, K. B., Nagle, D. S., and Blumberg, P. M. (1980): *Cell*, 19:1025-1232.
20. Duesberg, P. H. (1983): *Nature*, 304:219-225.
21. Emerit, I., Levy, A., and Cerutti, P. (1983): *Mutat. Res.*, 110:327-335.
22. Fischinger, P. J., Thiel, H. J., Lieberman, M., Kaplan, H. S., Dunlop, N. M., and Robey, W. G. (1982): *Cancer Res.*, 42:4650-4657.
23. Fisher, P. B., and Weinstein, I. B. (1980): In: *Molecular and Cellular Aspects of Carcinogens Screening Tests*, edited by R. Montesano, L. Bartsch, and L. Tomatis, pp. 113-131. IARC Scientific Publ., No. 27, IARC Press, Lyon.
24. Fisher, P. B., Bozzone, J. H., and Weinstein, I. B. (1979): *Cell*, 18:695-705.
25. Gattoni-Celli, S., Hsiao, W.-L., and Weinstein, I. B. (1983): *Nature*, 306:795.
26. Gensler, H. L., and Bowden, G. T. (1983): *Carcinogenesis*, 4:1507-1511.
27. Gilmore, T., and Martin, G. S. (1983): *Nature*, 306:487-490.
28. Goldfarb, M., Shimizu, K., Perucho, M., and Wigler, M. (1982): *Nature*, 296:404-409.
29. Hanania, N., Shaool, D., Harel, J., Wiels, J., and Trusz, T. (1983): *EMBO J.*, 2:1621-1624.
30. Hayashi, K., Fujiki, H., and Sugimura, T. (1983): In: *Cellular Interactions by Environmental Tumor Promoters*, edited by H. Fujiki et al., in press. Japan Scientific Societies Press, Tokyo.
31. Hayward, W. S., Neel, B. G., and Astrin, S. M. (1981): *Nature*, 290:475-480.
32. Hecker, E., Fusenig, N. E., Kunz, W., Marks, F., and Thielmann, H. W., editors (1982): *Carcinogenesis - A Comprehensive Survey, Vol. 7: Cocarcinogenesis and Biological Effects of Tumor Promoters*. Raven Press, New York.
33. Hennings, H., Shores, R., Wenk, M. L., Spangler, E. F., Tarone, R., and Yuspa, S. (1983): *Nature*, 304:67-69.
34. Hodgson, C. P., Elder, P. K., Ono, T., Foster, D. N., and Gertz, M. J. (1983): *Cell. Biol.*, 3:2221-2234.
35. Horowitz, A., Greenebaum, E., and Weinstein, I. B. (1981): *Proc. Natl. Acad. Sci. USA*, 78:2315-2319.
36. Horowitz, A., Fujiki, H., Weinstein, I. B., Jeffrey, A., Okin, E., Moore, R. E., and Sugimura, T. (1983): *Cancer Res.*, 43:1529-1535.
37. Hsiao, W., Gattoni-Celli, S., Kirschemeier, P., and Weinstein, I. B. (1984): *Mol. Cell. Biol.*, 4:634-641.
38. Ito, Y., Yanase, S., Tokuda, H., Kishishita, M., Ohigashi, H., Hirota, M., and Koshimizu, K. (1983): *Cancer Lett.*, 18:87-95.
39. Iwashita, S., and Fox, C. F. (1984): *J. Biol. Chem.*, 259:2559-2567.
40. Jacobs, S., Sayyoun, N. E., Saltiel, A. R., and Cuatracasas, P. (1983): *Proc. Natl. Acad. Sci. USA*, 80:6211-6213.
41. Kirschmeier, P., Gattoni-Celli, S., Dina, D., and Weinstein, I. B. (1982): *Proc. Natl. Acad. Sci. USA*, 79:273-277.
42. Kraft, A. A., and Anderson, W. B. (1983): *Nature*, 301:621-623.
43. Kuff, E. L., Feenstra, A., Lueders, K., Smith, L., Harvey, R., Hozumi, N., and Shulman, M. (1983): *Proc. Natl. Acad. Sci. USA*, 80: 1992-1996.
44. Lambert, M. E., Gattoni-Celli, S., Kirschmeier, P., and Weinstein, I. B. (1983): *Carcinogenesis*, 4:587-594.
45. Lambert, M., Pelligrini, S., Gattoni-Celli, S., and Weinstein, I. B. (1984): *Cold Spring Harbor Meeting on DNA Tumor Viruses*, abstract, in press. Cold Spring Harbor, NY.
46. Land, H., Parada, L. F., and Weinberg, R. A. (1983): *Nature*, 304:596-602.

47. Lavi, S., and Etkin, S. (1981): *Carcinogenesis*, 2:417-423.
48. Lee, L. S., and Weinstein, I. B. (1980): *Carcinogenesis*, 1:669-679.
49. Le Peuch, C. J., Ballester, R., and Rosen, O. M. (1983): *Proc. Natl. Acad. Sci. USA*, 80:6858-6862.
50. Lu, L. J. W., Randerath, E., and Randerath, K. (1983): *Cancer Letts.*, 19:231-239.
51. Macara, I. G., Marinetti, G. V., and Balduzzi, P. C. (1984): *Proc. Natl. Acad. Sci. USA*, in press.
52. Mulligan, R. C., and Berg, P. (1981): *Proc. Natl. Acad. Sci. USA*, 78:2072-2076.
53. Mufson, R. A., Okin, E., and Weinstein, I. B. (1981): *Carcinogenesis*, 2:1095-1102.
54. Newbold, R. F., and Overell, R. W. (1983): *Nature*, 304:648-651.
55. Nishizuka, Y. (1984): *Nature*, 304:648-651.
56. Payne, G. S., Bishop, J. M., and Varmus, H. E. (1982): *Nature*, 295:209-214.
57. Rechavi, G., Givol, D., and Canaani, E. (1982): *Nature*, 300:607-611.
58. Robertson, M. (1984): *Nature*, 300:149-152.
59. Ruley, H. E. (1983): *Nature*, 304:602-606.
60. Ryo, H., Shiba, T., Fukunaga, A., Kondo, S., and Gateff, E. (1984): *Gann*, 75:22-28.
61. Sharkey, N. A., Leah, K. L., and Blumberg, P. M. (1984): *Proc. Natl. Acad. Sci. USA*, 81:607-610.
62. Shen-ong, G. L. C., and Cole, M. D. (1984): *J. Virol.*, 49:171-177.
63. Shiba, T., and Saigo, K. (1983): *Nature*, 302:119-124.
64. Solomon, E. (1983): *Nature*, 309:111-112.
65. Stanbridge, E. J., Der, C. J., Doerson, C. J., Nishimi, Y., Peehl, D. M., Weissman, E., and Wilkinson, J. E. (1982): *Science*, 215:252-259.
66. Sugimoto, Y., Whitman, M., Cantley, I. C., and Erikson, R. I. (1984): *Proc. Natl. Acad. Sci. USA*, 81:2117-2121.
67. Sugimura, T. (1982): *Gann*, 73:499-507.
68. Temin, H. M. (1982): *Cell*, 28:3-5.
69. Tran, P. L., Castagna, M., Sala, M., Vassent, G., Horowitz, A. D., Schachter, D., and Weinstein, I. B. (1983): *Eur. J. Biochem.*, 130:155-160.
70. Weinberg, R. A. (1983): *Sci. Am.*, 249:126-142.
71. Weinstein, I. B. (1981): *J. Supramol. Struct.*, 17:99-120.
72. Weinstein, I. B. (1983): *Nature*, 302:750.
73. Weinstein, I. B., Gattoni-Celli, S., Kirschmeier, P., Hsiao, W., Horowitz, A., and Jeffrey, A. (1984): *Fed. Proc.*, 43:2287-2294.
74. Weinstein, I. B., Arcoleo, J., Backer, J., Jeffrey, A. M., Hsiao, W., Gattoni-Celli, S., and Kirschmeier, P. (1984): In: *Cellular Interactions of Environmental Tumor Promoters*, edited by H. Fujiki et al., in press. Japan Scientific Societies Press, Tokyo.
75. Weiss, R., Teich, N., Varmus, H., and Coffin, J., editors (1982): *Molecular Biology of Tumor Viruses. Second Edition, RNA Tumor Viruses.* Cold Spring Harbor Laboratory, Cold Spring Harbor, NY.
76. Werth, D. K., Niedel, J. E., and Pastan, I. (1983): *J. Biol. Chem.*, 258:11423-11426.
77. Wilson, V. L., and Jones, P. A. (1983): *Cell*, 32:329-346.

Carcinogenesis, Vol. 8, edited by M. J. Mass et al.
Raven Press, New York © 1985.

Multi-Event Model of Carcinogenesis: A Mathematical Model for Cancer Causation and Prevention

Kenneth C. Chu

Occupational Cancer Branch, National Cancer Institute, Bethesda, Maryland 20205

In carcinogenesis research, the investigation of skin carcinogenesis has led to many significant theoretical advances. Beginning in the 1940's, skin carcinogenesis was shown to involve two sequential processes: initiation (interpreted as the transformation of a normal cell to a transformed cell - called transformation in this paper), and tumor promotion (the development of an observable cancer from a transformed cell) (3,5,6,17,27,32).

In 1980, researchers reported that there may be at least three sequential stages in skin cancer in rodents (35). In a series of experiments involving the sequential administration of promoters and nonpromoters, it was shown that there are two sequential stages in tumor promotion. These studies showed that after an initiator was given, the order in which two chemicals were administered was critical to the appearance of tumors. There are chemicals that give tumors when they are given first and do not yield tumors when given the second agent. These have been called stage I promoters. Examples include 12-O-tetradecanoylphorbol-13-acetate (TPA), 4-O-methyl TPA, hydrogen peroxide, and calcium ionophore A23187 (36). On the other hand, there are chemicals that give tumors only when administered after stage I promoters. These are called stage II promoters. An example is mezerein (35).

More recently, carcinogenesis research has determined that there are chemicals (chemopreventive agents) that can block the tumorigenic action of different stage promoters. In a series of experiments, it has been shown that fluocinolone acetonide (FA) and tosyl phenylalanine chloromethyl ketone (TPCK) block the action of stage I promoters, while FA and retinoic acid block the action of stage II promoters (34).

Presently, the commonly used mathematical models for cancer, e.g., two-stage model (1) and multistage model (2), do not account for tumor promotion activities, such as stage I and II promoters or chemopreventive agents (45). The two-stage model of cancer, by definition, is inadequate to describe 3 or more stages in the carcinogenic process. The multistage model does not address the sequential aspects of the multistage nature of tumor promotion nor the role of chemoprevention. Rather the multistage model deals with the formation of a single transformed cell from a normal one (45).

The objective of this paper is to present a mathematical model to describe both cancer causation (the transformation and tumor promotion processes) and prevention (chemoprevention process). To accomplish this, the approach used expands the multistage model for cancer to account for the role of tumor promotion and chemoprevention.

METHODS

The model proposed for carcinogenesis is given in Fig. 1. Like the multistage model, a cell may undergo a series of changes or stages to become a transformed cell (2,14,45). However, unlike the multistage model, the cells at each stage may not only go to the next stage, but also may proliferate or die. Since the cell may undergo a number of different events, the model is termed the multi-event model (MEM) for cancer.

This formulation allows MEM to account for a number of carcinogenic phenomena not previously addressed by other models of carcinogenesis. First, MEM accounts for the role of stage promoters as chemicals that increase the proliferation of cells in individual stages. Second, the MEM accounts for the action of some chemopreventive agents such as substances that inhibit cell proliferation. Third, the MEM accounts for the natural history of cancerous lesions as well as the pathogenesis of chemically induced lesions, in terms of the stages in the formation of the malignant cell.

Formally, three cellular events are allowed to occur to cells in each stage in MEM: cell division, cell loss, and cell transition. In Fig. 1, $N_i(t)$ represents the number of cells which have the ability to divide at the ith stage at age t. The rate constant for cell division activities in the ith stage is given by $P_i(t)$, while the rate constant for cell loss activities in the ith stage is given by $D_i(t)$. The rate constant for cell transition from the ith to the $i + 1^{th}$ stage is given by $T_i(t)$. A set of differential equations can be set up to describe these processes. The equations and their solutions are given in the appendix (45).

The cell transition event represents the advancement of a cell in one stage to a progressively more malignant stage. The model assumes

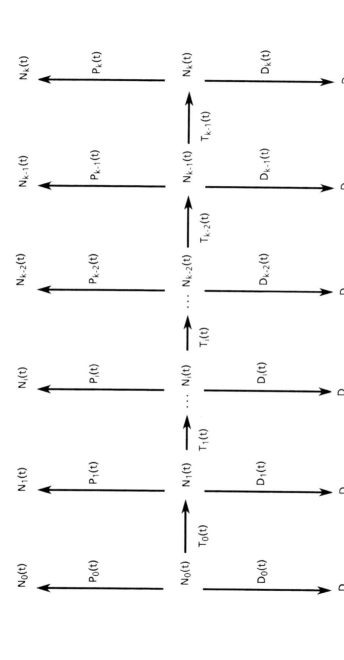

FIG. 1. Multi-event model for carcinogenesis.

that the cell transitions are irreversible, and the cells in each stage can reproduce daughter cells so that their characteristics are heritable. This assumption requires some clarification since it is known that when a transformation occurs, it may be repaired so that the effect is reversed. Experimental evidence indicates that transformed cells must undergo one replication in order to "fix" the transformed state (7,19). Thus, it is assumed that cells that have undergone a transition have not been repaired, and the transformation is fixed.

Another important event in the MEM is cell division, the cellular activities that cause the cells to reproduce. This fundamental event allows the number of cells in each stage of malignant transformation to increase independent of cell transition. This capability is not available in the multistage model.

An equally important event in the MEM is cell loss, the cellular activities that cause the cells to loose the ability to reproduce. This loss can occur because of cell death, elimination of cells from the body, or cell differentiation. The event, which is not available in the multistage model, is important since it provides a mechanism for decreasing the number of cells in a stage.

The inclusion of cell differentiation as a cell loss process is important. It is known that increased cell differentiation decreases the ability of cells to divide (30,31). Many believe that cell division is a necessary condition for a transition to occur (21,22,29,41,43). They believe that normal cells that are incapable of cell division do not cause cancer. For example, adult neurons do not divide and a tumor derived from neurons, neuroblastoma, is extremely rare in adults. Neuroblastomas tend to occur in early childhood when neurons are dividing during cell growth (26). As a consequence, since cell differentiation causes the cells to loose the ability to divide and to undergo cell transitions, differentiation is a cell loss activity.

If cell division activities in the ith stage ($P_i(t)$) are greater than cell loss activities ($D_i(t)$) (given cell transition activities are extremely rare) then there will be net cell proliferation, i.e., an increase in the number of cells at that stage. This formulation has some interesting implications. First, it is assumed that cells at each stage may be phenotypically similar to normal cells since methods to distinguish a single malignant cell from millions of normal cell are presently not known. When a number of cells are aggregated one can detect an abnormal effect, manifested as histopathologic abnormalities or clinical lesions. It is assumed that when a sufficient number of cells in a stage are produced, a unique abnormal effect, such as histopathologic entities or clinical lesions, will be observed. A consequence of this formulation is that since the cells in a stage account for the observation of a unique abnormal effect, the severity of the effect reflects the stages in the transformation process. For example, the sequential observation of hyperplasia, neoplastic nodule, and then carcinoma in rat liver (39) is considered as evidence for the multistage or multi-event nature of the carcinogenic process.

Second, the increase in the number of cells in a stage of malignant transformation may affect the transformation process. Since cell proliferation increases the number of cells in a stage the probability of a cell undergoing a transition to the next stage increases. The role of agents that stimulate proliferation, such as promoters, will be discussed in the section on the role of chemical agents.

If cell loss ($D_i(t)$) is greater than cell proliferation ($P_i(t)$), there is a decrease in the number of cells in that stage. This effect can be used to account for tumor regression and disappearance. For example, after an initiator is given, the administration of a promoter can cause a skin tumor. If the administration of the promoter is halted, the skin tumor can regress. In the MEM, this phenomenon would correspond to the promoter increasing the $P_i(t)$ rate so that $P_i(t)$ is greater than $D_i(t)$. The number of cells increases and a skin tumor becomes visible. After the cessation of the promoter, $D_i(t)$ becomes greater than $P_i(t)$, the number of cells decreases, and the tumor size decreases.

DISCUSSION

This discussion will include the relationship of the MEM to other models of carcinogenesis, insight regarding the progression to cancerous lesions from the MEM, and the MEM and its representation of the mechanisms of action of chemical carcinogens, tumor promoters and chemopreventive agents.

The Relationship of MEM to Other Cancer Models

The MEM is closely related to the multistage model. As stated earlier both use the same formulation of the transformation process. As a consequence, they draw similar conclusions about the factors that affect this process. If the MEM had zero rates for cell loss and proliferation for all stages but the last one, the resultant model would be effectively the same as the multistage model. In this sense, the multistage model is a special case of the MEM.

Recently, a two-stage transformation model was proposed (26). This basic model requires two stages - intermediate cells, then malignant cells (20,28,42). The model allows the intermediate cells to increase or decrese in number as well as to form malignant cells. In addition, this two-stage model uses the kinetics of the normal growth of tissues to help account for childhood as well as old age cancer incidences. This simple, yet elegant model has been most useful, particularly in accounting for a number of results in human genetics and cancer (26). If there were only two stages in the MEM model then the above two-stage model and the corresponding MEM could be viewed as equivalent. However, the two-stage model makes no allowance for the experimental evidence which distinguishes between stage I and II promoters (18).

The Progression of Cancerous Lesions and MEM

A natural outgrowth of the MEM formulation of cancer is an emphasis on the role of precancerous lesions. Since cells in each stage of the transformation process may proliferate and, at least theoretically, generate abnormal effects, a footprint for the progression of normal tissue to abnormal tissue to cancer may be obtained. Thus, a study of the progression of lesions is a critical factor in understanding the carcinogenic process.

There have been many studies on the progression of neoplastic lesions from their preneoplastic precursors (reviewed by 4,13,15,16). In skin carcinogenesis, it has been shown that normal cells proceed to promoter-dependent clones, to autonomous clones, to promoter-dependent papillomas, to autonomous papillomas, and finally to squamous cell carcinomas (11,12). In mammary cancer, progression of normal tissue to hormone dependent lesions to hormone independent (autonomous) lesions to malignant tumors has been demonstrated (15). In liver cancer in rats, the histopathologic progression from hyperplasia, neoplastic nodule, hepatocellular adenoma, hepatocellular carcinoma to metastatic carcinoma has been well documented (39). Another example is the large-scale mouse experiment on 2-acetylaminofluorene (23,24). The two target sites were the urinary bladder and liver. For each target site, there was a time progression of several degrees of hyperplasia, then adenoma and finally carcinoma.

These studies support the formulation in the MEM. The studies cited have at least two distinct precancerous lesions. The MEM implicitly assumes at least two intermediate stages in order to produce a three stage model. The MEM would interpret these data as evidence for at least three stages in a sequential multistage carcinogenic process. The studies indicate that precancerous effects showed progressive advancement to a malignant state. The MEM assumes the progressive advancement of a normal cell to a malignant cell. Since it is assumed that abnormal effects can only arise from the cells in a stage, the number of stages is always greater or equal to the number of unique abnormal effects.

Use of the MEM to Identify the Role of Chemical Agents

Since the MEM can be viewed as a general scheme for describing the total carcinogenic process, it can provide a conceptual framework for defining the role of the different types of chemical agents, such as initiators, promoters, complete carcinogens, chemoprevention agents, etc.

In the MEM, initiators and complete carcinogens affect the transition rates $(T_i(t))$. The transition probability can be modeled as $T_i = S_i + G_i C$, where S_i is the spontaneous transition rate, C is the effective concentration of the chemical agent and G_i is a proportionality constant (45). Previous work has indicated that there are carcinogenic agents that require a long latency period for the cancer to occur, such as β-naphthylamine, and benzidine. These carcinogens have been shown to act on the early stage of the transformation process i.e., T_0 or T_1 (14). Another group of carcinogens affect the transition rates of the later stages of the transformation process. These chemicals do not require a long latency period, e.g., arsenic (8,9,10).

In contrast to carcinogens that affect the transition rates, promoters may act by increasing the proliferation of cells. Promoters can act in several ways. There are promoters that increase the rate of cell division, $P_i(t)$, such a phenobarbital (33). Another type of promoter is one that acts by decreasing the rate of cell loss, i.e., decrease $D_i(t)$, such as TPA (37). It is postulated that these chemicals work by blocking the terminal differentiation of cells. Since terminal differentiation leads to cell loss, blocking terminal differentiation decreases the loss of cells. This action effectively causes an increase in the number of cells in the affected stage. In addition, the increase in cells increases the probability of a random transition. Thus, promoters, in this model, can cause irreversible effects. The irreversibility of some stages of tumor promotion has been well established by the work of Burns et al. (12). They demonstrated the irreversible formation of carcinomas from autonomous papillomas, and the irreversible formation of autonomous papillomas from one or more precursors in response to only TPA exposure.

It is tempting to classify carcinogenic agents into a scheme like this one. Some attempts have been made (25,40,44). Chemicals that are purported to act by affecting cell proliferation, such as promoters, have been called epigenetic agents, while those that are purported to affect the transition rates directly, such as initiators, have been called genotoxic agents. However, this classification assumes that 1) the actions of the agent are known, and 2) the agent is acting on only one event in one stage. The agent may be acting on more than one event or stage. It may affect a transition rate at one stage in the transformation process and affect a proliferation rate in another stage in the carcinogenic process. As stated earlier, promoters can cause irreversible changes, i.e., papillomas developing into carcinomas using only TPA (12). As a consequence, caution should be exercised in the development of mechanistic classification schemes.

Use of the MEM to Understand Chemopreventive Agents

The MEM can, not only account for types of carcinogenic agents, i.e., initiators and promoters, but also can describe the role of chemopreventive agents. Chemical agents that can prevent the formation of tumors are called chemopreventive agents. These agents may act by blocking the transformation process in a number of ways. First, they can act to block the action of carcinogens that affect the transition rates, i.e., ascorbic acid and vitamin A can act as scavengers of reactive carcinogens. Second, they can act to decrease cell proliferation of transformed cells or increase the rate of cell loss. For example, retinoids may increase the rate of cell differentiation allowing more cells to become differentiated and to become less prone to divide and to undergo a cell transition (38).

The fact that there are chemopreventive agents that selectively block the action of stage I and II promoters supports the sequential multistage nature of the tumor promotion process. In the MEM, this phenomenon corresponds to the stage I promoters acting to increase the proliferation rate of a stage, say i. Then stage I chemopreventive agents stop the effect of stage I promoters by increasing the cell loss rate above the proliferation rate in this stage. In a similar manner, stage II promoters act on the proliferation rate of the $i + 1^{th}$ stage while stage II chemopreventive agents act on cell loss rate for this stage. It is noted that these chemicals do not directly act on the cell transition process. Rather they affect the transition indirectly by increasing or decreasing the probability of a transition occurring by affecting the number of cells in the stage.

It is envisioned that MEM can be used as a conceptual framework for understanding and guiding research in cancer prevention and control, just as the multistage model has influenced research in etiology. The multi-event model offers a multistage mathematic model that is based on cellular events: transition, proliferation, and cell loss. These events are used to formulate a model that accounts for 1) the progression to cancer from precancerous lesions as well as the natural history of lesions, 2) tumor initiation, tumor promotion, and chemoprevention, and 3) the multistage nature of the transformation process.

ACKNOWLEDGEMENT

I would like to thank Charles C. Brown for numerous and informative discussions about this problem and possible solutions.

REFERENCES

1. Armitage, P., and Doll, R. (1957): *Brit. J. Cancer*, 11:161-169.
2. Armitage, P., and Doll, R. (1961): In: *Proceedings of the Fourth Berkeley Symposium on Mathematical Statistics and Probability, Vol. 4*, edited by J. Neyman, pp. 19-38. University of California Press, Berkeley.
3. Berenblum, I. (1941): *Cancer Res.*, 1:44-48.
4. Berenblum, I. (1974): *Carcinogenesis as a Biological Problem.* North Holland Publishing Company, New York.
5. Berenblum, I. and Shubik, P. (1947): *Brit. J. Cancer*, 1:379-391.
6. Berenblum, I. and Shubik, P. (1949): *Brit. J. Cancer*, 3:109-118.
7. Borek, C., and Sachs, L. (1968): *Proc. Natl. Acad. Sci. USA*, 59:83-85.
8. Brown, C. C., and Chu, K. C. (1982): In: *Environmental Epidemiology: Risk Assessment*, edited by R. L. Prentice and A. S. Whittemore, pp. 94-106. Society for Industrial and Applied Mathematics, Philadelphia.
9. Brown, C. C., and Chu, K. C. (1983): *Environ. Health Perspect.*, 50:293-308.
10. Brown, C. C., and Chu, K. C. (1983): *J. Natl. Cancer Inst.*, 70:455-463.
11. Burns, F. J., Vanderlaan, M., Sivak, A., and Albert, R. E. (1976): *Cancer Res.*, 36:1422-1427.
12. Burns, F. J., Vanderlaan, M., Snyder, E., and Albert, R. E. (1978): In: *A Comprehensive Survey, Vol. 2: Mechanisms of Tumor Promotion and Carcinogenesis*, edited by T. J. Slaga, A. Sivak, and R. K. Boutwell, pp. 91-96. Raven Press, New York.
13. Colburn, N. H. (1980): In: *Carcinogenesis - A Comprehensive Survey, Vol 5: Cocarcinogenesis and Biological Effects of Tumor Promoters*, pp. 33-56. Raven Press, New York.

14. Day, N. E., and Brown, C. C. (1980): *J. Natl. Cancer Inst.*, 64:977-989.
15. Foulds, L. (1969): *Neoplastic Development 1*. Academic Press, New York.
16. Foulds, L. (1975): *Neoplastic Development 2*. Academic Press, New York.
17. Friedewald, W. F., and Rous, P. (1944): *J. Exp. Med.*, 80:101-125.
18. Hicks, R. M. (1980): *Carcinogenesis*, 4:1209-1214.
19. Kakunaga, T. (1974): *Int. J. Cancer*, 14:736-742.
20. Kendall, D. G. (1960): *Biometrika*, 47:316-330.
21. Kennedy, A. R., Murphy, G., and Little, J. B. (1980): *Cancer Res.*, 40:1915-1920.
22. Little, J. B. (1981): *Radiat. Res.*, 87:240-250.
23. Littlefield, N. A., Farmer, J. H., and Gaylor, D. W. (1979): *J. Environ. Path. Toxicol.*, 3:17-34.
24. Littlefield, N. A., Greenman, D. L., and Farmer, J. H. (1979): *J. Environ. Pathol. Toxicol.*, 3:35-54.
25. Miller, E. C., and Miller, J. A. (1979): In: *Chemical Carcinogens, ACS Monograph 173*, edited by C. E. Searle, pp. 737-762. American Chemical Society, Washington, DC.
26. Moolgavkar, S. H., and Knudson, A. G., Jr., (1981): *J. Natl. Cancer Inst.*, 66:1037-1052.
27. Mottram, J. C. (1944): *J. Pathol. Bacteriol.*, 56:181-187.
28. Neyman, J., and Scott, E. (1967): *Fifth Berkeley Symposium on Mathematical Statistics and Probability*, pp. 754-776. University of California Press, Berkeley.
29. Oehlert, W. (1973): *Cell Tissue Kinet.*, 6:325-335.
30. Pierce, G. B. (1970): *Fed. Proc.*, 29:1248-1254.
31. Pierce, G. B., and Wallace, C. (1971): *Cancer Res.*, 31:127-134.
32. Rous, P., and Kidd, J. G., (1941): *J. Exp. Med.*, 73:365-384.
33. Schulte-Herman, R. (1974): *CRC Crit. Rev. Toxicol.*, 3:97-158.
34. Slaga, T. J. (1983): *Environ. Health Perspect.*, 50:3-14.
35. Slaga, T. J., Fischer, S. M., Nelson, K., and Gleason, G. L. (1980): *Proc. Natl. Acad. Sci. USA*, 77:3659-3663.
36. Slaga, T. J., Fischer, S.M., Weeks, C. E., and Klein-Szanto, A. J. P. (1981): *Rev. Biochem. Toxicol.*, 3:231-281.
37. Slaga, T. J., Sivak, A., and Boutwell, R. K., editors (1978): *Carcinogenesis - A Comprehensive Survey, Vol. 2: Mechanisms of Tumor Promotion and Cocarcinogenesis*. Raven Press, New York.
38. Sporn, M. (1980): In: *Carcinogenesis - A Comprehensive Survey, Vol. 5: Modifiers of Chemical Carcinogenesis*, edited by T. J. Slaga, pp. 99-109. Raven Press, New York.
39. Squire, R. A., and Levitt, M. (1975): *Cancer Res.*, 35:3214.
40. Stott, W. T., Reitz, R. H., Schumann, A. M., and Watanabe, P. G. (1981): *Food Cosmet. Toxicol.*, 18:567-576.
41. Tsuda, H., Sarma, D. S. R., Rajalaskshmi, S., Zubroff, J., Farber, E., Batzinger, R. P., Cha, Y., and Bueding, E. (1979): *Cancer Res.*, 39:4491-4496.
42. Tucker, H. G. (1961): *Fourth Berkeley Symposium on Mathematical Statistics and Probability*, Vol. 4, edited by J. Neyman, pp. 387-403. University of California Press, Berkeley.
43. Warwick, G. P. (1971): *Fed. Proc.* 30:1760-1765.
44. Weisburger, J. H., and Williams, G. M. (1981) *Science*, 214:401-407.
45. Whittemore, A., and Keller, J. B. (1978): *Soc. Ind. Appl. Math. Rev.*, 20:1-30.

STATISTICAL APPENDIX

Differential equations for multi-event model:

$$d\,N_0(t)/dt = [P_0(t) - T_0(t) - D_0(t)]\,N_0(t)$$

$$d\,N_1(t)/dt = N_0(t)\,T_0(t) + [P_1(t) - T_1(t) - D_1(t)]\,N_1(t)$$

$$d\,N_i(t)/dt = N_{i-1}(t)\,T_{i-1}(t) + [P_i(t) - T_i(t) - D_i(t)]\,N_i(t)$$

$$d\,N_K(t)/dt = N_{K-1}(t)\,T_{K-1}(t)$$

General solution to the differential equations (45):

Let $L_i(t) = \int_0^t R_i(s)\,ds$, where $R_i(s) = D_i(s) + T_i(s) - P_i(s)$ then,

$N_0(t) = N_0(0)\exp(-L_0(t))$ where $N_0(0)$ is the number of normal cells at $t = 0$ and

$$N_i(t) = \exp(-L_i(t)) \int_0^t T_{i-1}(\tau)\,N_{i-1}(\tau)\exp(L_i(\tau))\,d\tau \text{ for } i = 1 \text{ to } K-1$$

so that,

$$N_1(t) = \exp(-L_1(t)) \int_0^t T_0(\tau)\,N_0(\tau)\exp(L_1(\tau))\,d\tau$$

If the transition rates (T_i) are constant and small then

$$N_1(t) = \exp(-L_1(t))\,T_0 \int_0^t N_0(\tau)\exp(L_1(\tau))\,d\tau$$

If the $P_i(t)$ and $D_i(t) >> T_i(t)$ then $R_i(t) = D_i(t) - P_i(t)$

and if $L_i(t)$ is small for $i = 1$ to $K-1$ then $\exp(-L_i(t)) \simeq 1$ and

$$N_i(t) = T_{i-1} \int_0^t N_{i-1}(\tau)\exp(L_i(\tau))\,d\tau$$

and

$$N_1(t) = T_0 \int_0^t N_0(\tau)\exp(L_1(\tau))\,d\tau$$

Carcinogenesis, Vol. 8, edited by M. J. Mass et al.
Raven Press, New York © 1985.

Tumor Promotion and Tumor Progression

J. Carl Barrett

*Environmental Carcinogenesis Group, Laboratory of Pulmonary Function and Toxicology,
National Institute of Environmental Health Sciences,
Research Triangle Park, North Carolina 27709*

Identification of the factors which promote or enhance human respiratory tract carcinogenesis requires an understanding of the mechanisms by which chemicals and other environmental factors influence the later stages of neoplastic development. Our understanding of the post-initiation stages of carcinogenesis is aided by the knowledge that neoplastic transformation is a multistep process and that some agents act specifically as tumor promoters. This has led, however, to the generalizations that all substances that act in the later phases of carcinogenesis are tumor promoters and possibly act by common mechanisms. It is my intended purpose of this chapter to point out that these generalizations may be fallacious in certain systems and are an impediment to the elucidation of the mechanisms of the stages in neoplastic development. Specifically, I would like to point out that in the progression to malignancy, the development of cancers may be enhanced by agents which are not tumor promoters in the classical sense and hence there are mechanisms involved in the later stages of tumor development, which are distinct from those involved in tumor promotion.

The post-initiation phases of tumor development have been described in general terms as tumor promotion and tumor progression (22). It is important to know the relationship between these two processes, but this understanding depends in part on the acceptance of the definitions for these terms. The concept of tumor promotion has developed from experimental studies in which it was shown that sequential treatment of a target tissue with two chemicals (an initiator and a promoter), which are inactive alone, results in tumor formation (8,9). The concept of tumor progression is less well delineated and this term is used in different contexts. Foulds (15) has defined the concept of progression as "one of stepwise neoplastic development through qualitatively different stages . . . by way of permanent irreversible qualitative change in one or more of the characters" of the cells in the tumor. Foulds (15) emphasized that progression is a qualitative, irreversible change, not merely an extension of a lesion. Others have used the term tumor progression less rigorously to describe general population changes in a tumor at later stages without regard to specific qualitative changes. In the following discussion, I will use the term tumor progression, as defined by Foulds, to describe qualitative, permanent cellular changes, which occur in a developing cancer after initiation.

In the mouse skin model (8,9) it is easy to distinguish operationally tumor promotion as the formation of the papilloma and tumor progression as the development of the carcinoma from the papilloma. However, since promotion is defined on the basis of a phenomenon, not a mechanism, some potential overlap exists between promotion and progression. If the phenomenon of tumor promotion involves a qualitative, irreversible change in the initiated cells, then tumor progression (as defined by Foulds) occurs during tumor promotion. If tumor promotion is merely clonal expansion of the initiated cells then tumor progression occurs after tumor promotion as implied by the operational distinction mentioned above. To distinguish tumor promotion from tumor progression therefore requires definition of the mechanism of the former.

As discussed previously (4,13), there are two possible *cellular* mechanisms for tumor promotion:

1) Tumor promoters act only to amplify the number of initated cells relative to the normal cells resulting in the appearance of a visible lesion (i.e., tumor promotion is only a quantitative change in cellular populations) (23,34).

2) Tumor promoters modulate the initiated cell to a state which allows subsequent clonal proliferation of these cells relative to the normal cells in the tissue (i.e., tumor promotion is a qualitative plus a quantitative change in the initiated cells).

There is evidence that certain tumor promoters can cause a qualitative modulation of the initiated cells. In the mouse skin model different stages of tumor promotion have been identified (9,16,32). These experiments demonstrate that croton oil or 12-O-tetra-decanoylphorbol-13-acetate (TPA) can effect changes in initiated cells which allow them to be amplified by compounds ("second stage promoters"), which are inactive or weak promoters by themselves (32). For example, mezerein, which is as potent as TPA in inducing a variety of phenotypic effects on cells, is active only as a second stage promoter. Also, different inhibitors of promotion can be shown to be effective in inhibiting only the first or the second stages of promotion (33). These results suggest that potent promoters can modulate or convert (9) initiated cells qualitatively to allow them to amplify or proliferate into a clone of tumor cells.

The nature of first stage promotion is unclear. A single dose of TPA is effective for first stage promotion and the effect of this treatment can be irreversible at least for 1-2 months (17,30-33). These two characteristics are more similar to the phenomenon of initiation than promotion (36). Thus, first stage promotion may represent a progression of the initiated cells, i.e. a co-initiation change necessary for promotion. The possible mutagenic activity of TPA could possibly play a role in this stage (6,12,21); however, most of the reported chromosome or DNA damaging effects are induced by second stage as well as first stage promoters (6,12). The possible exception is the induction of mitotic aneuploidy (21), but this effect, observed in yeast, has not been confirmed in mammalian cells. The first stage of promotion can also be explained by the epigenetic induction of a new cellular phenotype, such as induction of an embryonic cell type (32,33).

The key feature of any model of tumor promotion is the amplification of the initiated cell *vis-à-vis* the non-initiated cell resulting in clonal expression of a tumor. The importance of this mechanism in tumor promotion of mouse skin is strongly supported by the observations that 1) all known mouse skin tumor promoters are hyperplastic agents (3,9), and 2) regenerative hyperplasia by wounding or abrasion is sufficient to cause tumor promotion (1,2). It has been stated that hyperplasia and tumor promotion are unrelated (3). However, correlative studies of these two effects are often difficult to interpret because the hyperplastic response to a single treatment of promoter is related to tumor formation after many months of treatment. These studies assume that the hyperplasia after a single treatment or multiple treatments is similar. This is clearly not the case (3,28,29). In mouse skin treated with the TPA, there is a potentiation of hyperplastic response with additional TPA treatments (26). With other promoters (14) and with other species (29), this potentiation is not observed and sometimes the epidermis adapts to the promoter and fails to respond hyperplastically (29). The differences in sustained hyperplasia with multiple TPA treatments can also be related to different sensitivities of different strains of mice to tumor promotion (28).

It is important to realize that hyperplasia and amplification of the initiated cell are not necessarily related. In fact, stimulation of growth of the entire epidermis would not allow expansion of the initated cell unless the initiated cell is altered in its differentiation potential and therefore is amplified relative to the non-initiated cell, many of which terminally differentiate after stimulation to proliferate. Studies by Yuspa and coworkers (20,37) support this hypothesis for mouse skin carcinogenesis. Amplification of initiated cells in other organs might occur by a specific stimulation of growth of initiated cells or by a differential inhibition of growth of the normal cells (13). Neither of these mechanisms would be associated with general hyperplasia of the tissue.

Thus, I would like to emphasize that a key feature of tumor promotion, regardless of the experimental system, is the clonal amplification of the initated cells. This can result from hyperplasia, specific growth stimulation, or differential toxicity. Since tumor promotion is a phenomenon rather than one specific mechanism, this term will continue to be used to describe a multitude of mechanisms by which tumors are enhanced. However, in classifying and identifying chemicals by mechanism it would be useful to make a distinction between agents which act primarily to enhance clonal expansion, such as tumor promoters, and agents which act primarily to enhance the progression of cells by inducing qualitative changes in a subpopulation of the cells which are then clonally selected.

This distinction can be illustrated by the mouse skin tumor model. The initiation-promotion system describes only the development of benign papillomas. A further progression of the cells to the malignant stage (carcinomas) has to occur for the model to describe the complete process of carcinogenesis. The progression of papillomas to carcinomas in mouse skin appears independent of tumor promoter (TPA) exposure, but is enhanced by subsequent exposure to mutagenic agents (11,18,30). Thus, the later stage of tumor progression can be distinguished clearly from the process of tumor promotion on the basis of the lack of response of the former to tumor promoters. This is strong evidence that multiple mechanisms are involved in the later stages of neoplastic development.

Potter (24,25) has stressed this mechanistic difference. He has suggested that "promotion acts by facilitating the spontaneous occurrence of a second mutation by expanding the population of initiated cells" (25). The hypothesis would predict that a second application of a mutagen, for example an initiator, would increase the progression of the cells to the malignant state. This hypothesis has been tested in mouse skin and other tissues and is consistent with the observed results (25). Potter has termed this experimental protocol initiation-promotion-initiation or I-P-I. Potter (25) has thus applied the term "initiator" to a compound that initiates the later steps in a multistep model of carcinogenesis. The further changes caused by this initiator "might be seen as 'progression', while the active agent would remain an 'initiator'" (25). While I am in complete agreement with this interpretation, the choice of terminology is highly unfortunate. Firstly, it is confusing. In describing results with this experimental protocol, one will have to be careful to distinguish the initial "initiator" from the final "initiator." But more importantly this terminology implies that the mechanisms of the initiation and progression processes are the same. Dr. Potter has suggested that these two processes may represent two sequential mutations (25); using the same term, initiator, for both processes reemphasizes this conclusion. However, different types of mutational change may be involved in carcinogenesis (5). Therefore, two mutations could be involved, but these could be different types of mutations induced by different types of mutagens. For example, initiation may be caused by a point mutation and tumor progression by gene amplification, genetic transpositions or aneuploidy. Specific mutagens may induce only one of these types of mutations (4,5) and therefore only be active at one stage of the neoplastic process. To leave open the possibility that the later, qualitative steps in progression may be due to different types of mutational events or even non-mutational, heritable events, I strongly urge that different terms be adopted for the processes of initiation and progression, both of which are distinct from tumor promotion. A new term is needed to emphasize these mechanistic differences. A logical choice of terms would be initiator, promoter, and "progressor."

An example of an agent that may be a specific progressor is arsenic. Sufficient evidence exists that arsenic is a human carcinogen, and yet insufficient evidence exists that it is carcinogenic in animals (19); it does not have activity as an initiator or a promoter (7). These seemingly disparate results could be explained if arsenic is a progressor. In fact, the human data indicate that arsenic influences a late stage in carcinogenesis (10). Arsenical compounds lack mutagenic activity in gene mutation assay (27) but are active as a clastogens (35), indicating that they have a specific type of mutagenic activity.

In conclusion, in an assessment of the factors that may enhance respiratory tract and other forms of carcinogenesis in humans, one must consider that a multitude of factors will be invovled. Some of the factors may act by facilitating the clonal expansion of initiated or premalignant cells (e.g., tumor promoters). These factors may be highly specific and selective in this action (e.g., hormones) or non-specific, such as wounding or regenerative hyperplasia after toxic injury. Other agents will act to facilitate the progression of the initiated or premalignant cells (i.e., as tumor progressors). These agents may be complete carcinogens, including initiators, or chemicals that lack initiating activity. Tumor progressors as well as initiators may be different types of mutagens or epigenetic carcinogens that induce heritable changes in gene expression.

REFERENCES

1. Argyris, T. S. (1980): *J. Invest. Dermatol.*, 75:360-362.
2. Argyris, T. S., and Slaga, T. J. (1981): *Cancer Res.*, 41:5193-5195.
3. Barrett, J. C., and Sisskin, E. E. (1980): In: *Carcinogenesis: Fundamental Mechanisms and Environmental Effects*, edited by B. Pullman and P. O. P. Ts'O, pp. 427-439. D. Reidel Publishing Co., Dordrecht.
4. Barrett, J. C., and Thomassen, D. G. (1984): In: *Methods of Estimating Risk in Human and Chemical Damage in Non-Human Biota and Ecosystems*, SCOPE, SGOMSEC2, IPCS Joint Symposia 3, edited by V. B. Vouk, G. C. Butler, D. G. Hoel, and D. B. Peakall, in press. John Wiley and Sons, Chichester.
5. Barrett, J. C., Thomassen, D. G., and Hesterberg, T. W. (1983): *Ann. N.Y. Acad. Sci.*, 407:291-300.
6. Birnboim, H. C. (1982): *Science*, 215:1247-1249.
7. Boutwell, R. K. (1963): *J. Agric. Food Chem.*, 11:381-384.
8. Boutwell, R. K. (1964): *Prog. Exp. Tumor Res.*, 4:207-250.
9. Boutwell, R. K. (1974): *CRC Crit. Rev. Toxicol.*, 2:419-443.
10. Brown, C. C., and Chu, K. C. (1983): *J. Natl. Cancer Inst.*, 70:455-463.
11. Burns, F. J., Albert, R. E., and Altshuler, B. (1984): In: *Mechanisms of Tumor Promotion, Vol. II: Tumor Promotion and Skin Carcinogenesis*, edited by T. J. Slaga, pp. 17-40. CRC Press, Inc., Boca Raton, FL.
12. Emerit, I., and Cerutti, A. (1982): *Proc. Natl. Acad. Sci. USA*, 79:7509-7513.
13. Farber, E. (1981): In: *Cancer - A Comprehensive Treatise*, 2nd Edition, edited by F. F. Becker, pp. 485-506. Plenum Publishing Company, New York.
14. Frei, J. V. (1977): *J. Natl. Cancer Inst.*, 59:299.
15. Foulds, L. (1969): *Neoplastic Development, Vol. 1*. Academic Press, London.
16. Furstenberger, G., Berry, D. L., Sorg, B., and Marks, F. (1981): *Proc. Natl. Acad. Sci. USA*, 78:7722-7726.
17. Furstenberger, G., Sorg, B., and Marks, F. (1983): *Science*, 220:89-91.
18. Hennings, H., Shores, R., Wenk, M. L., Spangler, E. F., Tarone, R., and Yuspa, S. H. (1983): *Nature*, 304:67-69.
19. International Agency for Research on Cancer (1980): *IARC Monographs on the Evaluation of Carcinogenic Risk of Chemicals to Humans. Some Metals and Metal Compounds (Arsenic, Beryllium, Chromium, and Lead), Vol. 23*, pp. 39-141. IARC, Lyon.
20. Kulesz-Martin, M. F., Loehler, B., Hennings, H., and Yuspa, S. H. (1980): *Carcinogenesis*, 1:1039-1047.
21. Parry, S. M., Parry, E. M., and Barrett, J. C. (1981): *Nature*, 294:263-265.
22. Pitot, H. C. (1978): *Fundamentals of Oncology*. Marcel Dekker, Inc., New York.
23. Potter, V. R. (1980): *Yale J. Biol. Med.* 53:367-384.

24. Potter, V.R. (1981): *Carcinogenesis*, 2:1375-1379.
25. Potter, V. R. (1984): *Cancer Res.*, 44:2733-2736.
26. Raick, A. N., Thumm, K., and Chivers, B. R. (1972): *Cancer Res.*, 32:1562-1568.
27. Rossman, T. G., Stone, D., Molina, M., and Troll, W. (1980): *Environ. Mutagen.*, 2:371-379.
28. Sisskin, E. E., Gray, J., and Barrett, J. C. (1982): *Carcinogenesis*, 3:403-407.
29. Sisskin, E. E., and Barrett, J. C. (1981): *Cancer Res.*, 41:346-350.
30. Slaga, T. J. (1984): In: *Mechanisms of Tumor Promotion, Vol. II: Tumor Promotion and Skin Carcinogenesis*, edited by T. J. Slaga, pp. 1-16. CRC Press Inc., Boca Raton, FL.
31. Slaga, T. J. (1984): In: *Mechanisms of Tumor Promotion, Vol. II: Tumor Promotion and Skin Carcinogenesis*, edited by T. J. Slaga, pp. 189-196. CRC Press, Inc., Boca Raton, FL.
32. Slaga, T. J., Fischer, S. M., Nelson, K., and Gleason, G. L. (1980): *Proc. Natl. Acad. Sci. USA*, 77:3659-3663.
33. Slaga, T. J., and Klein-Santo, A. J. P., Fischer, S. M., Weeks, C. F., Nelson, K., and Major, S. (1980): *Proc. Natl. Acad. Sci. USA*, 77:2251-2254.
34. Trosko, J. E., and Chang, C. C. (1980): *Med. Hypotheses*, 6:455-468.
35. Wan, B., Christian, R. T., and Soukup, S. W. (1982): *Environ. Mutagen.*, 4:493-498.
36. Weinstein, I. B. (1981): *Cancer*, 47:1133-1141.
37. Yuspa, S. H., and Morgan, D. L. (1981): *Nature*, 293:72-74.

Carcinogenesis, Vol. 8, edited by M. J. Mass et al.
Raven Press, New York © 1985.

Relevance of Tumor Promotion to Carcinogenesis in Human Populations

Ann R. Kennedy

Department of Cancer Biology, Harvard School of Public Health, Boston, Massachusetts 02115

There are now many examples of agents which will enhance or promote the development of lung cancers, as has been reviewed in detail (17). A particularly striking example of tumor enhancement in the lung comes from our own work with ^{210}Po, an α-emitting radionuclide which is present in cigarettes and the lungs of cigarette smokers (17). While a low dose of ^{210}Po α-radiation does not induce lung cancer by itself, it can be greatly potentiated by a series of saline instillations to the lung such that 20-40% of the exposed animals develop tumors (21,29). Although the mechanism for enhancement in tumorigenesis is unknown, we have observed that saline instillations serve as a nonspecific stimulus to cell proliferation in the lung (29). Recent research of ours suggests that cell proliferation is absolutely essential for the occurrence of malignant transformation (19,20).

Cigarette smoking in human populations appears to act as a promoting agent for the respiratory tract. It is known, for example, that people who stop smoking have a decreased risk of getting lung cancer compared to those who continue to smoke (7); such a "reversible" effect is a classical characteristic of promoting agents (33). Another example of cigarette smoke acting as a promoter for lung carcinogenesis comes from studies of the uranium mining populations. Data implicating radiation as the cause of lung cancer in underground miners come from studies in Central Europe (23), Newfoundland (8), and the Colorado Plateau region in the United States (24). The results of earlier studies in the Colorado Plateau (24) indicated that lung cancer arose primarily in the white miners who smoked cigarettes; the incidence of lung cancer in American Indian uranium miners, most of whom did not smoke cigarettes, and the non-cigarette smoking white uranium miners, was not significantly elevated. Very recent studies have indicated that the American Indian uranium miners, and the nonsmoking white miners, now have an elevated risk of lung cancer (1,14,28); it has been suggested that cigarette smoking served as a promoting agent for lung cancer development in the smoking white mining population (14). These are exactly the results expected for a promoting agent operating in human carcinogenesis. Promoting agents have the ability to produce more tumors, and reduce the latent period for tumor development, compared to the expectation following exposure to the carcinogenic agent alone (27); the cigarette-smoking white mining population had a higher incidence of lung cancer, and tumors appeared earlier in time, when compared to the nonsmoking uranium-mining population.

The dose-response curve for the incidence of lung cancer *vs* dose of radiation for the smoking white mining population is clearly linear (3). The presence of a promoting agent in radiation carcinogenesis often results in a linear curve, in both *in vivo* (12) and *in vitro* (22) experimental studies, while the curve expected for radiation treatment alone (in the systems cited above) is a quadratic or linear-quadratic curve. The conclusion reached by the most recent report from the Committee on Biological Effects of Ionizing Radiation (4) is that for low linear energy transfer radiation, the dose-response curve for most radiation-induced human cancer is best represented by a linear-quadratic form. Radiation-induced breast cancer in females is a highly notable exception, both for human (4,32) and animal (6) data, due to its linear dose response; this linear dose response could be due to the endogenous promotion by hormones in breast tissue. It is known that hormones can greatly influence carcinogenesis in experimental animals (2,13); hormones such as estrogen can greatly increase the incidence of cancer (2). It has been proposed that the sex hormones, such as estrogens, may act like tumor promoting agents in their ability to enhance the cancer incidence (31). Many of the effects of tumor promoting agents on cultured cells are also considered similar to hormonal actions (5,34). Like the reversible actions of tumor promoting agents *in vivo* and *in vitro*, many tumors in animals, such as mouse mammary tumors, are under hormonal controls in that removal of a necessary hormone can cause tumor regression (30). For human cancer, it has been reported that women who take estrogen as a therapy for postmenopausal problems have a greatly increased risk of developing cancer and that there is a rapid decline in risk following the discontinuation of estrogen use (16). Again, such a reversible effect is what would be expected of a promoting agent operating in human carcinogenesis. Endogenous hormonal promotion in the breast could easily account for the fact that the female breast is the most sensitive human organ to the induction of cancer by ionizing radiation (4,32).

The only other human organ with a radiosensitivity comparable to that of the female breast for the induction of cancer is the thyroid (4, 32). Like the dose response for radiation-induced human breast cancer in females, the dose-response curve for radiation-induced human thyroid cancer is also linear (4,25). It is known that thyroid hormones can greatly enhance the incidence of thyroid cancers in experimental animal carcinogenesis (2,10,15). Similarly, increased levels of thyroid-stimulating hormone result in an increase in the incidence of human thyroid neoplasia (11). Thus, endogenous hormonal promotion may well play a role in the genesis of thyroid cancer. In human populations, it has been observed that the risk of developing radiation-induced thyroid cancer is considerably higher in : 1) females (4), 2) those having a Jewish ethnic background (4), and 3) those who have emigrated from Morocco or Tunisia (26); these data suggest that factors other than the radiation exposure play a very large role in the genesis of this disease. It is thought that the sexual difference is "related to the fluctuating hormonal status in females, with significantly greater variations in the pituitary-thyroid axis and in secretion of thyroid-stimulating hormone than in males" (4, p. 302). The greater relative risk among the Jewish population could be due to genetic susceptibility; however, all of the increased risk factors considered together suggest that promotional factors, some of which may be present in the diet of "emigrating" populations, may be the most important determinants of whether cancer will result from the random distribution of energy by ionizing radiation. Clearly, diet is one of the major determinants of the cancer incidence in human populations (9), and many promotional factors are known to be present in the human diet.

Whether or not promotion exists in the induction of human cancer is still unknown; however, I have given some examples here which indicate that promotion may play a major role in carcinogenesis in human populations. There is no question that promotion occurs in experimental animal systems, as has been reviewed extensively elsewhere, and in the inducation of carcinogen-induced transformation *in vitro*, as has been recently reviewed (18). It would indeed be surprising if the phenomenon of promotion did not exist in human carcinogenesis.

ACKNOWLEDGEMENTS

The author's research in the area of this review is supported by NIH Grants CA 22704, CA 34680 and ES 00002.

REFERENCES

1.   Archer, V. E., Gillam, J. D., and Wagoner, J. K. (1976): *Ann. N.Y. Acad. Sci.*, 271:280-293.
2.   Berenblum, I. (1974): *Carcinogenesis as a Biological Problem*, pp. 133-141. North Holland Publishing Co., Amsterdam.
3.   Biological Effects of Ionizing Radiation - Committee Report I. (1972): *The Effects on Populations of Exposure to Low Levels of Ionizing Radiation*, p. 154. National Academy Press, Washington, DC.
4.   Biological Effects of Ionizing Radiation - Committee Report III. (1980): *The Effects on Populations of Exposure to Low Levels of Ionizing Radiation*. National Academy Press, Washington, DC.
5.   Blumberg, P. M. (1980, 1981): *In Vitro Studies on the Mode of Action of the Phorbol Esters, Potent Tumor Promotoers: Parts 1 and 2. CRC Critical Rev. Toxicol.*, 8:153-197, 199-234.
6.   Bond, V. P., Cronkite, E. P., Lippincott, S. W., and Shellabarger, C. J. (1960): *Radiation Res.*, 12:276-285.
7.   Cairns, J. (1978): *Cancer: Science and Society*, pp. 146-147. W. H. Freeman and Co., San Francisco.
8.   de Villiers, A. J., and Windisch, J. P. (1964): *Br. J. Ind. Med.*, 21:94-109.
9.   Doll, R., and Peto, R. (1981): *J. Natl. Cancer Inst.*, 66:1192-1308.
10.   Doniach, I. (1974): *Brit. J. Cancer*, 30:487-495.
11.   Foster, R. S., Jr. (1975): *Amer. J. Surg.*, 130:608-611.
12.   Fry, R. J. M., Ley, R. D., Grube, D., and Staffeldt, E. (1982): In: *Carcinogenesis, Vol. 7: Cocarcinogenesis and Biological Effects of Tumor Promoters*, edited by E. Hecker, N. E. Fusenig, W. Kunz, F. Marks, and H. W. Thielmann, pp. 155-165. Raven Press, New York.
13.   Furth, J. (1975): In: *Cancer, A Comprehensive Treatise, Vol. 1*, edited by F. F. Becker, pp. 75-120. Plenum Press, New York.
14.   Gottlieb, L. S., and Husen, L. A. (1982): *Chest*, 81:449-452.
15.   Hall, W. H. (1948): *Brit. J. Cancer*, 2:273-280.
16.   Jick, H., Watkins, R. N., Hunter, J. R., Dinan, B. J., Madsen, S., Rothman, K. J., and Walker, A. M. (1979): *New Engl. J. Med.*, 300:218-222.
17.   Kennedy, A. R., and Little, J. B. (1978): In: *Pathogenesis and Therapy of Lung Cancer*, edited by C. C. Harris, pp. 189-261. Marcel Dekker, Inc., New York.
18.   Kennedy, A. R. (1984): In: *Mechanisms of Tumor Promotion, Vol. III, Tumor Promotion and Carcinogenesis In Vitro*, edited by T. J. Slaga, pp. 13-55. CRC Press, Inc., Boca Raton, FL.
19.   Kennedy, A. R., Cairns, J., and Little, J. B. (1984): *Nature*, 307:85-86.
20.   Kennedy, A. R., and Little, J. B. (1984): *Radiation Res.*, in press.
21.   Little, J. B., McGandy, R. B., and Kennedy, A. R. (1978): *Cancer Res.*, 38:1929-1935.
22.   Little, J. B., and Kennedy, A. R. (1982): In: *Carcinogenesis, Vol. 7: Cocarcinogenesis and Biological Effects of Tumor Promoters*, edited by E.

Hecker, N. E. Fusenig, W. Kunz, F. Marks, and H. W. Thielmann, pp. 243-257. Raven Press, New York.

23. Lorenz, E. (1944): *J. Natl. Cancer Inst.*, 5:1-15.
24. Lundin, F. E., Wagoner, J. K., and Archer, V. E. (1971): *Radon Daughter Exposure and Respiratory Cancer: Quantitative and Temporal Aspects.* NIOSH and NIEHS Joint Monograph No. 1. National Technical Information Service, Springfield, VA.
25. Maxon, H. R., Thomas, S. R., Saenger, E. L., Buncher, C. R., and Kereiakes, J. G. (1977): *Amer. J. Med.*, 63:967-978.
26. Ron, E., and Modan, B. (1982): In: *Radiation Carcinogenesis: Epidemiology and Biologic Significance*, edited by J. D. Boice and J.F. Fraumeni. Raven Press, New York.
27. Ryser, H. J. P. (1971): *New Engl. J. Med.*, 285:721-734.
28. Samet, J. M., Kutvirt, D. M., Waxweiler, R. J., and Key, C. R. (1984): *New Engl. J. Med.*, 310:1481-1484.
29. Shami, S. G., Thibodeau, L. A., Kennedy, A. R., and Little, J. B. (1982): *Cancer Res.*, 42:1405-1411.
30. Süss, R., Kinzel, V., and Scribner, J. D. (1973): *Cancer, Experiments and Concepts.* Springer-Verlag, New York.
31. Troll, W. (1976): In: *Fundamentals in Cancer Prevention*, edited by P. N. Magee, S. Takayama, T. Sugimura, and T. Matsushima, pp. 41-55. University Park Press, Baltimore, MD.
32. U.N. Report, United States Scientific Committee on the Effects of Atomic Radiation. (1977): *Sources and Effects of Ionizing Radiation.* Report to the General Assembly, with annexes.
33. Weinstein, I. B. (1978): *Bull. N.Y. Acad. Med.*, 54:366-383.
34. Weinstein, I. B., Yamasaki, H., Wigler, M., Lih-Syng, L., Fisher, P. B., Jeffrey, A., and Grunberger, D. (1979): In: *Carcinogens: Identification and Mechanisms of Action*, edited by A. C. Griffin and C. A. Shaw, pp. 399-418. Raven Press, New York.

Carcinogenesis, Vol. 8, edited by M. J. Mass et al.
Raven Press, New York © 1985.

Enhancement and Promotion in Respiratory Cancer

John Higginson

Universities Associated for Research and Education in Pathology, Inc.,
Bethesda, Maryland 20814

The concept of multistage carcinogenesis in animals was developed by 1940 (2), and it is now widely recognized that factors operating prior, during, and after initiation may play significant roles in modulating chemical and viral carcinogenesis in human cancer. There is widespread controversy concerning the terminology and mechanisms of these modulating factors, especially promotional factors. Carcinoma of the lung was one of the first human cancers in which evidence of promotion was deduced and which has been widely studied in relation to cigarette smoking, based first on experimental studies and later on epidemiological data (1). Early epidemiological evidence also suggested that multistage mechanisms were operative in cancers of the liver and prostate (13).

It may not always be possible to determine at what stage or by what mechanism a specific modulating factor may act based only on epidemiological studies, but the data may provide guidelines (5). Thus, a compound which has an inhibitory effect on ciliary action might enhance an initiator non-specifically, in contrast to a promoting agent which might operate specifically at the cellular level in the later stages of carcinogenesis. The distinction, on an epidemiological basis, between early and late stage factors and their different impacts in lung and other cancers have been reviewed by a number of authors.

LUNG CANCER

Cigarette Smoking

The role of promotion in lung cancer was suggested early by Wynder and co-workers following experiments which showed strong promoting as well as initiating activity in cigarette tar. Later epidemiological studies (5,6,8) provided supportive evidence that lung carcinogenesis was a multistage process. Curves derived from data on smokers and ex-smokers are considered consistent with promoting or enhancing activity in cigarettes. Thus, the effects of cigarette smoking freeze after cessation and the rate approaches background. The risk is also higher for small amounts smoked for a long time rather than large amounts smoked for a shorter time. The promoting effect of cigarettes may be predominant in causing lung cancer and may have great impact on individuals exposed to other respiratory carcinogens.

At present, the data are insufficient to allow conclusive comments on passive smoking (4), but it would appear logical that exposure to smoking may have impact.

OCCUPATIONAL CANCER

Asbestos and Sharp Fibers

The multiplicative effect of asbestos and tobacco has been confirmed in a number of studies. Thus, while asbestos exposure alone may increase the relative risk of lung cancer by a factor of 4 to 5 in non-smokers and cigarette smoking alone by ten-fold, the combined risk is around fifty-fold. It appears that the excess relative risk is approximately proportional to accumulative asbestos exposure and independent of age at which exposure starts, which suggests a late-stage effect (5).

There is relatively little evidence that asbestos itself has a genotoxic effect in the bronchi; it does not react with DNA and shows no evidence of strong initiating action in non-smokers. A reduction in lung cancer incidence in asbestos workers follows cessation of smoking, which suggests there is no increase in initiated cells. Accordingly, it is assumed that activity is primarily promotive. In contrast, in mesothelioma induction, asbestos appears to have a strong early or initiating effect and its effect is dependent on duration since first exposure, whether brief or prolonged (5).

The exact mechanism of sharp fiber lung carcinogenesis is unknown, but possibly such fibers could trigger oncogene activity indirectly through a non-genotoxic effect as opposed to direct DNA damage. There is some evidence that other modulating factors, for instance size of fibers, are involved in the case of chrysotile-induced mesetheliomas in factory workers. Slight increases in lung cancer risk have been reported with other man-made mineral fibers (11), but the data are inconclusive.

Other Factors

Chloromethyl Ethers

The relative risk is reported higher in younger workers and continues after exposure stops, suggesting an early stage effect. Smoking data are insufficient (5).

Nickel

For lung cancer any interpretation of the available data would appear premature due to the distorting effects of increasing lung cancer incidence in cohorts since 1910 (5,7).

Ionizing Radiation

The increase in cancer in uranium miners is well known. The role of radon may be initiating but a promoting role for tobacco is also present.

Arsenic

The exact role of arsenic in human lung cancer is not yet clarified apart from the significant increase that occurs in workers exposed to high levels of the metal. However, some studies suggest it acts in the late stages of induction (5).

Dusty Occupations

The role of dust in human lung cancer is poorly understood and, for example, no reported increases of cancer have been reported in coal miners with pneumoconiosis. Many such studies, however, are not adequately controlled for level of cigarette smoking. The report of Hammond and Garfinkel (10) does suggest some effect for dusty occupations in the United States.

Air Pollution

Today there is general concensus that if ambient air pollution has a role in lung cancer, it may only operate in the context of cigarette smoking (3,9). The report of Hammond and Garfinkel (10) shows no evidence of differences in incidence between dirty or clean cities. In Utah, no difference was found in lung cancer rates between rural and urban environments for Mormons. This contrasted to non-Mormons and suggested that the urban/rural difference in non-Mormons was predominantly due to tobacco.

Infections

In old scars, for instance in tuberculosis, tumorlets develop and may provide a source for later carcinoma development.

Individual Susceptibility and Diet

Although individual susceptibility to cigarette smoke was linked to the activity of benzo(a)pyrene hydroxylase, the evidence remains inconclusive. The role of vitamin A deficiency is still uncertain.

Experimental Data

Studies on the role of promotion and enhancement in lung cancer have largely been carried out using surrogate systems such as mouse skin with a large variety of agents. Studies have been made on the role of enhancement of mouse adenomas by agents such as viruses. Whereas some of the later have been positive, it is not clear to what extent they are relevant to the human situation.

UPPER RESPIRATORY TRACT CANCERS

Nose and Para-Nasal Sinuses

Snuff has been implicated in causing cancer of the nose and paranasal sinuses in North America and in Africa. The mechanism is unknown since snuff contains both promoters and initiators.

The role of hard woods in causing adenocarcinoma of the sinuses has been reported in a number of studies (11). Again, it is not clear whether this is a promoting or an initiating action, but the possibility of an irritant effect of such particles acting as a promoting factor cannot be excluded.

Occupational Hazards

Cancer of the nose and nasal sinuses have been reported with chromium and nickel (7). Other reported agents include mustard gas, isopropyl alcohol, and gas manufacturing. Since the absolute risk for nickel increases with age at first exposure and remains relatively constant following cessation of exposure, Day and Breslow (5) conclude that the metal acts at a late stage, but in most studies, the number of reported cases is small.

Cigarette Smoking

Although the role of cigarette smoking as a strong promoter for lung cancer is well known, it is of interest that there is no evidence of an increase in the frequency of nose or nasopharyngeal cancer in smokers. There is no satisfactory explanation for this observation.

Formaldehyde

It has been suggested that in rats the effects of formaldehyde may possibly be promotive or act through non-specific mechanisms. No evidence of an effect has been reported in humans.

Dust

Dust and other particles are suspected as co-carcinogens in nasal cancer.

Nasopharynx

Cancer of the nasopharynx is rare except in certain population groups, notably, in China, the Far East, North Africa and certain Mediterranean communities. It is generally accepted that there is a strong hereditary susceptiblity to the neoplasia, but the nature of the factor is not understood. A relationship with certain HLA profiles has been found (12). There has been an extensive search for external chemical agents acting as initiators, but so far none have been conclusively identified. Considerable research has been done on the potential role of EB virus as an initiating factor. Although EB virus has been identified in tumor cells and the possibility of a multistage process involving viral infection combined with hereditary susceptibility appears possible, it remains to be confirmed.

Larynx

This cancer occurs in heavy cigarette smokers, and there is possibly a slight increase in individuals exposed to asbestos. In both cases, it would appear that the action would be similar to that in lung cancer, but the effect of cigarette smoking is much less carcinogenic. In many laryngeal cancers, alcohol has been implicated as a possible promoter.

CONCLUSIONS

There is strong supportive evidence for multistage carcinogenesis in lung carcinoma especially the promoting and/or enhancing role of cigarette smoking. In many cases, the data are insufficient, however, and it is not possible to discuss each stage in terms of reversibility. The evidence for cancers of other parts of the respiratory tract is less convincing but is highly probable for some sites and agents.

REFERENCES

1. Armitage, P., and Doll, R. (1961): *Brit. J. Cancer*, 11:161-169
2. Berenblum, I. (1978): In: *Carcinogenesis - A Comprehensive Survey, Vol. 2: Mechanisms of Tumor Promotion and Cocarcinogenesis*, edited by T. J. Slaga, A. Sivak, and R. K. Boutwell, pp. 1-10. Raven Press, New York.
3. Cederlof, R., Doll, R., Fowler, B., Friberg, L., Nelson, N., and Vouk, V. (1978): *Environ. Health Perspect.*, 22:1-15.
4. Correa, P., Pickle, L. W., Fontham, E., Lin, Y., and Haenszel, W. (1983): *Lancet*, 595-597.
5. Day, N. E., and Breslow, N. E. (1984) *Cancer Surveys*, in press.
6. Day, N. E., and Brown, C. C. (1980): *J. Natl. Cancer Inst.*, 64:977-989.
7. Doll, R., Morgan, L. G., and Speizer, F. E. (1970): *Brit. J. Cancer*, 24:623-632.
8. Doll, R., and Peto, J. (1976): *Brit. Med. J.*, 2:1525-1536.
9. Doll, R., and Peto, R. (1981): *The Causes of Cancer*. Oxford University Press, New York.
10. Hammond, E. C., and Garfinkel, L. (1980): *Prev. Med.*, 9:206.
11. International Agency for Research on Cancer (1981): *IARC Monographs on the Evaluation of the Carcinogenic Risk of Chemicals to Humans: Wood, Leather and Some Associated Industries, Vol. 25*. IARC, Lyon, France.
12. Olsen, J. H., and Jensen, O. M. (1984): *Scand. J. Work Environ. Health*, 10:17-24.
13. Wynder, E. L., Hoffmann, D., McCoy, D., Cohen, L., and Reddy, B. (1978): In: *Carcinogenesis - A Comprehensive Survey, Vol. 2: Mechanisms of Tumor Promotion and Cocarcinogenesis*, edited by T. J. Slaga, A. Sivak, and R. K. Boutwell, pp. 59-77. Raven Press, New York.

Carcinogenesis, Vol. 8, edited by M. J. Mass et al.
Raven Press, New York © 1985.

Relevance of Enhancement to Human Respiratory Tract Carcinogenesis

Roy E. Albert

Institute of Environmental Medicine, New York University Medical Center, New York, New York 10016

One difficulty in discussing the relevance of enhancement to human respiratory tract carcinogenesis is that there is confusion over the terminology that relates to the processes that enhance carcinogenesis. The terms initiation, promotion, and cocarcinogenesis are operational in nature and were originally defined according to the way in which agents were administered: concurrently for co-carcinogens and sequentially for initiators and promoters, in that order. The term initiation is frequently used to connote the early stage of the carcinogenic process and promotion commonly refers to the process of completing the conversion of the initiated state to malignancy. However, the term progression is often used in the same sense as promotion, i.e., moving the initiated state toward malignancy. Moreover, promotion, as a term referring to the completion of the carcinogenic process, is confusing because the action of a promoting agent completing the carcinogenic process is obviously different from the way in which a "complete carcinogen" carries out the carcinogenic process: a promoting agent, for example in the mouse skin, induces benign tumors which take a very long time to become cancers in contrast to the "complete carcinogen" which mostly produces cancers with very little intervention of the benign tumor stage. Hence, before addressing the question of the relevance of enhancement to human carcinogenesis, it is appropriate to attempt to define the kinds of enhancement processes that we can recognize today on mechanistic grounds.

Enhancement is the general term for any process that increases the expected yield of spontaneous or carcinogen-induced tumors. Enhancement is discussed here in relation to initiating carcinogens, i.e., those which are mutagens. There are noninitiating carcinogens but the issue of enhancement of such agents is not dealt with here. Initiating carcinogens induce neoplastic transformations at the cellular level that range from promotion-dependent initiations (regressible and nonregressible) to autonomous malignancies. The autonomous cell transformations have the capability of growing into tumors; the promotion-dependent transformations require promoting agents to become grossly visible tumors.

MECHANISMS OF ENHANCEMENT

As shown in Table 1, enhancement of initiating carcinogens can be described in three categories.

TABLE 1. Modes of enhancement

1.	Dose enhancement (action on carcinogen)
	↑ Carcinogen retention in target tissue (lung particulates)
	↑ Metabolic conversion to active carcinogen (enzyme inducers)
2.	Initiation enhancement (action on target cells)
	↑ Target cell population (hyperplastic agents)
	↑ Mutagenic effects (proliferation)
3.	Post-initiation enhancement (action on transformed cells)
	↑ Clonal expansion (promoters)
	↑ Progression toward malignancy (initiator)

Dose Enhancement

The action of enhancement is to increase the effective dose of the active form of the carcinogen in the target tissue. There are 2 kinds of processes that can be identified as dose enhancement: (1) where an enhancing agent increases the retention of the carcinogen in the target tissue, as with ferric oxide particles in combination with benzo(a)pyrene in the induction of lung cancer in rodents, and (b) when the enhancing agent alters metabolic process in such a way as to increase the yield of active metabolites from a precursor carcinogen as with cytochrome P450 enzyme activation.

Initiation Enhancement

This is a category of processes in which the enhancing agent affects the target cells in their response to the initiating action of the carcinogens. There are two kinds of processes that are identifiable in this context: (a) Expansion of the target cell population where the hyperplastic effect of the enhancement increases the number of target cells, and hence, the number of initiated cells. This effect is probably limited to epithelial tissues and may be important in withdrawal of the hyperplastic agent during the carcinogenic process, leading to a regression of the hyperplastic state and a markedly reduced rate of tumor formation. This was seen, for example, in the ED_{01} study with acetylaminofluorene (National Center for Toxicological Research) when the data were analyzed for bladder tumors. It also may be operative in the decreased cancer rate upon cessation of cigarette smoking. (b) Enhanced DNA damage by initiating carcinogens can lead to a higher yield of initiated cells. This is seen with agents or measures that increase cell proliferation and cause DNA adducts to become fixed as mutations before they are removed. Another possible mode of action toward this end involves enzyme damage which impairs DNA repair or synthesis.

Post-Initiation Enhancement

This can occur by an action on cells which are already transformed to increase the yield of cancer. There are two kinds of process that are identifiable in this context: (a) Clonal expansion of early stages of neoplastic transformation to form benign tumors which then progress slowly toward malignancy. This is the characteristic action of promoting agents in the rodent skin and liver. (b) Increased rate of progression of early stages of transformation toward malignancy. This effect has been observed only with promotion-induced papillomas in the mouse skin by the administration of direct-acting initiating carcinogens.

RELEVANCE OF ENHANCEMENT TO
HUMAN CARCINOGENESIS

The only unambiguous examples of enhancement of respiratory tract carcinogenesis are the interactions of cigarette smoking with asbestos and radon. The mechanism of carcinogenic interaction by these three agents is unknown. They are not the consequences of promotion since there is no associated formation of benign tumors. Irritant agents in cigarette smoke may enhance the carcinogenic response by the induction of hyperplasia.

The occurrence of a benign tumor stage which progresses very slowly to malignancy in humans does raise the possibility of enhancement by promotion. Examples include thyroid cancer from adenomas (hormonal promotion) and colon cancer from polyps (promotion by bile salts).

Carcinogenesis, Vol. 8, edited by M. J. Mass et al.
Raven Press, New York © 1985.

Types of Enhancement of Carcinogenesis and Influences on Human Cancer

Gary M. Williams

*Naylor Dana Institute for Disease Prevention, American Health Foundation,
Valhalla, New York 10595*

Chemical induction of cancer appears to procede through several distinct steps which may be divided into two logically necessary and mechanistically distinct sequences - neoplastic conversion of the cell, and neoplastic development of a tumor (Fig. 1). Neoplastic conversion is the process in which a normal cell is converted to a neoplastic one. This corresponds to initiation as originally defined by Berenblum (2). Current knowledge indicates that this process results from alterations in the genome of the cell produced by the inducing carcinogen. The second sequence, neoplastic development, is the process of growth of the neoplastic cell (actually the descendent of the original neoplastic cell, in all probability) into a tumor and the progressive acquisition of abnormal properties by the tumor. The facilitation of growth of such suppressed (dormant or latent) neoplastic cells into tumors was regarded by Berenblum (2) as the basis of promotion and, thus, promotion is a component of the sequence of neoplastic development. Promotion is usually described as augmentation of carcinogenesis effected by a specific agent, but may also include permissive conditions allowing tumor development. The sequence of neoplastic development also comprises at least one other process. During the evolution of a neoplasm, it can acquire qualitatively new properties, a phenomenon known as tumor progression (9).

The overall process of carcinogenesis can be enhanced at several steps in either the sequence of neoplastic conversion or development. Often, enhancement is described purely in terms of the temporal relationship of exposure to a carcinogen and an enhancing agent. For example, an agent that produces enhancement when given after a carcinogen is often designated as a promoter. A more desirable approach would be a mechanistic categorization of enhancing effects according to the step in carcinogenesis affected. This has been attempted previously (40) and will be further developed in this paper.

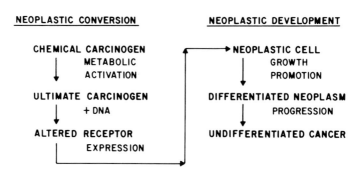

FIG. 1. Relationship of events in neoplastic conversion and neoplastic development.

TYPES OF ENHANCEMENT OF CARCINOGENESIS

There are at least three types of enhancement of carcinogenesis that can be distinguished on the basis of the properties and effects of the agents.

Syncarcinogenesis

The additive or synergistic effect of two or more carcinogens in neoplasm production is defined as syncarcinogenesis (20,27,28). Syncarcinogenesis can occur either when two carcinogens are administered concurrently, or when they are administered one after the other. To distinguish these two types, they have been designated as combination syncarcinogenesis and sequential syncarcinogenesis, respectively (40).

The enhancement of carcinogenesis resulting from syncarcinogenesis is phenomenologically identical to that resulting from multiple exposures, leading to either cocarcinogenesis or neoplasm promotion. In many studies of tumor enhancement, syncarcinogenesis is not explicitly distinguished from these other types of enhancement, apparently because of the frequent assumption that cocarcinogens and promoters are noncarcinogenic. Many promoters, however, are carcinogenic (4,9,37), requiring a distinction to be made. A potentially useful feature for this purpose is the fact that most carcinogens that have been shown to exert syncarcinogenic effects are of a type capable of forming reactive species that interact with DNA as well as other macromolecules (40). Such carcinogens are referred to as genotoxic (37,38). Reaction with DNA can lead to a variety of alterations in the genome which could be a basis for neoplastic conversion and accordingly, syncarcinogenesis produced by concurrent or sequential administration of two genotoxic carcinogens is likely to result from augmentation of the first sequence of carcinogenesis (Fig. 1). In support of this inference, in sequential syncarcinogenesis the order of administration of the two carcinogens can be reversed and separated by a significant interval and the effect still occurs (41). With cocarcinogenesis and promotion this is not the case.

Syncarcinogenesis was originally postulated to result from a summation of irreversible effects of the two carcinogens (20). As discussed, these irreversible effects appear to be the DNA alterations produced by the carcinogens. Thus, the principal mechanism of syncarcinogenesis appears to be summation of DNA damage (Table 1). Syncarcinogenesis on this basis is conceptually comparable to giving a greater dose of one genotoxic carcinogen leading to more neoplastic conversion. If summation of DNA damage is accepted as a basis for syncarcinogenesis, this effectively precludes non-genotoxic agents, i.e. cocarcinogens and promoters.

TABLE 1. Possible mechanisms of syncarcinogenesis

1. Summation of DNA damage produced by both agents.

2. Cocarcinogenic or promoting effects of one carcinogen.

DNA reactive carcinogens can display properties of cocarcinogens or promoters in addition to their genotoxic effects. Several studies have shown that administration of one carcinogen can inhibit repair of the DNA damage produced by a second one (18,22). This could also result in the accumulation of greater amounts of DNA damage leading to increased neoplastic conversion. Such an action has also been suggested for cocarcinogens. In sequential syncarcinogenesis, another basis for enhancement could be a promoting action of the second carcinogen on neoplastic cells generated by the first. Such promoting effects have been suggested to result from nongenotoxic metabolites of the carcinogen (38). The relative contribution of non-genotoxic effects is difficult to distinguish from summation of DNA damage in sequential carcinogen exposures. One possible approach to assess the promoting activity, as distinct from production of neoplastic conversion, of genotoxic carcinogens would be by determining their relative syncarcino-genic effect in two sequences of administration. Also, *in vitro* methods for the measurement of non-genotoxic effects are now available (33,38,39).

Cocarcinogenesis

Originally, cocarcinogenesis was broadly defined as the augmentation of neoplasm induction brought about by non-carcinogenic factors operating in conjunction with a carcinogen, designated as the initiating agent (2,31). Cocarcinogenesis thereby explicitly comprised several kinds of enhancement, including promotion. In common practice, however, cocarcinogenesis has been distinguished operationally from promotion as the enhancement of carcinogenicity resulting from application of a modifier either just before or together with a carcinogen, while promotion has referred to enhancement produced by an agent given after a carcinogen (34,37). According to this distinction, cocarcinogenesis would occur during the sequence of neoplastic conversion while promotion would take place in the sequence of neoplastic development. Enhancement of neoplastic conversion can be produced by an agent given after a genotoxic carcinogen at a time when the DNA damage produced by the carcinogen is still persistent (12,14). This apparently results from increased conversion of DNA damage to permanent genetic alterations and, thereby, increased neoplastic conversion. This effect should be considered a cocarcinogenic action unless proven otherwise. Therefore, to make the operational definition of cocarcinogenesis conform to a mechanistic distinction, it has been proposed to define cocarcinogenesis as the enhancement of carcinogenesis resulting from effects produced either immediately before or during carcinogen exposure or at a time after carcinogen exposure when chemical damage is still persistent (40).

A cocarcinogen by the definition stated cannot exert promotion, but carcinogenesis can be augmented by promoters when given together with a carcinogen. When the concurrent administration of a chemical with a carcinogen occurs over a lengthy period, any enhancement could be due to either a cocarcinogenic effect or to a promoting action on neoplastic cells that are arising from the carcinogen exposure. Unless it is clear that the agent has cocarcinogenic properties, it should be classified as a promoter. Nevertheless, some promoters can be cocarcinogenic and should be classified as promoters with cocarcinogenic activity to give emphasis to their more specific property.

The effects of chemical cocarcinogens have been less thoroughly studied than those of promoters (11,13,32). Cocarcinogens could operate through a variety of mechanisms to enhance neoplastic conversion (Table 2). Of these, increased carcinogen uptake, increased metabolic activation and enhanced conversion of DNA damage to permanent alterations are fairly well established. The other two require demonstration. Cocarcinogenesis could result from any of these effects alone or in combination. It must be emphasized that none of these mechanisms involves DNA damage by the chemical, or otherwise it would likely be a genotoxic carcinogen. Additionally, unlike syncarcinogens and promoters, cocarcinogens are noncarcinogenic.

TABLE 2. Possible mechanisms of cocarcinogenesis

1. Increased uptake of carcinogen.

2. Increased proportion of carcinogen metabolized to reactive products.

3. Depletion of competing nucleophiles.

4. Inhibition of rate or fidelity of DNA repair.

5. Enhancement of conversion of DNA lesions to permanent alterations.

Promotion of Neoplasia

Promotion was originally defined conceptually by Berenblum (2) as the encouragemnt of dormant neoplastic cells to develop into growing tumors. Operationally, the phenomenon is usually demonstrated as the enhancing effect on carcinogenesis by a modifier administered after a carcinogen (3). An important concept that requires greater attention is whether any enhancement of carcinogenesis by an agent administered subsequent to a carcinogen can be considered promotion or whether the phenomenon should be restricted to the facilitation of growth and development of dormant neoplastic cells as proposed by Berenblum.

In most "promotion" studies the second agent has been given shortly after a carcinogen, under which conditions unrepaired DNA adducts are likely to be present such that stimulation of cell proliferation can enhance neoplastic conversion of cells (Fig. 1) ultimately resulting in increased neoplasm formation. This represents, as discussed before, more of a cocarcinogenic effect, which is very different in nature from enhanced development of neoplastic cells. Also, as described, two carcinogens given in sequence can produce a syncarcinogenic effect, which is phenomenologically the same as initiation-promotion. Therefore, it is evident that designating an agent as a promoter simply based upon its enhancement of carcinogenesis when given after a carcinogen is imprecise. When the mechanism of enhancement is unknown, it is preferable to use a general term such as carcinogenesis enhancement.

In the early studies on neoplasm promotion in skin by croton oil or its active components, phorbol esters, it was demonstrated that application of the promoter before the initiating agent did not result in enhancement (2,3). While this generalization is not always true and depends to a large degree upon the experimental protocol (16), it is a useful biological property. Recently, the liver tumor promoter phenobarbital has been demonstrated not to enhance carcinogenesis when given before a genotoxic carcinogen (29, 41). Such differences in the effects of reverse sequence administrations distinguish promotion from syncarcinogenesis and should be done before an agent is accepted as a promoter.

Promotion was identified at a time when promoting agents were not rigorously tested for carcinogenicity and thus promoters were considered to be noncarcinogenic, although even the earliest studies on skin neoplasm promotion with croton oil and phorbol esters revealed a weak carcinogenic effect of these agents (34). It is now established that many agents with promoting activity will increase neoplasia without any other exposure when tested in appropriate protocols for long duration (4,9,15,37). Nevertheless, they do not seem to be able to produce DNA damage directly, and therefore have been categorized as a type of epigenetic carcinogen (37). It seems likely that their "carcinogenic" effects are due to a promoting action on cryptogenically-arising neoplastic cells, which must occur as the basis for the development of spontaneous neoplasms. The important difference between carcinogenic promoters and carcinogens that exert syncarcinogenesis is that the latter are genotoxic.

A number of cellular effects have been demonstrated for promoting agents (11,13,32). Those that could be the basis for the facilitation of growth of neoplastic cells into tumors are listed in Table 3. Promotion could be a consequence of any of these actions alone or in combination. These effects are non-genetic because of the restriction of promotion to effects on cells that are already neoplastic and hence do not require completion of neoplastic conversion.

Nevertheless, it is theoretically possible that an agent could produce genetic changes in neoplastic cells to render them more aggressive and thereby increase cancer development. In fact, it has been suggested that phorbol esters produce indirect genotoxicity mediated by reactive oxygen species (8,17). This effect, however, has not been shown to occur specifically in partially transformed cells to complete neoplastic conversion or to alter neoplastic cells to a phenotype with a greater growth advantage. Such reactive oxygen species could, nevertheless, produce membrane changes leading to promotion.

TABLE 3. Possible mechanisms of tumor promotion

1. Enhancement of expression of neoplastic phenotype
   (a) Inhibition of differentiation

2. Stimulation of cell proliferation
   (a) Cytotoxicity
   (b) Hormone effects

3. Alteration of cell membranes
   (a) Induction of proteases
   (b) Inhibition of intercellular communication

4. Immunosuppression

The mechanisms suggested for promotion in Table 3 are non-genotoxic, but it is also possible that genotoxic carcinogens may exert a promoting action through non-genotoxic effects. As discussed, this could contribute to syncarcinogenesis.

INFLUENCES OF ENHANCING FACTORS ON HUMAN CANCER

All three types of enhancement of carcinogenesis appear to influence the occurrence of human cancer. Syncarcinogenesis has not been definitely documented, but there are several situations in which it has probably occurred. Of particular importance is cigarette smoking which entails the inhalation of numerous genotoxic carcinogens (43). In principle, the enhancement by asbestos of lung cancer in cigarette smokers (26,30) could be an example of syncarcinogenesis; both agents are carcinogens. However, asbestos is not DNA-reactive (24) and displays other properties suggestive of a cocarcinogenic or promoting action. The high incidence of bladder cancer in workers engaged in the manufacture of dyestuff intermediates where exposures to several aromatic amines occurred (5) is probably attributable in part to syncarcinogenesis. These examples and the known potent interactions between genotoxic carcinogens in experimental models certainly indicates the need for extreme caution in the complex human situation.

There are several important examples of probable cocarcinogenic effects in humans. As discussed above, the augmentation of lung cancer by asbestos in cigarette smokers, although it could be considered a form of syncarcinogenesis, seems most likely to represent cocarcinogenesis. Recent studies have shown that in cell culture, asbestos enhances cell transformation (7) and mutagenicity (25) by benzo(a)pyrene. Since asbestos is known to adsorb polycyclics (19), it is probable that asbestos acts, at least in part, to transport certain types of carcinogens into cells. In addition, asbestos exerts several other effects (see 35), such as stimulation of cell proliferation, which are undoubtedly relevant to both its cocarcinogenic and possible promoting effects (21). Also, increased cancer of the upper alimentary tract in cigarette smokers who consume excess alcohol (see 10), appears to be attributable to a cocarcinogenic effect. Here, the basis seems to be the effect of alcohol on carcinogen absorption or metabolism. Another possible example of cocarcinogenesis is the high incidence of liver cancer seen in populations with endemic hepatitis and exposure to mycotoxins (see 6). Since the hepatitis B virus has been suggested to be oncogenic, this might be considered a type of syncarcinogenesis. On the other hand, hepatitis results in sustained liver cell proliferation during regeneration and this could render liver cells more susceptible to neoplastic conversion by mycotoxins or other environmental carcinogens.

Epidemiological studies suggest that tumor promoters play a major role in the etiology of human cancer. Chief among these promoting factors are cigarette smoke in enhancing (as well as initiating) lung cancer (43), dietary fat in enhancing colon and breast cancer, and possibly prostate and pancreas cancer (23). The relative contribution of cocarcinogenesis and promoting actions in these situations is not always evident. Nevertheless, studies of migrant populations that adopt lifestyle patterns associated with increased cancer rates strongly suggest that promotion resulting from exposure to new factors is of major importance.

CONCLUSIONS

Enhancement of carcinogenesis is a complex process, as has recently been discussed by Iversen and Astrup (15). There appear to be at least three distinct types of enhancement of experimental carcinogenesis that can be differentiated mechanistically (Table 4). Careful delineation of the exact mechanism of action of an enhancing chemical is important in the assessment of its likely impact on human cancer and strategies for intervention. For some well-defined promoting agents, their effects are highly dose-dependent, have a threshold and are reversible. For example, smoking cessation reduces the risk of lung cancer development probably because promoting phenomena are stopped (43). Likewise, cessation of pharmacologic estrogen exposure in post-menopausal women promptly lowers the occurrence of endometrial cancer (1). This would be accounted for by a promoting action of high levels of estrogen through mechanisms yet to be defined. On the basis of these observations, dietary intervention with a reduction of fat intake to 20% of total calories, from the customary 40% has been proposed as a means of lowering the risk of breast cancer development (42), and such a modification, together with increased consumption of fecal bulk-enhancing cereal fiber, has been advocated as an approach to lowering large bowel cancer risk (36).

TABLE 4. Distinction between types of multiple exposure
effects in chemical carcinogenesis

Process	Operational characteristics	Mechanistic characteristics
Combination syncarcinogenesis	Two carcinogens acting together	Both carcinogens genotoxic
Cocarcinogenesis	Enhancer acting before or together with carcinogen; or when carcinogen effects still persist	Enhancer facilitates neoplastic conversion; enhancer non-genotoxic and non-carcinogenic
Sequential syncarcinogenesis	Two carcinogens acting in sequence; sequence reversible	Both carcinogens genotoxic
Promotion	Enhancer acting after effects of carcinogen have been completed	Enhancer facilitates neoplastic development; enhancer may also be a carcinogen, but is non-genotoxic

REFERENCES

1. Austin, D. F., and Roe, K. M. (1982): *Am. J. Public Health*, 72:65-68.
2. Berenblum, I. (1974): In: *Carcinogenesis as a Biological Problem*, edited by A. Neuberger and E. L. Tatum. American Elsevier Publishing Company, Inc., New York.
3. Boutwell, R. K. (1974): *CRC Crit. Rev. Toxicol.*, 2:419-433.
4. Boyland, E. (1980): *IRCS J. Med. Sci.*, 8:1-4.
5. Case, R. A. M., Hosker, M. E., McDonald, D. B., and Pearson, J. T. (1954): *Brit. J. Ind. Med.*, 11:75-104.
6. Davis, W., and Rosenfeld, C., editors (1979): *Carcinogenic Risks/Strategies for Intervention.* IARC Scientific Publications, No. 25, International Agency for Research on Cancer, Lyon.
7. DiPaolo, J. A., DeMarinis, A. J., and Doniger, J. (1982): *J. Environ. Pathol. Toxicol.*, 5:535-543.
8. Emerit, I., and Cerutti, P. A. (1982): *Proc. Natl. Acad. Sci. USA*, 79:7509-7513.
9. Foulds, L. (1969): *Neoplastic Development.* Academic Press, New York.
10. Groupe, V., and Salmoiraghi, G. C., editors (1979): Alcohol and cancer workshop. *Cancer Res.*, 39:2816-2908.
11. Hecker, E., Fusenig, N. E., Kunz, W., Marks, F., and Thielmann, H. W., editors (1982): *Cocarcinogenesis and Biological Effects of Tumor Promoters.* Raven Press, New York.

12. Hirota, N., Moriyama, S., and Yokoyama, T. (1982): *J. Natl. Cancer Inst.*, 69:1299-1304.
13. International Symposium on Tumor Promotion. (1983): *Environ. Health Perspect.*, 50:3-368.
14. Ishikawa, T., Takayama, S., and Kitagawa, T. (1980): *Cancer Res.*, 40:4261-4264.
15. Iversen, O.H., and Astrup, E. G. (1984): *Cancer Invest.*, 2:51-60.
16. Iversen, O. H., and Iversen, U. M. (1982): *Brit. J. Cancer*, 45:912-920.
17. Kinsella, A. R., and Radman, M. (1978): *Proc. Natl. Acad. Sci. USA*, 75:6149-6153.
18. Kleihues, P., and Margison, G. (1976): *Nature*, 259:153-155.
19. Lakowicz, J. R., and Hylden, J. L. (1978): *Nature*, 275:446-448.
20. Nakahara, W. (1970): In: *Chemical Tumor Problems*, edited by W. Nakahara, pp. 287-330. Japanese Society for the Promotion of Science, Tokyo, Japan.
21. Nettesheim, P., Topping, D. C., and Tamasbi (1981): *Ann. Rev. Pharmacol. Toxicol.*, 21:133-163.
22. Pegg, A. E. (1978): *Nature*, 274:182-184.
23. Reddy, B. S., Cohen, L. A., McCoy, G. D., Hill, P., Weisburger, J. H., and Wynder, E. L. (1980): *Adv. Cancer Res.*, 32:238-345.
24. Reiss, B., Solomon, S., Tong, C., Levenstein, M., Rosenberg, S. H., and Williams, G. M. (1982): *Environ. Res.*, 27:389-397.
25. Reiss, B., Tong, C., and Williams, G. M. (1983): *Environ. Res.*, 31:100-104.
26. Saracci, R. (1977): *Int. J. Cancer*, 20:323-331.
27. Schmähl, D. (1970): In: *Chemical Tumor Problems*, edited by W. Nakahara, pp. 1-18. Japanese Society for the Promotion of Science, Tokyo, Japan.
28. Schmähl, D. (1980): *Arch. Toxicol.*, Suppl. 4, 29-40.
29. Schwartz, M., Bannasch, P., and Kunz, W. (1983): *Cancer Lett.*, 21:17-21.
30. Selikoff, I. J. (1977): In: *Origins of Human Cancer, Vol. 4, Human Risk Assessment*, edited by H. H. Hiatt, J. D. Watson, and J. A. Winsten, pp. 1765-1784. Cold Spring Harbor Laboratory, New York.
31. Sivak, A. (1979): *Biochim. Biophys. Acta*, 560:67-89.
32. Slaga, T. J., Sivak, A., and Boutwell, R. K., editors (1978): *Carcinogenesis, A Comprehensive Survey, Vol. 2, Mechnisms of Tumor Promotion and Cocarcinogenesis*, pp. 588. Raven Press, New York.
33. Trosko, J. E., Yotti, L. P., Dawson, B., and Chang, C. C. (19): In: *Short-Term Tests for Chemical Carcinogens*, edited by H. F. Stich, and R. H. C. San, pp. 420-427. Springer-Verlag, New York.
34. Van Duuren, B. L. (1969): *Prog. Exp. Tumor Res.*, 11:31-68.
35. Wagner, J. C., editor (1980): *Biological Effects of Mineral Fibres*, Vols. 1 and 2. International Agency for Research on Cancer, Lyon.
36. Weisburger, J. H., and Horn, C. L. (1982): *Bull. N.Y. Acad. Med.*, 58:296-312.
37. Weisburger, J.H., and Williams, G. M. (1980): In: *Toxicology the Basic Science of Poisons*, 2nd Edition, edited by J. Doull, C. D. Klaassen, and M. O. Amdur, pp. 84-138. MacMillan Publ. Co., Inc., New York.
38. Williams, G. M. (1980): *Ann. N. Y. Acad. Sci.*, 349:273-282.
39. Williams, G. M. (1981): *Food Cosmet. Toxicol.*, 19:577-583.
40. Williams, G. M. (1984): *Fund. Appl. Toxicol.*, 4:325-344.
41. Williams, G. M., and Furuya, K. (1984): *Carcinogenesis*, 5:171-174.
42. Wynder, E. L., and Cohen, L. A. (1982): *Nutr. and Cancer*, 3:195-199.
43. Wynder, E. L., and Hoffmann, D. (1976): *Semin. Oncol.*, 3:5 15.

Subject Index